# Current Clinical Urology

Eric A. Klein, MD, Series Editor
Professor of Surgery
Cleveland Clinic Lerner College of Medicine Head,
Section of Urologic Oncology
Glickman Urological and Kidney Institute
Cleveland, OH



More information about this series at http://www.springer.com/series/7635

Ronald Rabinowitz
William C. Hulbert • Robert A. Mevorach
Editors

# Pediatric Urology for the Primary Care Physician

Humana Press

*Editors*
Ronald Rabinowitz
Division of Pediatric Urology
Department of Urology
University of Rochester Medical Center
Rochester, NY, USA

William C. Hulbert
Division of Pediatric Urology
Department of Urology
University of Rochester Medical Center
Rochester, NY, USA

Robert A. Mevorach
Chesapeake Urology
Owings Mills
Maryland, MD, USA

ISSN 2197-7194 ISSN 2197-7208 (electronic)
ISBN 978-1-4939-5073-7 ISBN 978-1-60327-243-8 (eBook)
DOI 10.1007/978-1-60327-243-8
Springer New York Heidelberg Dordrecht London



Printed on acid-free paper

Humana Press is a brand of Springer
Springer is part of Springer Science+Business Media (www.springer.com)

*This book is dedicated to our loving wives Sally Rabinowitz, Leslie Hulbert, and Debra Mevorach and to all children with urologic conditions and their primary care physicians.*

# Preface

While there are pediatric urology texts for pediatric urologists and for general urologists, there are none for primary care physicians. This book is written specifically for the primary care physician, the initial contact for the many children with urologic conditions. The goal is to assist the primary care physician in the recognition of and participation in the care of children with these common problems. These include both congenital and acquired conditions. Management may involve medical and/or surgical intervention. The contributing authors were selected for their internationally recognized expertise and straightforward educational styles. It is our hope that this book will significantly help our primary care colleagues in the evaluation and management of children with genitourinary problems.


| | |
|---|---|
| Rochester, NY, USA | Ronald Rabinowitz, MD, FAAP, FACS |
| Rochester, NY, USA | William C. Hulbert, MD, FAAP, FACS |
| Maryland, MD, USA | Robert A. Mevorach, MD, FAAP, FACS |

# Acknowledgment

We wish to acknowledge and thank our academic secretary Lesia Vincent for her skill and dedication.

# Contents

# Contributors

**J. Christopher Austin, M.D.** Division of Urology, Oregon Health & Science University, Portland, OR, USA

**Nathan Ballek, M.D.** Lee's Summit, Missouri, MO, USA

**Stuart B. Bauer, M.D., F.A.A.P., F.A.C.S.** Children's Hospital Boston, Harvard Medical School, Boston, MA, USA

**Mark F. Bellinger, M.D.** The Children's Hospital of Pittsburgh, Pittsburgh, PA, USA

**Guy Bogaert, M.D., Ph.D.** Department of Urology, University Hospitals Gasthuisberg, Leuven, Belgium

**Luis Henrique Perocco Braga, M.D.** McMaster Children's Hospital, McMaster University, Hamilton, On (Ontario), Canada

**John W. Brock III, M.D., F.A.A.P., F.A.C.S.** Division of Pediatric Urologic Surgery at Monroe Carell Children's Hospital at Vanderbilt, Nashville, TN, USA

**Anthony A. Caldamone, M.D., F.A.A.P., F.A.C.S.** The Warren Alpert Medical School of Brown University, Providence, RI, USA

**Douglas A. Canning, M.D., F.A.A.P., F.A.C.S.** Division of Urology, The Children's Hospital of Philadelphia, University of Pennsylvania School of Medicine, Philadelphia, PA, USA

**Patrick C. Cartwright, M.D.** Department of Surgery, Division of Urology, University of Utah School of Medicine, Primary Children's Medical Center, Salt Lake City, UT, USA

**Marco Castagnetti, M.D.** Section of Paediatric Urology, Urology Unit, University Hospital of Padova, Padua, Italy

**Bartley G. Cilento Jr., M.D., M.P.H., F.A.A.P., F.A.C.S.** Department of Urology, Boston Children's Hospital, Boston, MA, USA

**Christopher S. Cooper, M.D., F.A.A.P., F.A.C.S.** Department of Urology, University of Iowa Hospitals and Clinics, Iowa City, IA, USA

**Shubha De, M.D.** Cleveland Clinic Foundation, Cleveland, OH, USA

**Marvalyn DeCambre, M.D., M.P.H.** Poplar Bluff Regional Medical Center, Poplar Bluff, MO, USA

**Steven G. Docimo, M.D., F.A.A.P., F.A.C.S.** Department of Pediatric Urology, Children's Hospital of Pittsburgh, University of Pittsburgh Medical Center, Pittsburgh, PA, USA

**H. Serkan Dogan, M.D.** Department of Urology, Pediatric Urology Division, Uludag University Faculty of Medicine, Bursa, Turkey

**Jack S. Elder, M.D., F.A.C.S.** Division of Pediatric Urology, Massachusetts General Hospital, Boston, MA, USA

**Pamela I. Ellsworth, M.D.** Division of Urology, UMassMemorial Medical Center, Worcester, MA, USA

**Fernando A. Ferrer Jr., M.D.** Department of Surgery, Division of Urology, University of Connecticut School of Medicine, Farmington, CT, USA

**Israel Franco, M.D., F.A.C.S., F.A.A.P.** Director of pediatric urology at Maria Fareri Children's Hospital, New York Medical College, Valhalla, NY, USA

**John P. Gearhart, M.D., F.A.A.P., F.A.C.S.** Division of Pediatric Urology, Johns Hopkins Hospital, The Brady Urological Institute, Baltimore, MD, USA

**Jordan Gitlin, M.D.** Hofstra Northshore-LIJ School of Medicine, New York, NY, USA

**Richard W. Grady, M.D.** Department of Urology, The University of Washington School of Medicine, Seattle, WA, USA

Division of Pediatric Urology, Children's Hospital & Regional Medical Center, Seattle, WA, USA

**Saul P. Greenfield, M.D.** Department of Pediatric Urology, Women and Children's Hospital of Buffalo, Buffalo, NY, USA

**Anne-Marie Houle, M.D., F.R.C.S.C., M.B.A.** Surgery Department, CHU Sainte-Justine, Montréal University, Chemin de la Côte Sainte-Catherine, Montréal, QC, Canada

**William C. Hulbert Jr., M.D., F.A.A.P., F.A.C.S.** Division of Pediatric Urology, Department of Urology, University of Rochester Medical Center, NY, USA

**Antoine E. Khoury, M.D., F.A.A.P., F.A.C.S.** Department of Urology, School of Medicine, University of California Irvine, Irvine, CA, USA

**Steve S. Kim, M.D.** Assistant Professor of Clinical Urology Keck School of Medicine, University of Southern California Children's Hospital Los Angeles, Division of Urology, Los Angeles, CA, USA

**Joel Koenig, M.D.** Division of Urology, Southern Illinois University School of Medicine, Springfield, IL, USA

**Martin A. Koyle, F.A.A.P., F.A.C.S.** Division of Urology, Hospital for Sick Children, Toronto, ON, Canada

**Yegappan Lakshmanan, M.D., F.A.A.P.** Children's Hospital of Michigan, Detroit, MI, USA

**Michael Leonard, M.D., F.R.C.S.(C).** Department of Urology, Children's Hospital of Eastern Ontario, Ottawa, ON, Canada

Department of Surgery, University of Ottawa, Ottawa, ON, Canada

**Daniel Lewinshtein, M.D.** Department of Urology, Montréal University, Quebec, QC, Canada

**James A. Listman, M.D.** Bernard and Millie Duker Children's Hospital at Albany Medical Center, Albany, NY, USA

**Armando J. Lorenzo, M.D., M.Sc., F.R.C.S.C., F.A.A.P., F.A.C.S.** Hospital for Sick Children, University of Toronto, Toronto, ON, Canada

**Kenneth G. Nepple, M.D.** Department of Urology, University of Iowa Hospitals and Clinics, Iowa City, IA, USA

**Max Maizels, M.D., F.A.A.P., F.A.C.S.** Division of Urology, Ann and Robert H. Lurie Children's Hospital, Northwestern University Feinberg School of Medicine, Chicago, IL, USA

**Gianantonio Manzoni, M.D., F.E.A.P.U., F.R.C.S.** Department of Pediatric Urology, Fondazione IRCCS Cà Granda, Ospedale Maggiore Policlinico, Milan, Italy

**Patrick McKenna, M.D., F.A.A.P., F.A.C.S.** American Family Children's Hospital, University of Wisconsin, Madison, WI, USA

**Robert A. Mevorach, M.D., F.A.A.P., F.A.C.S.** Chesapeake Urology, Owings Mills, Maryland, MD, USA

**Rosalia Misseri, M.D.** James Whitcomb Riley Hospital for Children, Indiana University School of Medicine, Indianapolis, IN, USA

**Hiep T. Nguyen, M.D.** Pediatric Urology, Cardon Children Medical Center, Banner Children's Specialists, Mesa, AZ, USA

**Thomas E. Novak, M.D.** Division of Urology, San Antonio Military Medical Center, San Antonio, TX, USA

**Joao Luiz Pippi Salle, M.D., Ph.D., F.A.A.P., F.R.C.S.C.** Division of Urology, Department of Surgery, Sidra Medical and Research Center, Doha, State of Qatar

**J. Todd Purves, M.D., Ph.D.** Medical University of South Carolina, Charleston, SC, USA

**Ronald Rabinowitz, M.D., F.A.A.P., F.A.C.S.** Division of Pediatric Urology, Department of Urology, University of Rochester Medical Center, Rochester, NY, USA

**Puneeta Ramachandra, M.D.** Division of Pediatric Urology, Children's Hospital Central California, Madera, CA, USA

**Waifro Rigamonti, M.D.** Paediatric Surgery and Urology Unit, Burlo Garofalo Hospital, Trieste, Italy

**Richard C. Rink, M.D.** James Whitcomb Riley Hospital for Children, Indiana University School of Medicine, Indianapolis, IN, USA

**Jonathan Ross, M.D.** Department of Pediatric Urology, University Hospitals Rainbow Babies and Children's Hospital, Cleveland, OH, USA

**Sherry S. Ross, M.D.** University of North Carolina, Chapel Hill, NC, USA

**H. Gil Rushton, M.D., F.A.A.P.** Children's National Medical Center, Washington, DC, USA

**Dawn D. Saldano, R.N., A.P.N., M.S.N.** Division of Urology, Ann and Robert H. Lurie Children's Hospital, Northwestern University, Feinberg School of Medicine, Chicago, IL, USA

**Scott Schurman, M.D.** Upstate Golisano Children's Hospital, Syracuse, NY, USA

**Robert D. Schwarz, M.D., F.R.C.S.C.** Department of Surgery, Division of Urology, Dalhousie University, Halifax, NS, Canada

**Curtis A. Sheldon, M.D.** Cincinnati Children's Hospital Medical Center, Cincinnati, OH, USA

**Linda Dairiki Shortliffe, M.D.** Pediatric Urology, Department of Urology, Stanford University Medical Center, Stanford, CA, USA

**Andres Silva, M.D.** University of Sao Paulo, School of Medicine, Almeida Prado, Butantã, São Paulo, SP, Brazil

**Warren Snodgrass, M.D.** Department of Urology, Pediatric Urology Section, Children's Medical Center and The University of Texas Southwestern Medical Center, Dallas, TX, USA

**Brent W. Snow, M.D.** Department of Surgery/Urology, Primary Children's Hospital, University of Utah School of Medicine, Salt Lake City, UT, USA

**Howard M. Snyder III, M.D.** Department of Pediatric Urology, The Children's Hospital of Philadelphia, Philadelphia, PA, USA

**Andrew A. Stec, M.D.** Division of Pediatric Urology, Johns Hopkins Hospital, The Brady Urological Institute, Baltimore, MD, USA

**Danielle D. Sweeney, M.D.** Pediatric Urology of Central Texas, Austin, TX, USA

**Thomas Tailly, M.D.** Department of Urology, University Hospitals Gasthuisberg, Leuven, Belgium

**Stacy T. Tanaka, M.D.** Division of Pediatric Urology, Monroe Carell Jr. Vanderbilt Children's Hospital, Nashville, TN, USA

**Serdar Tekgül, M.D.** Department of Urology, Pediatric Urology Division, Hacettepe University Faculty of Medicine, Ankara, Turkey

**Erica J. Traxel, M.D.** Cincinnati Children's Hospital Medical Center, Cincinnati, OH, USA

**Julian Wan, M.D.** Department of Urology, Division of Pediatric Urology, CS Mott Children's Hospital, Ann Arbor, MI, USA

**Pierre E. Williot, M.D.** Department of Pediatric Urology, Women and Children's Hospital of Buffalo, Buffalo, NY, USA

**Ilene Yi-Zhen Wong, M.D.** Academic Urology, King of Prussia, PA, USA

**Bertram Yuh, M.D.** Department of Pediatric Urology, Women and Children's Hospital of Buffalo, Buffalo, NY, USA

# Fetal Hydronephrosis

1

Andres Silva and Hiep T. Nguyen

## Introduction

### Ultrasound of the Fetal Genitourinary Tract

The incidence of identifying genitourinary abnormalities during prenatal ultrasound (US) screening is approximately 2–9 per 1,000 births, accounting for 17 % of all anomalies diagnosed prenatally. With the more common use of improved high-resolution US scanners, this incidence is rapidly increasing. The use of prenatal US allows children with congenital abnormalities of the genitourinary tract to be detected prior to developing signs and symptoms such as urinary tract infection, abdominal mass, hematuria, kidney stones, and pain. These children benefit from early diagnosis with the goal of preventing these complications and to preserve renal function when possible. However, not all findings on prenatal US represent pathology; many have no clinical significance. The dilemma is to be able to differentiate which children require intervention from those who do not. Specific findings on prenatal US can help to make this differentiation. Some important time points and US findings of the fetal urinary tract are listed in Table 1.1.

### Hydronephrosis: The Scope of the Problem

Prenatal hydronephrosis affects 1–2 % of all pregnancies and is one of the most common prenatally detected anomalies. Although the use of prenatal ultrasound as a screening tool for birth defects has not been shown to improve perinatal outcome, more patients are undergoing prenatal counseling for the discovery of prenatal hydronephrosis. Children diagnosed with this entity on routine ultrasound often undergo extensive prenatal imaging that may include serial ultrasound and magnetic resonance imaging (MRI). In addition, they also undergo numerous postnatal examinations including serial renal ultrasound, voiding cystourethrogram (VCUG), diuretic renogram, intravenous pyelogram, and MRI urogram. Although current prenatal testing is mostly noninvasive, much of the postnatal assessment is invasive and exposes the child to radiation or anesthesia that may be unnecessary. The diagnosis of antenatal hydronephrosis (ANH) causes significant parental anxiety and physician uncertainty with regard to prenatal and postnatal management. Consequently, the efficacy and social

A. Silva, M.D.
University of Sao Paulo, School of Medicine, Almeida Prado, Butantã, São Paulo, SP 05508-070, Brazil

H.T. Nguyen, M.D. (✉)
Pediatric Urology, Cardon Children Medical Center, Banner Children's Specialists, 1400 S. Dobson Road, Mesa, AZ 85202, USA
e-mail: htn7377@comcast.net

R. Rabinowitz et al. (eds.), *Pediatric Urology for the Primary Care Physician*, Current Clinical Urology,
DOI 10.1007/978-1-60327-243-8_1, © Springer Science+Business Media New York 2015

**Table 1.1** US key time points of the fetal GU tract

| |
|---|
| Fetal kidneys: |
| Ureteral bud formation at 5th week of gestation (weeks) |
| Urine formation at 5th–8th week |
| 5 $cm^3$/h at 20th week |
| 50 $cm^3$/h at 40th week |
| Can be visualized at 12th–13th week |
| Visualization of hydronephrosis at 12th–18th week |
| Distinct renal architecture at 20th week |
| Detailed examination is better in the second and third trimesters |
| Renal measurements: 12–40 weeks |
| AP diameter: 0.8–2.6 cm |
| Transverse diameter: 0.9–2.6 cm |
| Length: 1.0–2.7 cm |
| Fetal bladder: |
| Can be visualized at 14 weeks |
| Emptying of the fetal bladder can be seen at 15th week |
| Size: |
| 10 $cm^3$ at 30th week |
| 50 $cm^3$ at term |
| Amniotic fluid: |
| Early = transudate of amnion |
| Later = fetal urine + lung fluid-swallowing |
| Amniotic fluid volume: |
| 380 $cm^3$ at 20th week |
| 800 $cm^3$ at 28th week |
| 800 $cm^3$ at 40th week |
| Amniotic volume dependent on urine production at 16th week |
| Etiology of polyhydramnios (>1.5 L) |
| Esophageal obstruction |
| Multicystic kidney |
| Mesoblastic nephroma |
| Some obstructive processes |
| Etiology of oligohydramnios (<0.5 L) |
| Amnion nodosum |
| Amniotic fluid leak |
| Urinary tract obstruction |
| Consequences of oligohydramnios |
| Pulmonary hypoplasia |
| Potter's syndrome: flat nose, recessed chin, low-set ears, bowed legs, small chest, talipes equinovarus, and hypoplastic hands |
| Limb deformities |

health-care costs of routine prenatal ultrasound as a screening tool for potential postnatal health risks such as urinary tract pathologies remain undefined and quite controversial.

**Table 1.2** Classification system for prenatal hydronephrosis

| Date of detection | Degree of hydronephrosis | Pelvic diameter (mm) |
|---|---|---|
| Second trimester | Mild | 4–7 |
| | Moderate | 8–10 |
| | Severe | >10 |
| Third trimester | Mild | 7–10 |
| | Moderate | 10–15 |
| | Severe | >15 |

## Definitions

Hydronephrosis is used when describing the dilatation of renal pelvis (pelviectasis) and/or calyces (caliectasis). It can be physiologic and have no clinical consequences whatsoever or be caused by urinary tract pathologies such as obstruction or vesicoureteral reflux (VUR). It is important to identify the etiology of the hydronephrosis, because in itself it is merely a finding, not a diagnosis. The number of children diagnosed with prenatal hydronephrosis has increased in the past decade due to the more common use of fetal US imaging. Hydronephrosis presents in a spectrum, ranging from severe renal pelvic dilatation to small changes only noticeable to the trained eye. The anteroposterior (AP) diameter of the renal pelvis taken in the axial plane is the most commonly used measurement in defining prenatal hydronephrosis. It has been found to be the most simple and reliable parameter and is dependent on the gestational age of the fetus when the dilation is detected. While there remains controversy on the exact AP diameter considered being abnormal, there is a commonly accepted classification system (Table 1.2) used in describing prenatal hydronephrosis.

## Natural History

In most of the cases, the etiology of prenatal hydronephrosis is considered to be physiological. It will most likely resolve at the end of the pregnancy or within the first year of life. This spontaneous resolution may be due to several factors related to the maturation of the urinary tract. Fetal urine production is 4–6 times greater than after birth, due to the higher renovascular resistance, greater glomerular filtering rate (GFR), and lower concentrating ability. This high urine output can overwhelm the capacity of the collecting system, resulting in dilation. As the kidneys mature, the urine output decreases and the hydronephrosis improves. In addition, the collecting system is more compliant during fetal development compared to that after birth, due to the composition and orientation of elastin and collagen. As the collecting system matures, alterations in its composition allow for accommodation of greater volume of urine without significant dilation. Finally, dilation of the proximal collecting system can also result from partial or transient anatomical or functional obstructions, such as persistent ureteral folds or delays in normal peristalsis, that resolve during fetal development.

Sairam et al. reviewed 11,465 scans at 18–23 weeks and observed the resolution of prenatal hydronephrosis antenatally and after birth. When the AP diameter was less than 7 mm, all patients had spontaneous resolution of the prenatal hydronephrosis antenatally or shortly after birth. In contrast, approximately 45 % of those with AP diameter greater than 7 mm had resolution of the prenatal hydronephrosis. Other authors noted similar findings with approximately 30 % resolving antenatally and 50–60 % resolving postnatally.

## Differential Diagnosis

The etiology for prenatal hydronephrosis includes transient or physiologic hydronephrosis, ureteropelvic junction (UPJ) obstruction, VUR, ureterovesical junction (UVJ) obstruction, multicystic dysplastic kidney, and posterior urethral valves (PUV). Their incidences are listed in Table 1.3. Less common causes include ureterocele, ectopic ureter, duplex system, and urethral atresia. The degree of hydronephrosis observed on the first prenatal US is a good predictor of postnatal pathology. In a recent meta-analysis of the literature, we found that risk of postnatal pathology positively correlated with the degree of hydronephrosis, from 12 % in the mild group to 88 % in the severe group (Table 1.4). With regard to the specific diagnosis, all pathologies except for VUR were positively correlated with the increasing degree of prenatal hydronephrosis. This supports the observation that US is a poor predictor of reflux (i.e., high grade of reflux may be present despite the absence of hydronephrosis).

When the degree of prenatal hydronephrosis is not known, we found that the degree of hydronephrosis is also a good predictor of postnatal pathology. When evaluating 1,441 children with a history of prenatal hydronephrosis, the risk of postnatal pathology increases from 19 % in the no hydronephrosis group to 96 % in the severe group (Table 1.5). With regard to the specific

**Table 1.3** Differential diagnosis for PNH and their incidence

| Diagnosis | Incidence |
|---|---|
| Transient/physiologic | 50–70 % |
| UPJO | 20–40 % |
| VUR | 15–25 % |
| UVJO/megaureter | 1–20 % |
| MCDK | 2–5 % |
| PUB | 1–5 % |
| Ureterocele, ectopic ureter, duplex system, urethral atresia | Less common |

**Table 1.4** Predictive value of the prenatal US in the risk for postnatal pathology

| | Mild (%) | Mild-moderate (%) | Moderate (%) | Moderate-severe (%) | Severe (%) | Trend *p*-value |
|---|---|---|---|---|---|---|
| Any pathology | 12 | 39 | 45 | 72 | 88 | <0.001 |
| UPJ | 5 | 14 | 17 | 37 | 54 | <0.001 |
| VUR | 4 | 11 | 14 | 12 | 9 | 0.10 |
| PUV | 0.2 | 0.9 | 0.9 | 6.7 | 5.3 | <0.001 |
| Ureteral obstruction | 1 | 12 | 10 | 11 | 5 | 0.25 |
| Others | 1 | 2 | 3 | 6 | 15 | 0.002 |

**Table 1.5** Predictive value of the postnatal US in the risk for postnatal pathology

| | Normal (%) | Mild (%) | Mild-moderate (%) | Moderate (%) | Moderate-severe (%) | Severe (%) | Trend *p*-value |
|---|---|---|---|---|---|---|---|
| Any pathology | 19 | 30 | 44 | 62 | 92 | 96 | <0.05 |
| UPJ | 1 | 8 | 17 | 23 | 53 | 61 | <0.05 |
| VUR | 15 | 19 | 24 | 26 | 25 | 25 | <0.05 |
| Ureteral obstruction | 3 | 4 | 6 | 18 | 22 | 25 | <0.05 |
| Others | 1 | 1 | 2 | 2 | 1 | 2 | <0.05 |

**Table 1.6** Other prenatal US findings that suggest potential postnatal pathology

| | |
|---|---|
| Kidney: | Renal parenchyma—echogenicity and thickness |
| | Calyceal dilation |
| | Unilateral versus bilateral hydronephrosis |
| | Variation in the degree hydronephrosis |
| Ureter: | Ureteral dilation |
| Bladder: | Size and emptying |
| Urethra: | Posterior urethral dilation |
| Other: | Amniotic fluid volume |
| | Extra renal fluid |
| | Other anomalies |
| | Gender |
| | Overall growth and development |

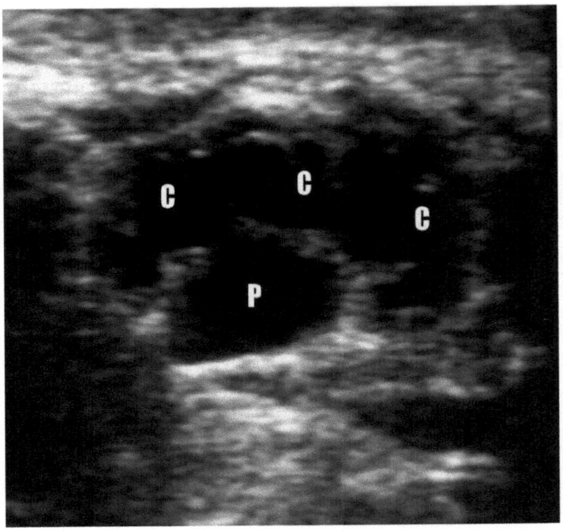


**Fig. 1.1** Fetal ultrasound of a UPJ obstruction. Coronal imaging through the right kidney demonstrating dilated calyces (C) and a dilated renal pelvis (P), suggestive of a right UPJ obstruction

diagnosis, all pathologies except for VUR were positively correlated with the increasing degree of prenatal hydronephrosis. With respect to VUR, there is a statistical difference in the normal and mild group compared to all other groups, but there was no positive trend with the increasing degree of hydronephrosis.

It is very important to describe the fetal hydronephrosis not only by its severity but also on other renal, ureteral, bladder, and urethral US findings (Table 1.6). The presence of bilateral hydronephrosis suggests the presence of PUV, VUR, bilateral UPJ obstruction, urethral aplasia, prune belly syndrome, or megacystis-megaureter complex. The association with hydroureter increases the risk of VUR, UVJ obstruction, or PUV. A thickened bladder that does not empty completely with an associated dilated urethra (keyhole sign) is highly suggestive of PUV. Oligohydramnios and renal parenchymal changes such as increased echogenicity and thinning suggest the presence of associated compromise in renal function.

## Ureteropelvic Junction Obstruction (UPJO)

Obstruction of urinary flow from the renal pelvis into the ureter is one of the more common causes of prenatal hydronephrosis, with an incidence ranging from 20 to 40 %. It is characterized on fetal US by the presence of renal pelvic dilatation and a normal bladder and the absence of a dilated ureter (Fig. 1.1). When occurring unilaterally, the amniotic fluid volume is unaffected. UPJ obstruction should be suspected in cases of moderate or severe dilatation. UPJ obstruction is unilateral in 70 % of the cases. It is usually sporadic, although familiar cases have been reported. The etiology of the obstruction can either be functional (i.e., abnormal peristalsis segment) or anatomic (i.e., caused by crossing vessels, fibrous bands, kinks, or polyps in the ureter).

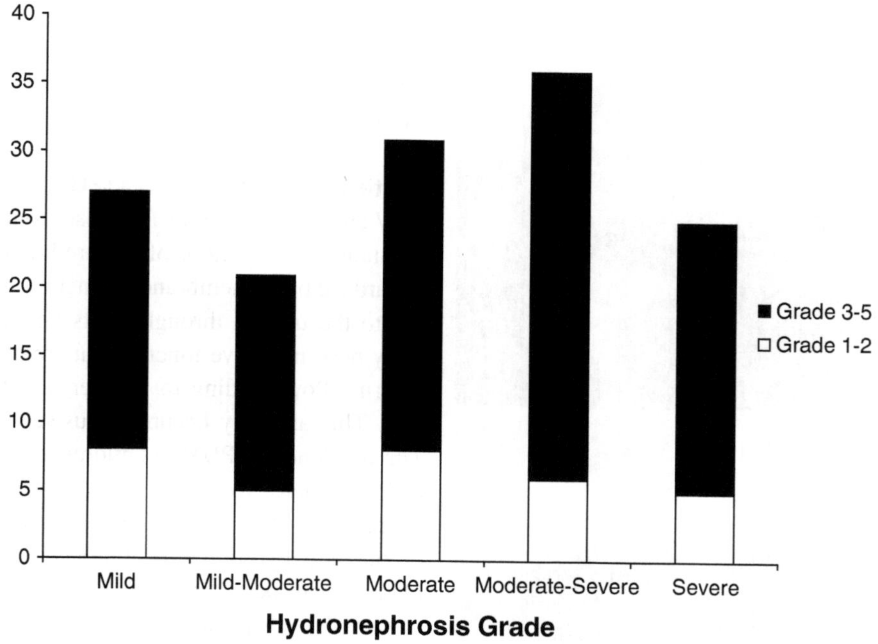


**Fig. 1.2** The incidence and grade of VUR in children with PNH

Functional obstruction occurs in most cases of UPJ obstruction that were detected in the evaluation for prenatal hydronephrosis.

## VUR

VUR occurs when urine flows from the bladder back to the kidney. The incidence of VUR in children with a history of PNH ranges from 15 to 25 %. On prenatal US, VUR is suggested when there is varying degree of hydronephrosis or hydroureteronephrosis during the scanning (Fig. 1.2). In a study performed in our institution, we observed that the degree of prenatal hydronephrosis did not correlate with the incidence or the grade of VUR (Fig. 1.3). However, the presence of a dilated ureter did increase the likelihood of VUR (odds ratio of 1.52). We could not identify any specific US or clinical predictors that can exclude VUR. Thus, there are no reliable findings to predict reflux on fetal US. The presence of significant hydroureteronephrosis, a large thin-walled bladder, and normal renal architecture and amniotic fluid in a male fetus may correspond to significant reflux, which has been termed as megacystis-megaureter association. VUR is bilateral in 60–70 % of the cases. It is the most commonly inherited anomaly of the genitourinary tract with a 33–40 % incidence in siblings.

## Ureterovesical Junction Obstruction (UVJO)/Megaureter

Obstruction at the level of the junction between the ureter and the bladder impairs urinary flow from the distal ureter into the bladder, resulting in dilation of the entire collecting system from the distal ureter to calyces. The incidence of UVJ obstruction/megaureter in children with a history of PNH ranges from 10 to 20 %. On fetal US, UVJ obstruction is suggested when there is dilation of renal pelvis and ureter to the level of the bladder (Fig. 1.4). This diagnosis should be considered when a significantly dilated ureter is visualized. It is not uncommon for the dilated ureter to be mistaken as fetal bowel. The etiology of UVJ obstruction/megaureter may be due to a deficiency of smooth muscle in the ureterovesical ureter, resulting in an adynamic distal segment that impedes normal peristalsis of urine through the ureter (primary) or due to extrinsic compression of the ureter by a thick bladder wall

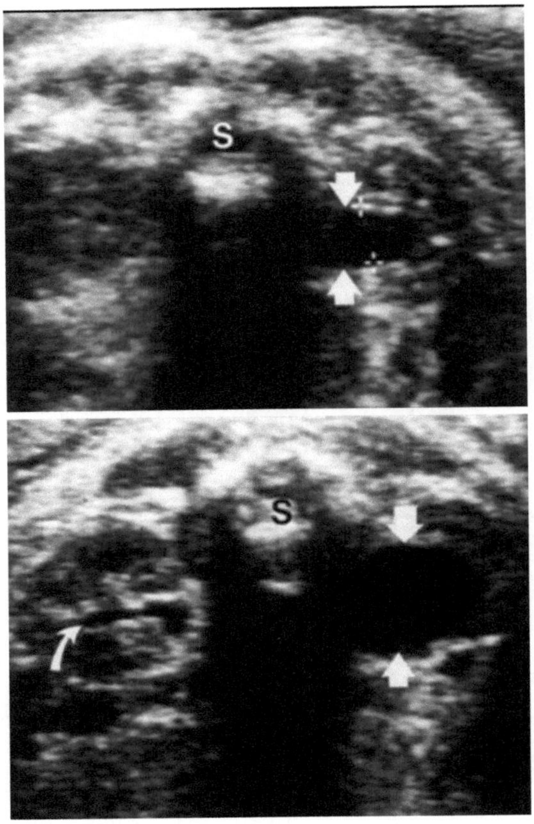


**Fig. 1.3** Fetal US of VUR. Transverse imaging through the right and left kidney demonstrates fluctuation in the degree of hydronephrosis (*arrows*) during the same examination, suggestive of VUR. S = Spine

in pathological states such as PUV or neurogenic bladder (secondary). UVJ obstruction/megaureter is bilateral in 10–25 % of the cases, and most cases are sporadic without a genetic component.

## Posterior Urethral Valves (PUV)

PUV are redundant folds that arise from the verumontanum on the floor of the urethra, extending toward the bulbomembranous junction and attaching to the urethra throughout its circumference. They have no active function but create a barrier to urine flow, leading to bladder outlet obstruction. This anomaly occurs exclusively in males. The incidence of PUV in children with a history of PNH ranges from 1 to 5 %. On fetal US, the diagnosis of PUV is suspected when there is uni- or bilateral hydroureteronephrosis, a thick wall bladder with persistent dilatation and a fusiform or pear-shaped appearance, and a dilated posterior urethra (keyhole sign) (Fig. 1.5). Increased renal echogenicity or cysts and varying degrees of oligohydramnios may be present. During the first trimester, echogenic kidneys and dilated renal pelves can be seen, though the amniotic fluid is usually normal since this fluid is not primarily of renal origin before 16 weeks. Variable US findings are seen due to the wide spectrum of severity of the disease. The etiology is hypothesized to be

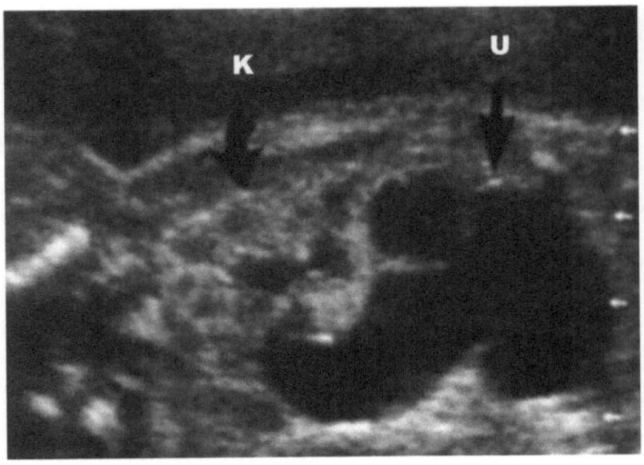


**Fig. 1.4** Fetal US of UVJ obstruction/megaureter. Transverse imaging of the left kidney (K) demonstrates a dilated ureter (U) with mild pelviectasis. Together these findings suggest the diagnosis of UVJ obstruction/megaureter

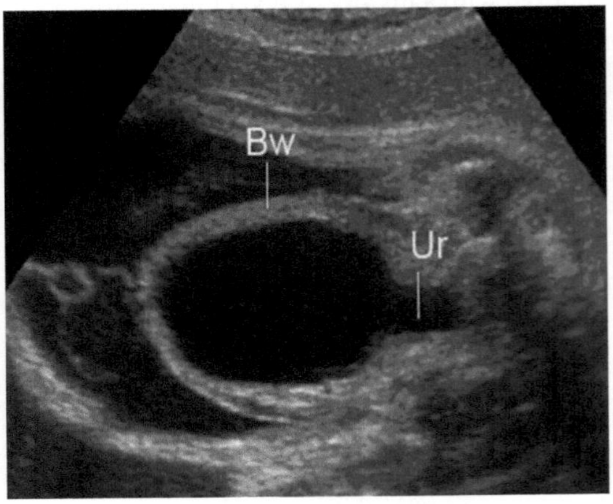


**Fig. 1.5** Fetal US appearance of PUV. Sagittal imaging through the bladder demonstrates a thick bladder wall (Bw) and a dilated proximal urethra (Ur)—keyhole sign, suggestive of PUV

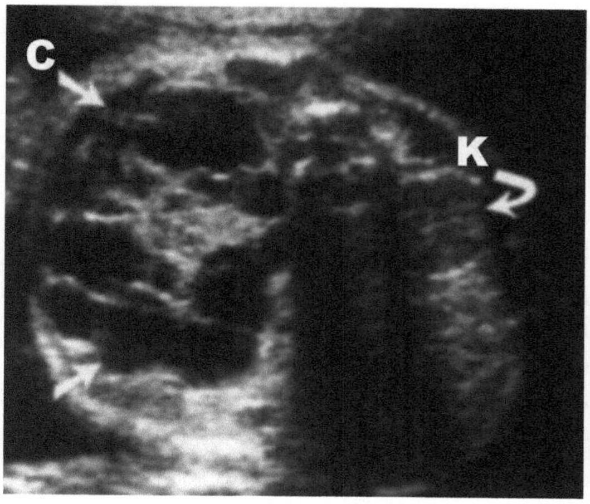


**Fig. 1.6** Fetal US of MCDK. Transverse imaging of the left and right kidney demonstrates a normal left kidney (K) and multiple noncommunicating cystic structures and little parenchyma in the right kidney, suggestive of MCDK

that the terminal ends of the Wolffian ducts mismigrate and are integrated into the urethral wall abnormally, resulting in obliquely oriented ridges that act as one-way valve, impeding urine flow from the bladder. Most cases of PUV are sporadic without a genetic component.

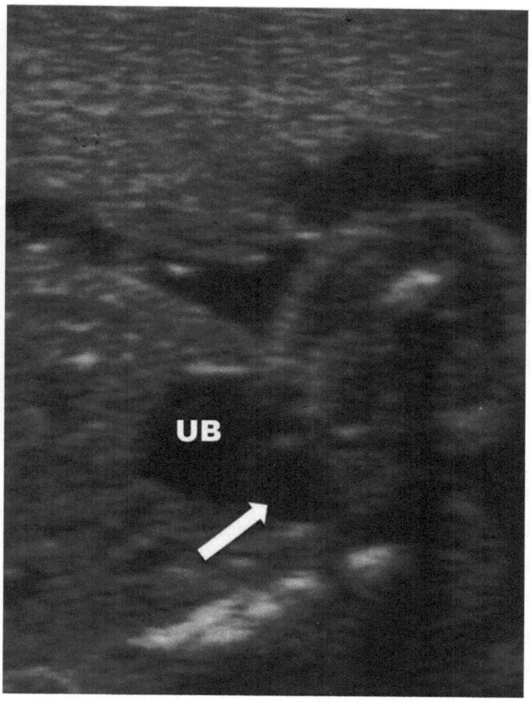


**Fig. 1.7** Fetal US of ureterocele. Transverse imaging through the bladder (UB) demonstrates a cystic structure (*arrow*) at its base, suggestive of a ureterocele

### Multicystic Dysplastic Kidney (MCDK)

MCDK is an anomaly of renal development, in which the renal parenchyma consists primarily of dysplastic elements (primitive ducts and metaplastic cartilage) with a preponderance of cysts encompassing the kidney. Not uncommonly, MCDK is mistaken for hydronephrosis on fetal US as. The incidence of MCDK in children with a history of PNH ranges from 2 to 5 %. On fetal US, the diagnosis of MCDK is suggested when a nonreniform structure with multiple noncommunicating fluid-filled cystic spaces without a central large cyst and little renal parenchyma is visualized in the renal fossa (Fig. 1.6). The etiology of MCDK is unknown, but it appears that it does not have a genetic component. VUR in the contralateral renal unit is found in 20–40 % of children with a unilateral MCDK.

### Ureterocele

A ureterocele is a cystic dilatation of the intravesical submucosal ureter, usually associated with an obstructed orifice that impairs urinary flow into the bladder. When associated with a duplicated system (80 % of the cases), the ureterocele is associated with the upper pole collecting system (Weigert-Meyer Law). The incidence of ureterocele in children with prenatal hydronephrosis is less than 1 %. On fetal US, the diagnosis of a ureterocele is suggested when there is a thin-walled cystic structure in the base of the bladder with associated upper pole hydroureteronephrosis (Fig. 1.7). The etiology is unknown but is hypothesized that it results either from an incomplete breakdown of the ureteral (Chwalla) membrane present at the time of ureteral bud arising from the mesonephric duct or from a delay in the establishment of the lumen of the ureteral bud. There does not seem to be a genetic component; however, ureteroceles are more commonly seen in females than males (5–7 to 1). VUR is commonly found in association with the ureterocele, 50–70 % in the ipsilateral lower pole and 10–30 % in the contralateral renal unit.

## Management of PNH: Which Patients Will Need Further Evaluation?

Once a fetal genitourinary abnormality is diagnosed, the management of the fetus is dependent upon the severity and the etiology of hydronephrosis and the gestational age at which it was diagnosed. When the hydronephrosis is severe (especially in bilateral cases) or is associated with oligohydramnios or echogenic kidneys, urgent referral should be made to help council the parents on diagnosis and management. Similarly, findings of bilateral hydroureteronephrosis, a thickened bladder wall, or dilated posterior urethra (suggestive of PUV) should be urgently evaluated. In most cases, the hydronephrosis is mild or moderate and is unilateral without associated changes in amniotic fluid or renal parenchymal abnormalities. Consequently, serial prenatal US should be performed to monitor for progression. There is no set recommendation on the frequency of US imaging but it may range from every 4–6 weeks.

### The Role of Fetal Intervention

Occasionally, in utero intervention may be required with the goal of preventing pulmonary hypoplasia (by restoring normal amniotic fluid), improving kidney and bladder function. The type of fetal intervention includes early delivery, open bladder decompression, vesicoamniotic shunts, and minimally invasive endoscopic and laparoscopic valve ablation and vesicostomy. All of these procedures have significant maternal and fetal risks; consequently, it has to be determined that the benefits of fetal intervention outweigh the risks before undertaking such procedures.

The indication for fetal intervention in fetuses with hydronephrosis is limited to those with evidence of severe bladder outlet obstruction with oligohydramnios but have a normal karyotype, have no other systemic anomalies, are singleton fetuses, and, most importantly, have favorable renal function. The use of serial fetal bladder aspiration and examination of urine components (β2-microglobulin, sodium, chloride, and osmolality) are the most helpful methods of evaluating fetal renal function. As glomerular filtration rate increases, the presence of urinary sodium and low molecular weight plasma proteins (β2-microglobulin) decreases. However, in the case of dysplastic kidneys, electrolytes and proteins cannot be retained. Good renal function is seen in fetuses with favorable urinary indices (Na $<100$, Cl $<110$, Osm $<210$, β2 microglobulin $<10$–20) by serial sampling over 3 days. Urine sodium $<100$ mEq/mL and echolucent kidney are associated with good outcome (81 % survival), while sodium levels $>100$ mEq/mL and echogenic kidneys have been associated with poor outcome (12 % survival).

### Postnatal Follow-Up

If the hydronephrosis resolved during pregnancy, further postnatal radiological evaluation may not be necessary. In children with a history of prenatal hydronephrosis that resolved during pregnancy, the incidence of VUR is less than 5 % and the incidence of urinary tract obstruction would be rare. However, the parents should be advised that if their child develops a urinary tract infection later on, he/she should be evaluated for VUR. In contrast, infants with history of prenatally detected hydronephrosis that did not resolve during pregnancy should undergo further postnatal follow-up. The postnatal US and a VCUG should be performed within several days after birth in children with a solitary kidney, severe bilateral hydronephrosis, and/or ureterocele. Serum electrolytes and creatinine should be obtained to evaluate renal function. If the diagnosis of PUV is suspected or confirmed, urinary drainage should be instituted as soon as possible.

In cases of moderate prenatal hydronephrosis that did not resolve or a history of prenatal hydronephrosis of unknown severity and a postnatal US that demonstrated moderate or worse grade of hydronephrosis, a postnatal US and a VCUG would be indicated since the incidence of clinically significant urinary tract pathology is high enough to outweigh the risks of performing

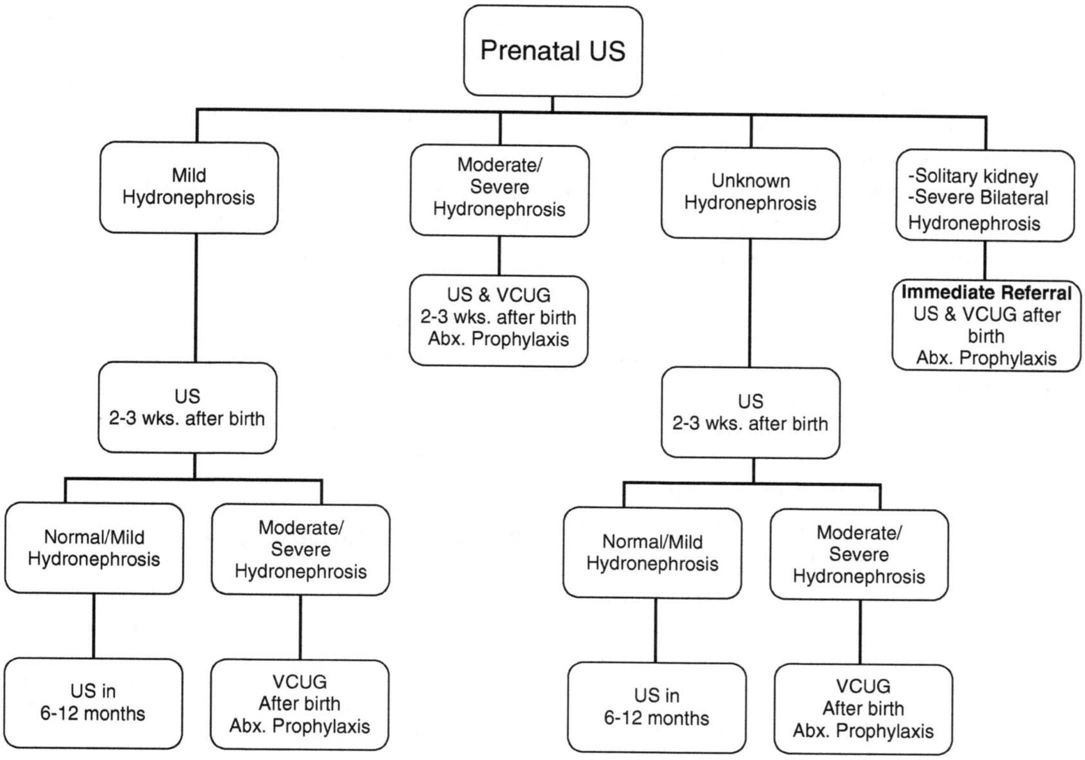


**Fig. 1.8** Suggested follow-up according to ultrasound findings

the radiologic tests. The US should be performed after 48 h since the degree of dilation may be significantly underestimated during the first few days of life, due to neonatal oliguria. The management of children with mild prenatal hydronephrosis and no or mild hydronephrosis on postnatal US is more controversial. In general, it is recommended that a follow-up US be performed. There is no standard recommendation on the timing of the US, but it is usually suggested that it will be performed 6 months to a year after birth. A follow-up postnatal US is recommended since significant urinary tract obstruction has been documented in children with a normal postnatal US. In addition, since the US is noninvasive and does not require exposure to radiation, it has minimal associated risks. The need for a VCUG in these children is highly debated. The incidence of VUR ranges from 5 to 20 %. VCUG requires exposure to radiation and placement of a urethral catheter, making the procedure more invasive than US. Consequently, some practitioners routinely performed VCUG in these children, while others do not and recommend a VCUG only if subsequent UTI occurs. These recommendations are summarized in Fig. 1.8.

## The Role of Antibiotic Prophylaxis

The advantages of using antibiotic prophylaxis in children with prenatal hydronephrosis have not been formally evaluated. It is expected that its use would prevent urinary tract infection and, consequently, prevent renal damage in the immature infant kidney. Some practitioners recommend antibiotic prophylaxis in all patients with confirmed postnatal hydronephrosis, while others only in cases with severe dilation. Oral amoxicillin (25 mg/kg once a day) is most commonly recommended during the first 3 months of life. Trimethoprim (2 mg/kg once a day) or nitrofurantoin (1–2 mg/kg once a day) may be utilized after 3 months of age. One practical approach would be to use antibiotic prophylaxis only when VUR or lower urinary tract obstruction (such as UVJ obstruction/megaureter, ureterocele, and PUV) is suspected. The rationale for this approach is that children with VUR and lower urinary tract obstruction are at higher risks of developing UTIs than those with transient/physiologic hydronephrosis or upper urinary tract obstruction.

## Antenatal Counseling

The diagnosis of prenatal hydronephrosis may cause significant parental anxiety with regard to its implication on renal function and fetal health and the need for prenatal and postnatal management. Consequently, it is important to assure the parents that prenatal hydronephrosis represents a spectrum of urinary tract anomalies with variable severity. The etiology of the hydronephrosis cannot be accurately determined by prenatal US. However, US findings such as AP size, the presence of oligohydramnios, and the onset on the dilatation may suggest its etiology and estimate the severity of the problem. In the majority of the cases (approximately 60 %), prenatal hydronephrosis is transient and has no significant clinical sequelae. Many will resolve during pregnancy or shortly after birth. Less than 5 % of the patients diagnosed with prenatal hydronephrosis require surgery for correction of VUR or urinary tract obstruction. Prenatal hydronephrosis may occur with subsequent pregnancy, occurring in 67 % of cases (relative risk of 6.1). Nevertheless, it is important to inform the parents about the importance of postnatal follow-up for diagnosis and appropriate management. It is possible in patients with mild prenatal hydronephrosis to avoid performing a VCUG; however, this must be done in selected cases with reliable families.

## Recommended Reading

Chitty LS, Masturzo B. Prenatal diagnosis of fetal renal abnormalities. In: Gearhart JP, editor. Pediatric urology. Philadelphia: Saunders; 2001. p. 58–91.

Craig AP. Perinatal urology. In: Walsh PC, editor. Campbell's urology, vol. 3. 8th ed. Philadelphia: Saunders; 2002. p. 1781–811.

Lee RS, Cendron M, Kinnamon DD, Nguyen HT. Antenatal hydronephrosis as a predictor of postnatal outcome: a meta-analysis. Pediatrics. 2006;118:586–93.

Shokeir AA, Nijman RJM. Antenatal hydronephrosis: changing concepts in diagnosis and subsequent management. BJU Int. 2000;85:987–94.

# Multicystic Dysplastic Kidney

# 2

Kenneth G. Nepple and Christopher S. Cooper

Multicystic dysplastic kidney (MCDK) is a nonfunctioning kidney that does not undergo normal differentiation and therefore has immature-appearing renal parenchyma with cystic dilations (Fig. 2.1). MCDK is often diagnosed on antenatal ultrasound, where MCDK is the second most common urinary tract abnormality after hydronephrosis. MCDK is almost always unilateral and slightly more frequent in boys and on the left side. MCDK is an uncommon entity with an incidence of 1 in 4,300 births [1]. However, knowledge of MCDK is important for diagnosing and managing these children.

In normal embryogenesis, the ureteric bud undergoes a series of divisions to form the collecting system of the kidney; however, in MCDK the ureteric bud is thought to have abnormal branching into the metanephric blastema resulting in cystic dilations that resembles a bunch of grapes [2]. The dysplastic renal parenchyma frequently occurs in association with an atretic ipsilateral ureter. The "dysplasia" in MCDK refers to renal tissue that fails to undergo the normal process of differentiation to mature functioning nephrons; therefore, the histopathologic appearance is of immature renal parenchyma and cysts of varying sizes. The diagnosis of "dysplasia" should not be confused with the use of "dysplasia" as premalignant in other conditions (e.g., cervical cancer), as the incidence of malignancy in MCDK is exceedingly low.

Key points to remember about MCDK:

- MCDK has essentially no function on renal scan, which is required in establishing the diagnosis.
- "Dysplasia" refers to the failure of development of renal tissue and not to precancerous or malignant dysplasia.
- The contralateral "normal" kidney has a significantly increased risk of vesicoureteral reflux.
- The typical natural history of MCDK is of progressive involution, and nephrectomy is rarely required.

## Presentation

The increased use of prenatal ultrasound imaging results in the early detection of most MCDK. Some children present with a palpable abdominal mass or following radiographic imaging at later ages during evaluation of urinary tract infection. Some children remain asymptomatic and are not diagnosed until a much later age. MCDK frequently involutes and some that are diagnosed in utero regress so that the child appears to have unilateral renal agenesis after birth. MCDK is very rarely diagnosed in adults, and thus many

K.G. Nepple, M.D. (✉) • C.S. Cooper, M.D., F.A.A.P., F.A.C.S.
Department of Urology, University of Iowa Hospitals and Clinics, 200 Hawkins Drive, Iowa City, IA 52242, USA
e-mail: Kenneth-nepple@uiowa.edu

R. Rabinowitz et al. (eds.), *Pediatric Urology for the Primary Care Physician*, Current Clinical Urology, DOI 10.1007/978-1-60327-243-8_2, © Springer Science+Business Media New York 2015

adults with a solitary kidney may have had an MCDK as a child.

MCDK is typically not associated with symptoms. However, MCDK may present as a palpable abdominal mass in a newborn, and the kidney can rarely be large enough to cause respiratory distress. MCDK is not typically associated with the development of urinary tract infection or hematuria, possibly because the function of the kidney is so low that little, if any, urine is actually produced by the kidney. The contralateral kidney typically has normal function, so presentation as acute renal failure is rare unless ureteropelvic junction obstruction is present in the contralateral kidney. Cardiac or neurologic conditions have not been consistently associated with MCDK.

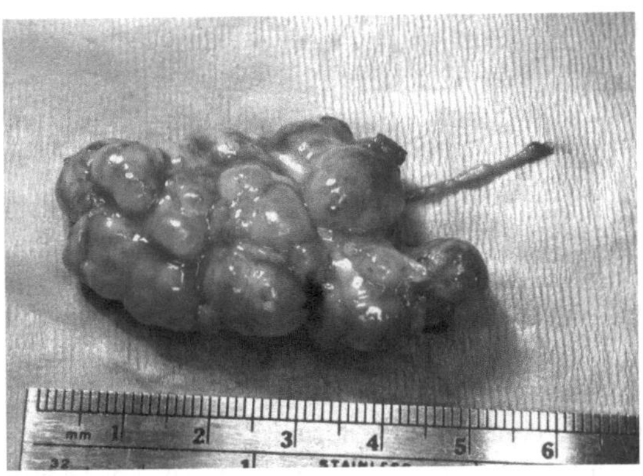

**Fig. 2.1** Nephrectomy specimen of MCDK

## Imaging Studies

The fetal kidney can be visualized on ultrasound at 18 weeks; however, the prenatal diagnosis is usually not made until the third trimester [3]. The antenatal diagnosis of MCDK may be considered based on appearance of the kidney on prenatal ultrasound which is of multiple noncommunicating cysts of various sizes. Because the anatomic detail of prenatal ultrasound is not precise, MCDK may also be labeled as antenatal hydronephrosis.

The postnatal ultrasound appearance of MCDK is of multiple noncommunicating cysts of various sizes that resemble a cluster of grapes (Fig. 2.2). The cysts on ultrasound appear as numerous anechoic (black) circular areas of variable size. The MCDK can be either enlarged or atrophic, and there is loss of the normal reniform shape and an absence of normal renal parenchyma. The contralateral kidney frequently undergoes compensatory hypertrophy resulting in a larger than normal size. Although infrequently obtained, a CT scan of MCDK demonstrates a cystic kidney with

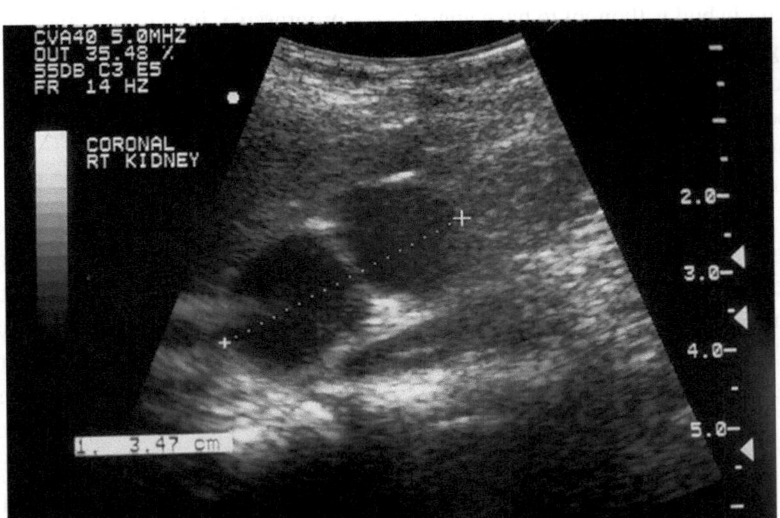


**Fig. 2.2** Ultrasound appearance of MCDK with noncommunicating cysts and no parenchyma

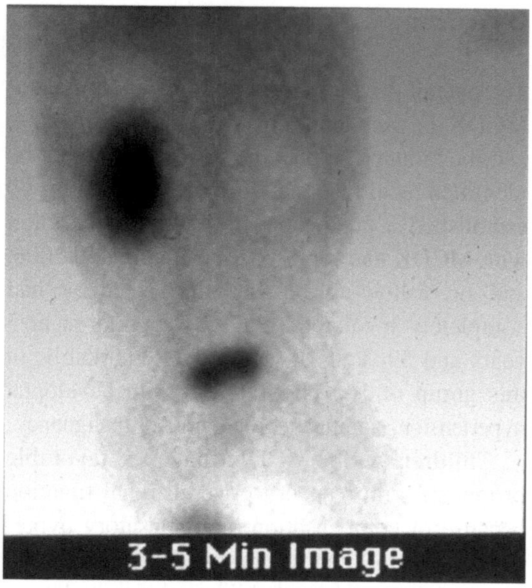


**Fig. 2.3** Renal scan demonstrating no function of a right MCDK with an absence of radioisotope uptake, while uptake (*black area*) is seen in the left kidney with excretion to the bladder

**Table 2.1** Diagnostic workup of MCDK

| |
|---|
| • History and physical exam |
| • Blood pressure measurement |
| • Serum creatinine |
| • Urinalysis, urine culture |
| • Renal ultrasound |
| • Renal scan (DMSA) |
| • VCUG |

decreased parenchymal thickness and images following administration of intravenous contrast show decreased uptake and excretion in the affected kidney.

A renal scan is performed, usually within the first 3 months of life, to confirm the absence of function in the affected kidney and to rule out the diagnosis of a kidney affected by a severe uretero-pelvic junction obstruction. A renal scan is a nuclear medicine radionuclide study that utilizes intravenous injection of a radioisotope (dimercaptosuccinic acid [DMSA] or mercaptoacetyltriglycine [MAG-3]) that is taken up and excreted by normally functioning kidneys and provides minimal radiation exposure. In MCDK the kidney shows no or minimal function on renal scan (Fig. 2.3), in contrast to kidneys with hydronephrosis which show functioning parenchyma. Table 2.1 outlines the diagnostic workup.

## Differential Diagnosis

Several other entities should be considered in the differential diagnosis of MCDK. The modality of choice when evaluating cystic disease of the kidney is ultrasound. Most of the differential diagnoses may be excluded based on the interpretation of radiographic images by an experienced radiologist or urologist.

MCDK at times may be difficult to differentiate from severe hydronephrosis, which is the most common cause of a palpable abdominal mass in an infant. In hydronephrosis, the overall reniform shape of the kidney is maintained, but the renal collecting system (calyces and renal pelvis) is dilated and can give an appearance suggestive of multiple cysts. However, the "cysts" in hydronephrosis communicate with the renal pelvis. In contrast, with MCDK, the normal shape of the kidney is lost, cysts are non-communicating, and the collecting system is not visualized. On renal scan, a severely hydronephrotic kidney will usually show some function, in contrast to a nonfunctioning MCDK.

MCDK also must be differentiated from other forms of cystic kidneys. Simple renal cysts may occasionally be found in children and warrant follow-up ultrasound. Wilm's tumor tends to be solitary and encapsulated, which can be differentiated from MCDK based on radiographic appearance. Polycystic kidney can be broken into two groups: autosomal recessive (typically diagnosed in the perinatal period) and autosomal dominant (diagnosed based on evaluation for known family history or in adulthood as most children are asymptomatic). The pathogenesis for MCDK is different than that of polycystic kidney. In MCDK the ureteric bud does not branch normally and results in dysplasia of the entire kidney, while in autosomal recessive polycystic kidney the architecture is destroyed by cystic deformation from dilated collecting ducts, while the collecting system and reniform shape of the kidney remain normal. In the autosomal dominant variant, the dilation is in all portions of the nephron. Polycystic kidney disease is due to genetic mutations and involves both kidneys.

MCDK that has atrophied and involuted must also be differentiated from an atrophic kidney secondary to a different etiology, such as recurrent pyelonephritis or damage secondary to high-grade vesicoureteral reflux. Kidneys with reflux nephropathy may have poor function and renal dysplasia, but there are no associated cysts.

## Associated Urinary Tract Abnormalities

About 15 % of MCDK will have vesicoureteral reflux into the dysplastic kidney, and 15–40 % of children with MCDK have vesicoureteral reflux in the "normal" contralateral kidney [4, 5]. Nineteen percent of children in the MCDK study group had contralateral reflux [5]. We routinely obtain voiding cystourethrogram (VCUG) in all children diagnosed with MCDK; however, some suggest that the initial VCUG can be deferred in children with a normal ultrasound of the contralateral kidney [5]. Prophylactic antibiotics and conservative management are used when vesicoureteral reflux is present in the contralateral kidney, and if breakthrough infections occur, urologists should have a lower threshold for operative intervention due to reflux into a solitary functioning kidney.

Contralateral ureteropelvic junction obstruction can be present in up to 12 % of children with MCDK, which is increased over the risk in the general population [4]. Because the contralateral kidney provides the entire renal function in children with MCDK, those with ureteropelvic junction obstruction can present with acute renal failure.

The risk of future urinary tract infection may at times be used as an indication for nephrectomy, but the true risk of urinary tract infection or pyelonephritis in MCDK is low. One report found only 5 % of children with MCDK had a urinary tract infection during follow-up [6].

## Outcome

The overall prognosis for children with unilateral MCDK is excellent. The MCDK can involute, and the kidney can become so small it cannot be identified by ultrasound. The MCDK study group established a prospective follow-up of children with MCDK and reported their findings in 2006, and on follow-up ultrasound the kidney had completely involuted in 47 % of children at 5 years and 59 % at 10 years [5]. Remarkably, in this group of 165 children, no child developed hypertension, significant proteinuria, or malignancy.

Children with MCDK have a favorable prognosis with respect to overall renal function because of compensation (compensatory hypertrophy) by the contralateral kidney. One study reported that in 81 % of children the contralateral kidney enlarged to greater than 2 standard deviations compared to normal kidney size, and in children followed for 10 years in the MCDK registry, the mean glomerular filtration rate was 86 mL/min/1.73 $m^2$ (range, 48–125), with only 2 of 31 having an abnormal glomerular filtration rate of <60 [5]. Another report of 80 children found that all children had normal renal function and no proteinuria despite having only one functional kidney [6]. However, we have taken care of a boy who was born with MCDK and severe hydronephrosis of the contralateral kidney who went on to require renal transplant despite prompt treatment of the obstructed functioning kidney in the neonatal period.

Hypertension is a reported infrequent effect of MCDK thought to be renin secreted from ischemic areas of the dysplastic kidney [1]. A systematic review found only 6 cases of hypertension in 1,115 children (0.5 %), which is similar to the risk of hypertension in the general pediatric population [7]. Hypertension has been used as an indication for nephrectomy; however, cases have been reported of hypertension that persists even after nephrectomy [8].

A major concern of parents with regard to children with MCDK is the development of malignancy. While rare case reports of the development of Wilm's tumor in less than 10 children with MCDK have been reported [1, 9], the concerns for potential malignancy development have not been substantiated by recent reviews. A systematic review of 26 cohort studies found no report of malignancy in 1,041 children [10], and one subsequent large series of 165 patients reported no malignancy identified [5]. One study performed flow cystometry in tissue from 30 MCDKs and found no abnormalities in the number of chromosomes present [11].

## Management

All children with MCDK should be referred to a urologist or nephrologist. The management of MCDK has been an area of controversy. The appropriate subsequent follow-up for MCDK remains controversial and heavily debated, with a recent trend toward nonsurgical management and less frequent observation.

Most MCDKs can be managed conservatively with radiographic follow-up, rather than operatively. Nephrectomy remains indicated for cases of respiratory or gastrointestinal compromise (abdominal distension or poor feeding), suspicious solid renal mass, or hypertension. Some parents may seek nephrectomy due to parental anxiety or kidneys that fail to involute during follow-up. In one large series, nephrectomy was required in less than 7 % of children with MCDK [5]. In cases where nephrectomy is required, a laparoscopic approach is feasible if not excluded due to young patient age or large kidney size. Open nephrectomy can be performed through a small incision because cysts can be aspirated intraoperatively to leave only a small kidney for removal. Nephrectomy is generally well tolerated in children with low risk of complications and short hospital stay. In cases where the MCDK is refluxing, a nephroureterectomy may be indicated.

In the management of children with MCDK, some propose that one issue supporting nephrectomy over observation is that insurance companies may be more likely to offer standard insurance rates to a person with an absent kidney as opposed to someone with MCDK. In a survey of the life insurance industry, La Salle reported that 15 % would issue life insurance to a child with MCDK that was observed versus 71 % if treatment had been a nephrectomy [12].

## Follow-Up

A consensus among pediatric urologists for radiographic follow-up of MCDK has not been reached. Previous surveillance regimens with frequent ultrasound were based on the false assumption that the development of Wilm's tumor was common in children with MCDK. Our typical recommended plan is radiographic follow-up every 12–18 months until kidney involution, after which radiographic follow-up can be discontinued. Others have recommended less frequent surveillance ultrasound at 2 and 5 years of age and then every 5 years [5]. A consensus has also not been reached regarding the length of follow-up required, with various groups recommending imaging to age 8, adulthood, or complete involution. One group recently commented that follow-up ultrasound provides no clinical benefit and increases parental anxiety and recommended no radiographic follow-up [13]. However, in those children who have contralateral renal pelvic dilation, follow-up ultrasound should be obtained more frequently due to the concern for development of ureteropelvic junction obstruction.

Blood pressure should be measured at clinic visits to assess for hypertension. While our group recommends continued blood pressure follow-up in all children, others have recommended that children with complete involution of the kidney, normal blood pressure, normal creatinine, and normal urinalysis can be discharged from long-term follow-up [5]. Children with MCDK have a solitary functioning contralateral kidney and should be counseled to avoid activities that would place that kidney at risk. This would include avoidance of contact sports and high-risk activities.

## References


1. Gordon AC, Thomas DF, Arthur RJ, Irving HC. Multicystic dysplastic kidney: is nephrectomy still appropriate? J Urol. 1988;140(5 Pt 2):1231–4.
2. Bisceglia M, Galliani CA, Senget C, Stallone C, Sessa A. Renal cystic diseases: a review. Adv Anat Pathol. 2006;13(1):26–56.
3. Avni EF, Thoua Y, Lalmand B, Didier F, Droulle P, Schulman C. Multicystic dysplastic kidney: natural history from in utero diagnosis and postnatal followup. J Urol. 1987;138(6):1420–4.
4. Glassberg KI. Renal dysgenesis and cystic disease of the kidney. In: Wein AJ, Kavoussi LR, Novick AC, Partin AW, Peters CA, editors. Campbell-Walsh urology, vol. 4. 9th ed. Philadelphia: Saunders; 2007. p. 3305–58. Chap. 114.
5. Aslam M, Watson AR. Unilateral multicystic dysplastic kidney: long term outcomes. Arch Dis Child. 2006;91(10):820–3.
6. Weinstein A, Goodman TR, Iragorri S. Simple multicystic dysplastic kidney disease: end points for subspecialty follow-up. Pediatr Nephrol. 2008;23(1):111–6.
7. Narchi H. Risk of hypertension with multicystic kidney disease: a systematic review. Arch Dis Child. 2005;90(9):921–4.
8. Snodgrass WT. Hypertension associated with multicystic dysplastic kidney in children. J Urol. 2000;164(2):472–3; discussion 473–4.
9. Homsy YL, Anderson JH, Oudjhane K, Russo P. Wilms tumor and multicystic dysplastic kidney disease. J Urol. 1997;158(6):2256–9; discussion 2259–60.
10. Narchi H. Risk of Wilms' tumour with multicystic kidney disease: a systematic review. Arch Dis Child. 2005;90(2):147–9.
11. Jung WH, Peters CA, Mandell J, Vawter GF, Retik AB. Flow cytometric evaluation of multicystic dysplastic kidneys. J Urol. 1990;144(2 Pt 2):413–5; discussion 422.
12. LaSalle MD, Stock JA, Hanna MK. Insurability of children with congenital urological anomalies. J Urol. 1997;158(3 Pt 2):1312–5.
13. Onal B, Kogan BA. Natural history of patients with multicystic dysplastic kidney-what followup is needed? J Urol. 2006;176(4 Pt 1):1607–11.

# Renal Agenesis and Associated Anomalies

3

Mark F. Bellinger

An absent kidney is one of the most common congenital anomalies of the urinary tract. While bilateral renal agenesis is a lethal anomaly that may rarely be seen by primary care physicians, unilateral renal agenesis (URA) is commonly quite innocuous, may be discovered only by serendipity, and may have consequences not evident until many years after birth.

## Bilateral Renal Agenesis

Bilateral renal agenesis is an uncommon and catastrophic anomaly, which is almost universally fatal, usually presenting as a stillbirth or as death within the first 24–48 h after birth from severe respiratory failure due to pulmonary hypoplasia. The clinical characteristics of children with bilateral renal agenesis (Potter's syndrome) have been well-described as: low birth weight, Potter's facies (prominent inner canthal folds with a prominent skinfold beneath the eyes, a broad, blunted nose, a prominent depression between the lower lip and chin, low-set ears, a bell-shaped chest, bowed and clubbed legs, dry loose-appearing skin, and large claw-like hands). This constellation of phenotype may appear in a variable clinical spectrum and appears to be the consequence of severe oligohydramnios. About 75 % of infants with Potter's syndrome are male, and the genitalia and vas deferens are normal in most cases [1].

The initial radiographic evaluation of infants with bilateral renal agenesis usually consists of an abdominal ultrasound examination only.

Care for those infants who are not stillborn is primarily supportive, as a child who survives with ventilatory support will die of renal failure relatively quickly in the majority of cases.

Genetic counseling and sibling ultrasound screening are appropriate in cases of bilateral renal agenesis. Although the exact inheritance pattern is unknown, there is some evidence to suggest an autosomal dominant inheritance with high penetrance. It is not unusual to find parents or siblings with undiagnosed URA or other congenital urinary anomalies.

## Unilateral Renal Agenesis

The true incidence of URA is most likely significantly underestimated because of the usual lack of clinical findings or symptoms associated with this anomaly. It has been estimated that the incidence is between 1 in 1,100 and 1 in 1,500 births, with a male predominance of almost 2:1. URA has been associated with several genetic syndromes including the DiGeorge, Fraser, Kallmann, trisomy C and D, and cat-eye syndromes, among others. Many cases have been discovered serendipitously on prenatal ultrasound examination.

M.F. Bellinger, M.D. (✉)
The Children's Hospital of Pittsburgh,
501 Guyasuta Road, Pittsburgh, PA 15215, USA
e-mail: markbellinger@mac.com

R. Rabinowitz et al. (eds.), *Pediatric Urology for the Primary Care Physician*, Current Clinical Urology,
DOI 10.1007/978-1-60327-243-8_3, © Springer Science+Business Media New York 2015

The clinical significance of URA may be related directly to one of three clinical scenarios: (1) problems related to the contralateral kidney that may lead to obstruction, renal insufficiency, or urinary infection, (2) genital anomalies related embryologically to URA, and (3) trauma or other insult to the solitary kidney.

In order to understand the spectrum of potential clinical scenarios that may be associated with URA, it is imperative to have some basic understanding of the development of the kidney and genital structures and of the close embryological relationship between the two.

The development of the genital and urinary systems is closely interwoven. As a result of this intimacy, defects in renal development may have a tremendous impact upon the embryogenesis of genital structures. In addition, the fact that anomalies of renal development may occur at different stages of embryogenesis has the potential to produce variable defects in genital development and thus a spectrum of clinically silent anomalies. These internal genital anomalies, although innocuous in childhood, may become clinically significant in adolescence or adulthood.

The formation of a functioning kidney requires the joining of two disparate embryological entities: the metanephric mesoderm (metanephric blastema) and the ureteral bud. In the development of each structure and the process of coalescence, any number of embryological misadventures may lead to renal agenesis and thus a spectrum of genital anomaly.

The ureteral bud develops as an outgrowth from the mesonephric duct. The mesonephric duct is a remnant of the development of the primitive mesonephric kidney, a structure which never functions in the human. However, the mesonephric duct in the male becomes the vas deferens and seminal vesicle. If the mesonephric duct fails to form properly, anomalies of these seminal structures will result, in addition to the fact that the ureteral bud will not form. Agenesis of the ureteral bud negates the possibility of formation of a kidney since the ureteral bud, which forms the ureter, the renal pelvis, and the collecting ducts, must grow to join with the metanephric blastema. These ureteral bud structures, which are the conduits by which urine is transported, must unite with nephrons which are developing concomitantly in situ in the metanephric blastema. Thus, if either the ureteral bud or the mesonephric blastema is absent or dysgenetic, formation of a normal, functioning kidney will not occur.

Embryogenesis of the mullerian duct occurs in immediate contiguity with the mesonephric duct. It appears that development of the mullerian duct is induced by the development of the mesonephric duct itself. The mullerian duct forms the ipsilateral fallopian tube and coalesces in the midline with its contralateral mirror image to form the uterus and upper portion of the vagina. Anomalous development of the mesonephric duct thus may have severe consequences on development of the uterus, ipsilateral fallopian tube, and upper vagina [2]. Commonly seen anomalies include uterus didelphys, commonly with the ipsilateral hemiuterus and upper vagina being hypoplastic and/or noncanalized and thus obstructed when menstruation begins. Clinically and radiographically, these anomalies may not become evident until puberty.

The increasing use of prenatal ultrasound screening over the last 30 years has led to the appreciation of another etiology of URA: involution of a multicystic dysplastic kidney. Multicystic renal dysplasia is a common cause of renal cystic disease. Serial ultrasound studies have confirmed that a large number of cystic kidneys may undergo spontaneous involution both prenatally and postnatally. Involution in most cases results in diminution in the size of the cystic kidney until it is undetectable by ultrasound and other imaging studies. It is thus assumed that an unknown number of patients with unilateral renal "agenesis" may have in fact had a kidney that did form, with subsequent spontaneous involution. The end result for the patient's renal function will be the same in either embryologic scenario: a solitary functioning kidney. However, since a multicystic kidney implies the development of a mesonephric duct and ureteral bud, the concern about anomalous development of the mullerian structures should be eliminated when involution of a multicystic kidney can be documented. Unfortunately, without a prenatal study showing conclusively

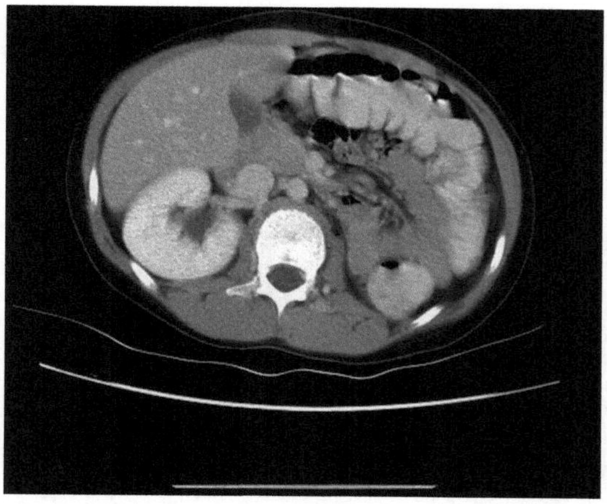

**Fig. 3.1** Abdominal CT with contrast showing a normal right kidney. The left kidney is absent, and the left colon is located in a medial and posterior location in the renal fossa

that a multicystic kidney was present, the true etiology of renal agenesis must remain speculative, and concern about the potential for late-presenting mullerian anomalies cannot be eliminated.

URA is predominantly a clinically silent anomaly. In the majority of cases, this anomaly will be a serendipitous finding during abdominal imaging of the fetus, infant, or child for various and sundry reasons. Males have a higher incidence of URA, and the left kidney is slightly more likely to be absent than the right.

Imaging studies may suggest or confirm the presence of URA. Plain abdominal radiographs may suggest renal agenesis when the gas pattern suggests that the splenic flexure of the colon is displaced medially and posteriorly into the left renal fossa (left renal agenesis) or when the hepatic flexure is positioned in the right renal fossa (right renal agenesis). These of course are only soft signs that require further imaging to confirm renal absence. On occasion, abdominal ultrasound, computed tomography (CT), radionuclide imaging, or other imaging study may conclusively demonstrate the absence of one kidney (Figs. 3.1 and 3.2). It should always be remembered that the absence of a normally placed kidney in the renal fossa may occur in the presence of an ectopic kidney (lumbar or pelvic kidney or cross-fused renal ectopia) and that adequate imaging should be performed to rule out renal ectopia.

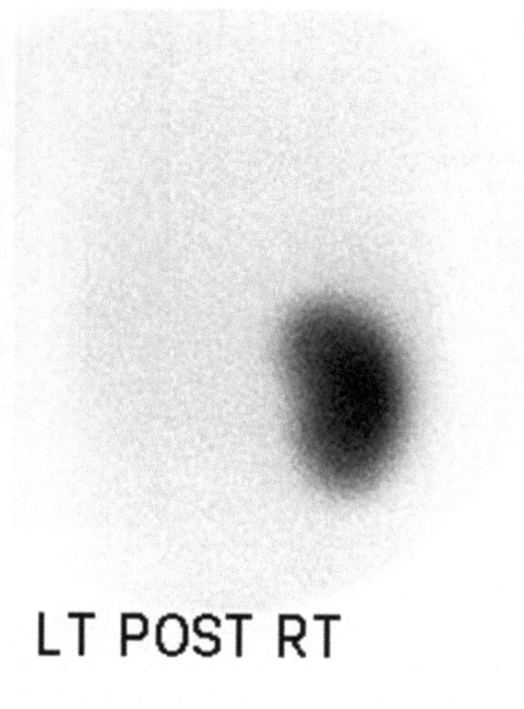


**Fig. 3.2** DMSA (Technetium-99 m dimercaptosuccinic acid) scan, posterior view. The right kidney is normal, and the left kidney is absent

In the case of an involuted multicystic kidney, a small remnant of cystic kidney may be evident on CT or MRI imaging. The presence of a cystic ipsilateral pelvic mass in an adolescent with URA may indicate an obstructed mullerian structure (i.e., bicornuate uterus with an obstructed segment). Conversely, imaging of the upper urinary tract in the presence of internal genital anomalies may confirm the presence of ipsilateral renal agenesis. In some cases, URA may be associated with an ipsilateral ureterocele or cystic intravesical or retrovesical mass representing an embryological remnant of the ureteral bud or wolffian duct (Fig. 3.3). In any event, the finding of what appears to be URA on any imaging study should indicate the need for pediatric urological consultation so that the need for further imaging can be determined. This is preferable to simply ordering more imaging studies that may not be indicated.

Renal length measurements may be helpful in the diagnosis of URA. Since contralateral renal

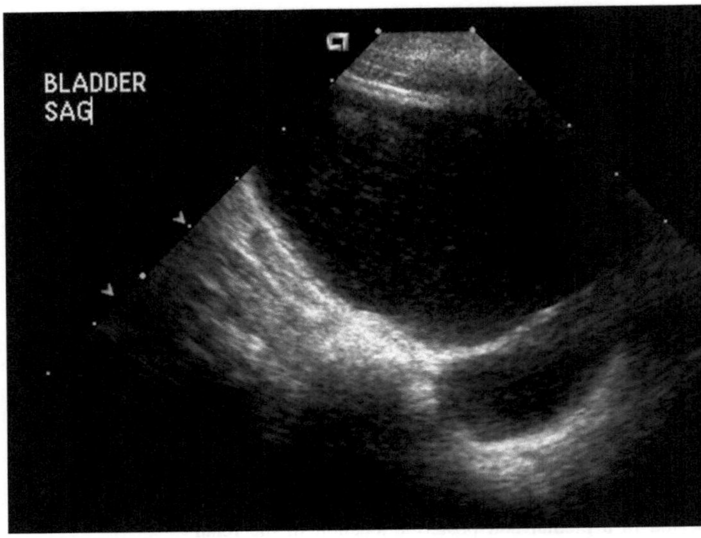


**Fig. 3.3** Pelvic ultrasound in a male infant. The bladder is seen at the upper midportion of the scan, with a cystic retrovesical lesion below the bladder to the left side of the image. This is a retrovesical cyst associated with an absent left kidney

hypertrophy is seen in the absence of one renal unit, renal length measurement is an important consideration in this diagnosis. It should be remembered, however, that other clinical entities, including duplication of the collecting system, may be associated with increased renal length.

Physical findings associated with URA are limited. The finding of a pelvic mass on abdominal or pelvic examination in an adolescent may be an indication of internal genital malformation or obstruction associated with an absent kidney. Similarly, the absence of a vas deferens or epididymis may signal concern about URA or anomaly. Vaginoscopy may demonstrate abnormality, and cystoscopy may demonstrate an absent ureteral orifice and ipsilateral trigonal absence or hypoplasia. It should always be remembered, however, that an absence of the ureteral orifice in the bladder does not rule out the possibility of the kidney being present and draining via an extravesical ectopic ureter.

Management of a patient with URA consists of diagnosis and assessment of baseline renal function, observation with occasional reevaluation, and management of any expected or unexpected complications of the embryological anomaly. Given the potential for a spectrum of anomaly, it is appropriate to obtain pediatric urological consultation when URA is documented. Evaluation, as noted above, consists of thorough and appropriate imaging to insure the diagnosis of URA and to rule out associated anomalies. It is appropriate to assess the function of the contralateral kidney with serum BUN and creatinine levels. The family should be aware that any clinical findings that may indicate a problem with the solitary functioning kidney (pain, hematuria, urinary tract infection…) should be evaluated fully. In particular, in infants and young children, the finding of significant urinary tract infection may indicate the need for voiding cystourethrography to assess for the presence of vesicoureteric reflux into the solitary kidney. Girls with URA, even when pelvic sonograpy in childhood is normal, should be followed with serial pelvic ultrasound examination beginning in the prepubertal period and continuing past menarche. This follow-up is indicated for prospective evaluation of the possibility that gynecological consequences of URA will become evident only after menarche.

One question that eventually arises when URA or absence is documented relates to the potential for renal injury, in particular in respect to the potential for renal trauma during participation in contact sports. Historically the recommendation for children and adolescents with a solitary kidney has been to avoid contact sports.

Recent studies have documented that, in fact, renal injuries related to participation in organized sporting activities are indeed uncommon, and, in fact, cycling injuries are a far more common cause of renal trauma than contact sport-related injury [3]. It would appear reasonable to caution families that children who suffer injury of any type (trauma, infection, or other insult) to a solitary kidney may be placed in jeopardy for renal dysfunction or loss. However, participation in organized sports in most cases need not necessarily be restricted, with the caveat that, at the high school level and beyond, the use of flank or kidney protection may be a conservative approach to minimizing the potential for renal injury in contact sports.

## References

1. Bauer S. Anomalies of the upper urinary tract. In: Campbell-Walsh urology. 9th ed., vol. 4. Philadelphia: Saunders, 2007:3269–3276.
2. Magee M, Lucey D, Fried F. A new embryological classification for uro-gynecologic malformations: the syndromes of mesonephric duct induced mullerian deformities. J Urol. 1979;121:265–7.
3. Grinsell M, Showalter S, Gordon K, Norwood V. Single kidney and sports participation: perception versus reality. Pediatrics. 2006;118:1019–26.

# 4 Renal Duplication Anomalies

Michael Leonard

## Introduction

Complete renal duplication is a condition in which there are two discrete renal moieties each with its own renal pelvis and ureter. The incidence of ureteral duplication in unselected autopsy series is 0.8 %. Most duplication anomalies are uncomplicated, do not result in clinical problems, and do not merit urological consultation. However, if the duplication anomaly is associated with an upper pole moiety (UPM) ectopic ureter or ureterocele or lower pole moiety (LPM) vesicoureteric reflux or ureteropelvic junction obstruction, urological consultation is recommended. Clinically relevant duplication anomalies are seen twice as commonly in females, with no side predilection. There is a genetic predisposition to renal duplication anomalies, as 1/8 of parents or siblings of an affected child are similarly afflicted.

M. Leonard, M.D., F.R.C.S.(C) (✉)
Department of Urology, Department of Surgery, Children's Hospital of Eastern Ontario, University of Ottawa, 401 Smyth Road, Ottawa, ON, Canada, K1H 8L1
e-mail: mleonard@cheo.on.ca

## Embryology of the Kidney and Ureter

During embryologic development, three different fetal kidneys are formed: pronephros, mesonephros, and metanephros. The former two completely regress and disappear, while the latter forms the kidney.

The mesonephric (Wolffian) duct appears at 24 days of gestation. Shortly thereafter its distal end joins the primitive cloaca, and it becomes a hollow tubular structure. At 28 days of gestation, a sprout from the distal portion of the Wolffian duct, called the ureteric bud, interacts with the metanephric blastema and triggers a mutual stimulus for the development of the kidney and ureter. Abnormalities with this interaction are regarded as the cause for renal and ureteral anomalies, and renal duplication is one of them. Complete renal duplication occurs when two distinct ureteric buds emanate from the Wolffian duct. The most caudal of these buds is associated with the LPM of the kidney, while the cranial bud is associated with the UPM. The ureteric buds are then absorbed into the developing bladder trigone and migrate cranially and laterally. Since the most caudal bud is absorbed first, it has more time to migrate cranially and laterally, resulting in the LPM orifice being more cranial and lateral on the trigone than the UPM orifice, which is more caudal and medial. This relationship is known as the Weigert-Meyer law, and there are very rare

R. Rabinowitz et al. (eds.), *Pediatric Urology for the Primary Care Physician*, Current Clinical Urology, DOI 10.1007/978-1-60327-243-8_4, © Springer Science+Business Media New York 2015

exceptions to this rule. The ectopic ureteric bud may interact defectively with the metanephric blastema resulting in a moiety which is dysplastic and poorly functional. This is particularly common with upper pole moieties associated with ectopic ureters and ureteroceles.

## Clinical Presentation and Investigation

As mentioned previously, many patients with uncomplicated renal duplication anomalies do not present with urological problems and may come to light as an incidental finding on abdominal ultrasound performed for an unrelated reason. Clinically relevant duplication anomalies may present in varied ways. Antenatally detected hydronephrosis in the fetus on ultrasound assessment is a common mode of presentation. Patients may also present with urinary tract infection/urosepsis, recurrent flank pain with nausea and vomiting (ureteropelvic junction obstruction—UPJO), urinary incontinence or purulent vaginal discharge (ectopic ureter in a female), or recurrent epididymitis (ectopic ureter in a male).

Investigation usually starts with a renal ultrasound and may also require the performance of a voiding cystourethrogram (VCUG) or renal scan depending on the pathology detected. Newer imaging modalities, such as MRI, have been found useful in selected cases.

## Anomalies Associated with Upper Pole Moiety

There are two major anomalies associated with the UPM of a duplex system: ectopic ureter and ureterocele.

(a) Ectopic Ureter

The UPM ureteric bud may branch more craniad than normal from the Wolffian duct and thus enter the trigone later than it usually would or even continue to be attached to the Wolffian duct. This results in a ureter that inserts into the bladder neck or urethra in either sex. In boys it may also insert to the ejaculatory duct, vas deferens, or seminal vesicle. In girls, the ureter may enter the Gartner's duct and rupture into the vagina or introitus. It may also rarely insert into the cervix or uterus. Presentation may include antenatal hydronephrosis, urinary tract infection, or urinary incontinence in a girl with an otherwise normal voiding pattern. Rarely a girl may present with recurrent purulent vaginal discharge. Males do not present with incontinence, as the ectopic ureter inserts to the urinary tract proximal to the external sphincter complex. However, males may present with acute epididymitis as the ectopic ureter may insert into the reproductive tract. The physical examination may be normal, especially in infants detected as having an UPM ectopic ureter by antenatal hydronephrosis. In such patients a flank mass may occasionally be palpable. If presenting with a urinary tract infection, there may be concurrent flank tenderness to palpation or percussion. An enlarged, erythematous, and tender hemiscrotum would be consistent with epididymitis in a male. Careful examination of the introitus in the female may reveal the slow continual dribbling of urine from an ectopic ureter inserting to the urethra or vagina. Investigation should include a renal ultrasound in all children. The UPM is usually hydronephrotic and associated with a tortuous hydroureter. Those presenting with urinary tract infection also require a VCUG to rule out reflux, as in some cases UPM ureters ectopic to the bladder neck or proximal urethra reflux. A renal scan is usually obtained to assess the function of the UPM, which is often minimal due to underlying dysplasia. In most cases an UPM heminephrectomy is performed to remove the poorly functioning UPM and as much of the associated ectopic ureter as possible. A stump of ectopic ureter is left behind and generally does not result in problems. In the rare instance the UPM has good function, its ureter may be joined to the LPM ureter or reimplanted into the bladder to reintegrate it into the urinary tract.

(b) Ureterocele

Ureterocele is a cystic dilatation of the distal ureter, which may be contained entirely within the bladder (intravesical) or may extend into the bladder neck or urethra (ectopic). Duplex systems are more commonly associated with ectopic ureteroceles and single systems with intravesical ureteroceles. Duplex system ectopic ureteroceles are more common in girls and more commonly left sided and may be bilateral in 10 % of cases. Patients may present with antenatally detected hydronephrosis, urinary tract infection/urosepsis, bladder outlet obstruction, or prolapse through the urethral orifice (females only). Physical findings mimic those discussed for ectopic ureter, with the exception of scrotal findings. Additionally, in a female infant, the ureterocele can rarely prolapse through the urethra resulting in a mass at the introitus. Investigation comprises a renal ultrasound and VCUG. The ultrasound demonstrates a hydronephrotic UPM associated with a dilated tortuous hydroureter, which culminates in a bubble-like appearance in the bladder (Fig. 4.1). There may also be ipsilateral LPM hydronephrosis, and indeed contralateral hydronephrosis, particularly in the setting of bladder outlet obstruction. Vesicoureteric reflux (VUR) is seen in 50 % of LPM ipsilateral to the ureterocele and in 20 % of contralateral ureters. Renal scans are often obtained to assess the degree of UPM function and/or obstruction by the ureterocele. Like ectopic ureters, the UPM function is often poor when associated with a ureterocele. Management depends on the acuity of patient presentation, presence of VUR, and UPM function. If a patient presents with urosepsis not responding to antibiotics or prolapse of the ureterocele through the urethral orifice, emergency drainage is required. In more elective circumstances, management varies greatly from endoscopic incision through upper pole heminephrectomy to complete reconstruction (upper pole heminephrectomy with ureterocele excision and LPM ureteric reimplantation).

## Anomalies Associated with Lower Pole Moiety

### VUR

Vesicoureteric reflux is the most common urinary tract abnormality associated with duplex systems and complete ureteral duplication. As

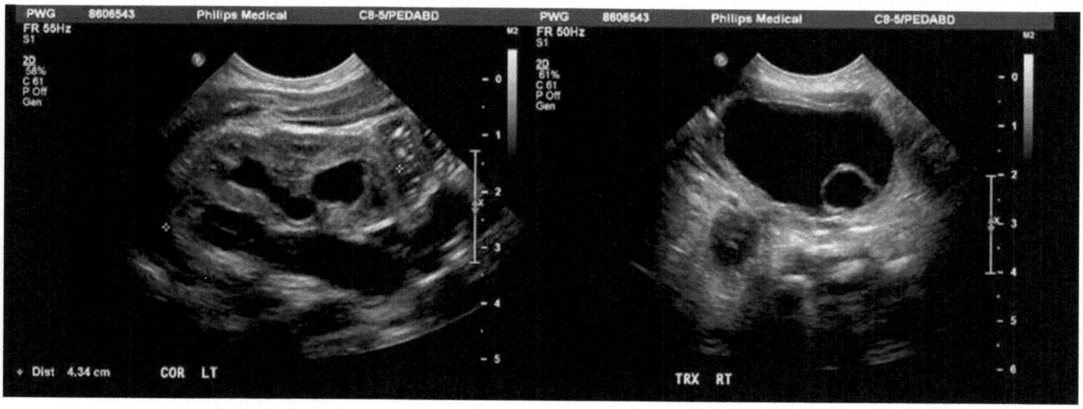


**Fig. 4.1** One-month-old boy with left renal duplication, hydroureteronephrosis of the upper unit, and ureterocele inside the bladder

mentioned in the Embryology section, the Weigert-Meyer law explains the differences observed in the ureteral orifice location and submucosal tunnel length of the distal ureters in complete renal duplication. As the LPM ureter inserts more proximally and laterally on the bladder trigone, it has a shorter submucosal tunnel length and consequently a suboptimal anti-reflux mechanism. The UPM ureter rarely refluxes, and this is attributed to its distal location on the trigone, which confers a longer submucosal tunnel and a more effective flap-valve mechanism. VUR is diagnosed by VCUG or nuclear cystogram. The typical VCUG image of VUR to the LPM in a complete duplication will show the "drooping lily" appearance of the collecting system: fewer calices than expected in a single system with the upper calices in a more horizontal axis. Reflux to the LPM in a duplex kidney may be associated with hydronephrosis, recurrent urinary infection, and in severe cases thinning of the LPM parenchyma. Physical examination is nonspecific for the presence of VUR and would be expected to be normal in a child who is asymptomatic. Management for reflux in a duplex collecting system is similar to that for VUR in a single collecting system, with antibiotic prophylaxis being the first choice in most cases. Surgery is reserved for more severe grades of reflux associated with breakthrough urinary infections and/or progressive renal scarring with loss of ipsilateral renal function. Reported data shows the same rate of resolution of reflux to LPM of duplex systems when compared with VUR to a single system. When surgical treatment is elected, reimplantation of both ipsilateral ureters and heminephrectomy of the LPM are options. The choice is mainly dictated by the amount of functioning parenchyma in the LPM and the severity of dilation of the ureters. More recently, endoscopic sub-ureteral injection of bulking substances for correction of VUR has shown acceptable rates of cure in duplex systems.

## UPJO

UPJO is the most common congenital obstruction in a single system; however the incidence of UPJO in duplex collecting systems is less frequent (2 %) and most commonly affects the LPM. Obstruction of the UPJ is rarely seen in the UPM. It may present with antenatal hydronephrosis, flank pain, recurrent urinary infection, or kidney stones. Physical findings are nonspecific and may range from a normal examination to a patient with severe upper quadrant and flank tenderness ipsilateral to the obstruction. UPJO may be an intrinsic primary congenital malformation of the ureter, but in duplex collecting systems, it is often associated with crossing vessels of the renal pedicle or high-grade VUR. Severe VUR to the LPM may cause significant ureteral dilation with secondary kinking of the UPJ, resulting in obstruction. UPJO of the lower moiety may be associated with different degrees of dilation of the collecting system and impairment of the urinary drainage. Usually the LPM ureter is not dilated, unless there is a concomitant severe grade of VUR, which would be documented by VCUG. UPJO of the LPM is suspected by an US that shows a dilated collecting system in the lower portion of a duplex kidney. Dilation of the urinary system is not always associated with obstruction of the kidney, whereas renal scarring and diffuse thinning of the parenchyma on the US may represent an indirect sign of kidney damage. The presence of obstruction is assessed using a diuretic renal scan, which provides the differential renal function of both kidneys, the differential function of the UPM and LPM of the duplex system, and the drainage curves of both kidneys and ipsilateral moieties to allow for assessment of obstruction. A significant obstruction with compromise of the relative LPM function is an indication for surgical correction, which may be accomplished by an open or laparoscopic pyeloplasty. Severe UPJO of a nonfunctioning LPM is best managed with heminephrectomy of the LPM and excision of as much ureteral length as possible if VUR is present.

## Recommended Reading

Belman AB, King LR, Kramer S. Clinical pediatric urology. 4th ed. London: Martin Duntz; 2002.

Ben-Ami T, Gayer G, Hertz M, et al. The natural history of reflux in the lower pole of duplicated collecting systems: a controlled study. Pediatr Radiol. 1989;19(5):308–10.

Decter RM. Renal duplication and fusion anomalies. Pediatr Clin North Am. 1997;44(5):1323–41.

Gonzales F, Canning DA, Hyun G, Casale P. Lower pole pelvi-ureteric junction obstruction in duplicated collecting systems. BJU Int. 2006;97(1):161–5.

Wein AJ, Kavoussi LR, Novick AC, Partin AW, Peters CA. Campbell-Walsh urology. 9th ed. Philadelphia: W.B. Saunders; 2007.

# 5 Ureteropelvic Junction Obstruction in the Pediatric Population

Danielle D. Sweeney and Steven G. Docimo

## Introduction

Ureteropelvic junction obstruction (UPJO), defined as the functionally significant impairment of urinary transport from the renal pelvis to the proximal ureter, is the most common cause of hydronephrosis in newborns and young children [1]. Left untreated, this condition may cause progressive dilation of the renal collecting system, with deterioration of renal function and loss of renal unit. UPJO has a diverse presentation, as it may be a primary congenital abnormality diagnosed prenatally, or secondarily acquired, and not apparent until late adolescence or adulthood. This chapter will focus on primary UPJO with review of the current methods of diagnosis and treatment options, as well as the authors' approach to managing this condition.

D.D. Sweeney, M.D. (✉)
Pediatric Urology of Central Texas, Austin, TX, USA
e-mail: danielledsweeney@gmail.com

S.G. Docimo, M.D., F.A.A.P., F.A.C.S.
Department of Urology, The Children's Hospital of Pittsburgh, The University of Pittsburgh Medical Center, 3705 Fifth Avenue, G205 DeSoto Wing, Pittsburgh, PA 15213, USA

## Etiology and Epidemiology

The etiology of UPJO cannot be isolated to just one source. In children, UPJO is usually primary or congenital in nature, related to developmental abnormalities of the ureteropelvic junction or caused by extrinsic compression from anatomic variants. Less commonly it can be linked to secondary causes such as infection, vesicoureteral reflux (VUR), recurrent stone passage, or iatrogenic strictures from previous surgery.

Causes of primary intrinsic UPJO include an aperistaltic segment of the ureter from abnormalities of the ureteral musculature, congenital ureteral strictures due to excessive collagen deposition at a narrowed site, and ureteral fibroepithelial polyps [2] (Fig. 5.1). Primary extrinsic causes include high insertion of the ureter into the renal pelvis, ureteral kinking, and most frequently, vessels to the lower pole of the kidney that pass anterior to the ureteropelvic junction and intermittently cause obstruction (Fig. 5.2).

The incidence of UPJO is approximately 1:500 with a male to female ratio of 2:1 [3]. It is more common on the left side than the right side and is reported to be bilateral in 10–40 % [3]. Associated anomalies, primarily of urologic origin, are common in those with congenital UPJO. VUR, albeit low grade, is found in 40 % of patients, renal dysplasia or multicystic dysplastic kidney disease is present in 10 %, unilateral kidney agenesis in 5 %, and VATER (Vertebral Anal Tracheal Esophageal Renal) syndrome in 20 % [1].

R. Rabinowitz et al. (eds.), *Pediatric Urology for the Primary Care Physician*, Current Clinical Urology,
DOI 10.1007/978-1-60327-243-8_5, © Springer Science+Business Media New York 2015

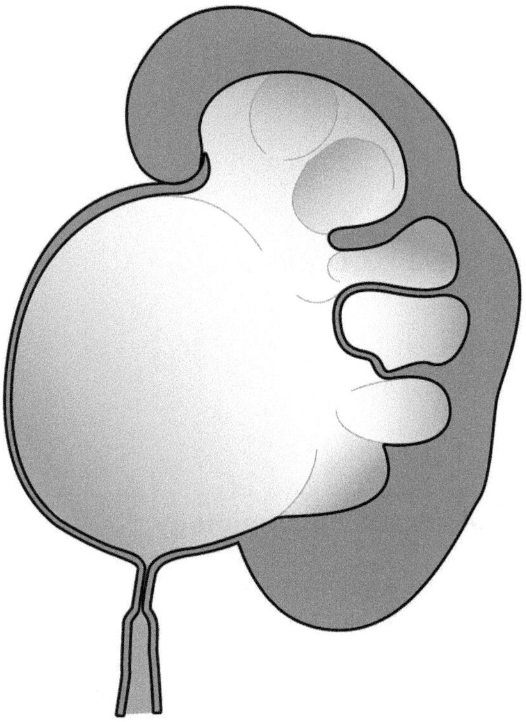

**Fig. 5.1** Primary intrinsic UPJO with a pathologic narrowed ureter at the ureteropelvic junction

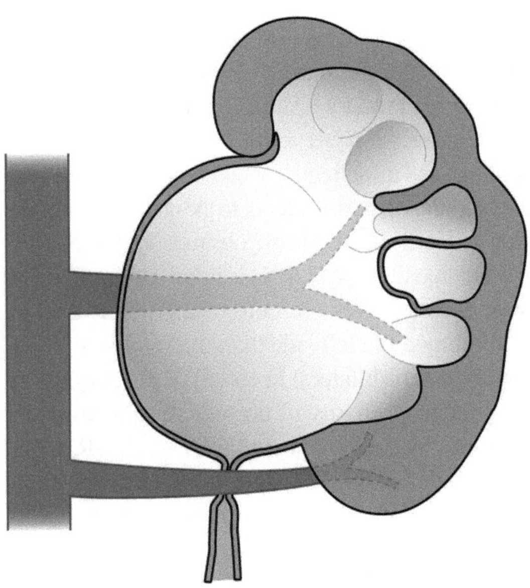

**Fig. 5.2** Primary extrinsic UPJO from vessels to the lower pole of the kidney

## Presentation

The presentation of UPJO can be as varied as the etiologies of the disease. In the infant population, hydronephrosis is usually diagnosed prenatally with the use of maternal ultrasonography. These infants are typically asymptomatic at the time of delivery; however, approximately 10–30 % are found to have UPJO on postnatal evaluation [1]. In the absence of prenatal screening, infants with hydronephrosis can also present with an abdominal mass, feeding difficulties, failure to thrive, or sepsis.

In older children, presentation is typically characterized by a symptomatic episode of abdominal or flank pain and nausea and vomiting, called a Dietl's crisis. Cyclic vomiting alone can also be a sign of intermittent UPJO; however this symptom complex is often misdiagnosed as gastrointestinal in origin. Less common presentations include urinary tract infection, hematuria, nephrolithiasis, and rarely hypertension. With the increased use of radiographic imaging, incidental diagnosis of asymptomatic UPJO is also prevalent.

## Evaluation and Diagnosis

The evaluation of UPJO in the infant or child varies with presentation. The evaluation of infants with prenatally diagnosed hydronephrosis will be initiated at the time of birth. For older children, the evaluation of possible UPJO commences with their first Dietl's crisis or clinically significant event.

### Ultrasonography

For infants that have been diagnosed prenatally with hydronephrosis, a renal ultrasound should be obtained neonatally to reassess the dilatation of the renal collecting system.

Renal ultrasonography does not diagnose obstruction or predict resolution; however it can correlate with a clinically relevant obstructive process. When the anterior-posterior diameter of the renal pelvis is >15 mm, it is suggestive of the

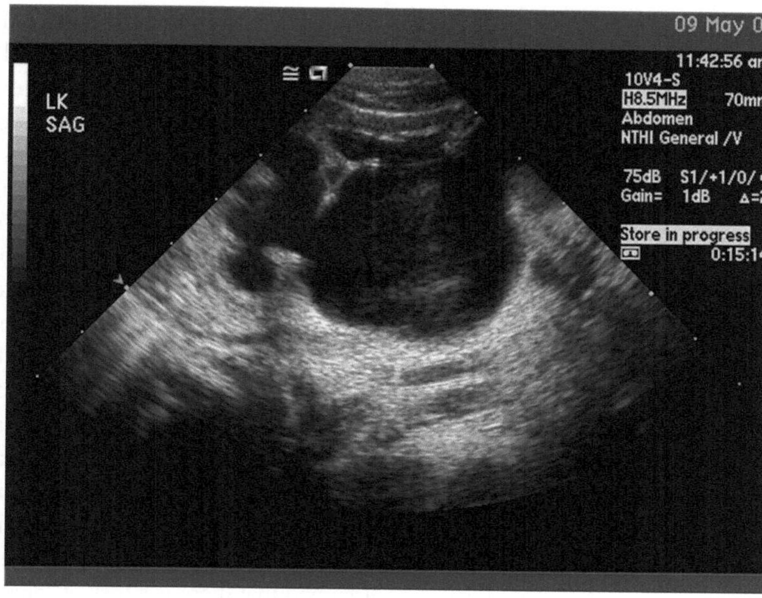


**Fig. 5.3** Typical appearance of UPJO on ultrasound. Note dilated renal pelvis and calyces

presence of obstruction, as is a trend of worsening hydronephrosis over time (Fig. 5.3). Renal size should be measured in the affected kidney and contralateral kidney over a period of time. As obstruction worsens, there tends to be an overall decrease in function and growth of the affected kidney with a compensatory hypertrophy of the contralateral healthy kidney.

Ultrasonography is also a useful tool in older children who present acutely. We commonly give our patients with a history of intermittent abdominal pain a prescription for a renal ultrasound, to be obtained at the time of an acute episode. This modality is a relatively simple, noninvasive test that can monitor dilation over time. It can easily be done in the office setting.

## Computed Tomography

Computed tomography (CT) has not been the first-line imaging modality for the diagnosis of hydronephrosis or UPJO in children, particularly infants. This is primarily due to the radiation exposure risk of CT and the relative ease and accuracy of renal ultrasonography. However, many older children with UPJO, who present with nonspecific complaints of abdominal pain or nausea and vomiting, are evaluated with a CT scan to evaluate other possible causes of their symptoms such as appendicitis or bowel obstruction. Therefore, it is important to know the typical CT scan appearance of UPJO. Significant hydronephrosis is noted without the presence of a dilated ureter (Fig. 5.4). CT can be beneficial in defining retroperitoneal anatomy, particularly aberrant lower pole crossing vessels to the kidney. When performed with IV contrast, an overall functional assessment of the kidney can also be made; however the benefits of this modality often do not outweigh the radiation risk or cost of the study. CT as a primary imaging study should be evaluated on an individual basis after the risks and benefits have been considered.

## Intravenous Pyelogram

Intravenous pyelography (IVP) has fallen out of favor in the work-up of hydronephrosis and suspected UPJO due to its high radiation exposure and the ease and accuracy of other imaging modalities such as ultrasonography. IVP can still be useful in those cases with unclear anatomy and a confusing clinical picture. The ideal timing for this study would be during an acute episode of obstruction.

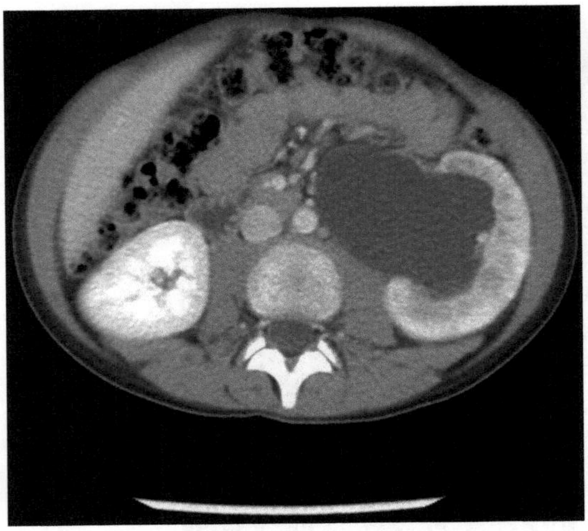

**Fig. 5.4** CT appearance of UPJO obstruction. Note dilated renal pelvis and normal caliber ureter

## Voiding Cystourethrogram

A voiding cystourethrogram (VCUG) should be performed in all children with prenatally diagnosed hydronephrosis to evaluate for the presence of VUR even if UPJO is suspected as the cause of collecting system dilatation. VUR is present in 40 % of children with UPJO, although it is usually low grade [1]. Infants with prenatal hydronephrosis should be started on prophylactic antibiotics at the time of birth, until the VCUG has confirmed the absence of VUR.

## Diuretic Radionuclide Renography

Radionuclide renography is an objective study that is able to suggest the diagnosis of obstruction by analyzing quantitative data regarding differential renal function. When performed in conjunction with the administration of a diuretic, this test is able to assess the velocity of washout of the radioisotope from each kidney, hence a direct measurement of renal collecting system emptying. Initially, this test was performed with technetium-99 m diethylenetriaminepentaacetic acid (DTPA), an agent that is exclusively filtered by the glomeruli with an extraction excretion of 20 %, which provides an indirect measurement of GFR glomerular filtration rate (GFR) in nondilated kidneys [4]. This agent has largely been replaced by mercaptoacetyltriglycine (MAG3), which is excreted mostly by the proximal renal tubules and provides an indirect means of measuring estimated renal plasma flow. MAG3 radionuclide renography tends to provide more accurate functional information than DTPA radionuclide renography, particularly in dilated renal collecting systems, and has become the study of choice at most institutions.

The measurement of the excretory curve of the renogram will correlate with the efficiency of emptying of the renal pelvis. In an obstructed system, the radioisotope is not as effectively cleared from the kidney. Furosemide is usually given to promote diuresis and emptying. When the kidney does not respond to the diuretic, it is assumed that there is a loss of renal function and/or significant renal obstruction [4].

The technique and ultimately the results of the test are extremely operator dependent, and unfortunately there is no universal protocol for performing this study; therefore results can vary from center to center. The relative standard would be to perform this test in a well-hydrated child with a catheter draining the bladder, as a full bladder can lead to VUR in the susceptible ureter, or poor emptying in an otherwise unobstructed system. The administration of the diuretic can vary depending on the protocol used. It is our preference that the diuretic be administered 20–30 min after the renogram (F +20–30) or when the renal pelvis is filled with contrast, whichever is later. Following administration of the diuretic, the time to washout suggests the degree of obstruction.

The analysis of the drainage curve should take into consideration the technique and the time to diuretic administration. A general standard in analyzing the curve is to report the time it takes for the radioisotope activity to decrease by 50 % (T ½). If the T ½ is less than 10 min, the study is determined to be normal. When the T ½ is between 10 and 20 min, the study is equivocal, and if the T ½ is greater than 20 min, the kidney reportedly is obstructed (Fig. 5.5). Caution must be observed when taking these results at absolute face value, as the technique, the drainage curves, and the clinical condition of the child must be taken into consider-

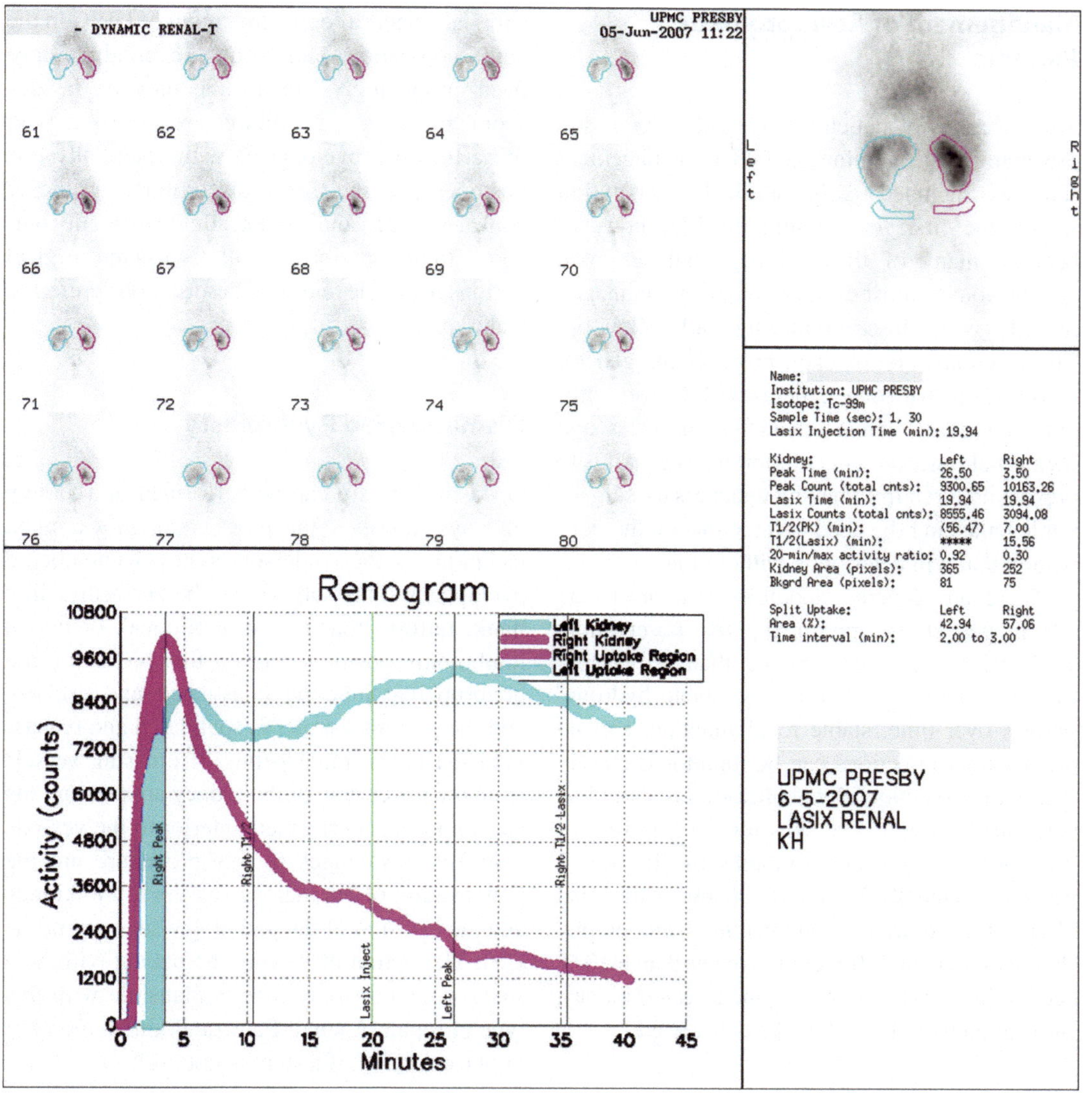


**Fig. 5.5** Drainage curve of MAG3 diuretic radionuclide renography

ation in the analysis. It should be noted that diuretic renography should not generally be performed in infants less than a month of age, as false-positive results may be obtained with an immature kidney.

## Pressure Flow Study

A pressure flow study is an invasive test that measures the intrapelvic pressure during infusion of a fluid into the renal pelvis and the subsequent decrease in intrapelvic pressure over time. This is termed the pressure decay. The pressure decay represents the efficiency of urine transport as well as the relative compliance and volume of the collecting system [1]. A rapid pressure decay indicates a non-obstructed system, while a slow pressure decay demonstrates obstruction. Pressure flow studies are not routinely performed in the pediatric population and are usually used in equivocal clinical situations after a prior repair.

## Management of Asymptomatic Patients

This category of patients is typically diagnosed prenatally or in infancy. Older management schemes included early surgical intervention within the first few months of life; however because many of these kidneys will improve spontaneously, most of these infants are managed initially with close monitoring and follow-up. There is some controversy; however the general consensus is that some patients will recover without intervention while others will progress and their renal function will deteriorate. The goal is to prevent children from having unnecessary surgery while balancing the need to intervene on the population that will deteriorate without intervention.

There are general guidelines that determine which patient is appropriate for observation. Typically patients with greater than 40 % split function of the affected kidney, stable hydronephrosis over time, stable renal function, and no urinary tract infections can be monitored closely without intervention. Renal ultrasounds should be performed every 3–4 months for the first year of life, followed by every 6 months for the next 2 years then annually. If there is a change in the renal ultrasound, diuretic radionuclide renography should be obtained. If there is greater than a 10 % decline in overall function of the affected kidney, surgical intervention should be considered.

## Management of Symptomatic Patients

Patients with less than 40 % function of the affected kidney, those with progressing hydronephrosis on serial exams, or those that present clinically with colic, hematuria, stones, or infection should undergo operative intervention for the management of UPJO.

Open dismembered pyeloplasty has been the gold standard treatment of UPJO for decades, with contemporary success rates greater than 90 % [5]. However, the paradigm has begun to shift, and more minimally invasive techniques for treatment of this condition in children have been sought. Laparoscopic pyeloplasty is an accepted surgical standard for the treatment of UPJO in the adult population, and results in children have been promising. Recent outcomes of laparoscopic pyeloplasty in children are consistent with those for open pyeloplasty, with potentially less postoperative incisional discomfort, a quicker convalescence, and an excellent cosmetic outcome. In this section we will discuss the surgical options available and then describe our preferred technique.

## Dismembered Pyeloplasty

Open pyeloplasty can be performed in a variety of ways; however the most commonly applied technique is the Anderson-Hynes dismembered pyeloplasty. This surgery can be performed in a flank, retroperitoneal, transperitoneal, or dorsal lumbotomy position. During this procedure the ureteropelvic junction is isolated and excised, and the proximal ureter is spatulated and reanastomosed to the renal pelvis. If crossing vessels from the lower pole of the kidney are present, the anastomosis is performed anterior to the vessels. Two key advantages to this procedure are the preservation of anomalous vessels to the kidney and the excision of the pathologic segment of the UPJ. The option of leaving the patient without a stent or nephrostomy tube is plausible with this type of repair. A small Penrose drain is often left in place for 24 h if a stent is not utilized.

## Laparoscopic Pyeloplasty

With the desire to find less-invasive treatment options, there has been a recent interest in the development of minimally invasive surgical options for pediatric patients. The first pediatric series of transperitoneal laparoscopic dismembered pyeloplasty in the literature was reported in 1999, and since that time a variety of techniques and approaches have been described [5]. The technique overall is the same as the open dismembered pyeloplasty, in that the diseased segment is excised and the proximal ureter is spatulated and reapproximated to the renal pelvis. Transperitoneal, retroperitoneal, and robotic approaches have all been reported, with advocates for each procedure. In the end, the approach used should be based on the experience and comfort of the operating surgeon. Success rates for this procedure have been reported in the literature to be comparable to the open technique [5]. At our institution, we primarily perform transperitoneal laparoscopic dismembered pyeloplasty in children with UPJO, greater than 4 months of age, in need of operative repair. In our series we have not had any major complications, and in 90 patients our overall success rate is greater than 95 %.

Robotic-assisted laparoscopic pyeloplasty has been reported in the pediatric urology literature [6]. The benefit of performing the repair robotically assisted is that it allows three-dimensional visualization and 6° of wrist movement, making suturing more intuitive and lowering the learning curve. However, the use of the robot requires additional and larger ports as compared to standard laparoscopy, and the overall cost of equipment and training is much higher. In addition, the robot is not universally available.

## Endoscopic Procedures

Endoscopic procedures for the correction of UPJO are commonly performed in adults, however with lower success rates than open or laparoscopic pyeloplasty. This application has not been found to be useful as a primary treatment option for children. Endopyelotomy (endoscopic incision through the narrowed area) may be performed in either an antegrade or retrograde manner and can be useful in children who have failed open or laparoscopic pyeloplasty.

## Complications and Follow-Up

Complications from pyeloplasty, open or laparoscopic, are fairly uncommon. Early complications include urinary tract infection and prolonged urinary leakage from the anastomosis. This is usually treated with placement of a ureteral stent and/or Foley catheter drainage. Late complications include lack of improvement or worsening hydronephrosis, continued pain, urinary tract infections, or worsening renal function. In rare occasions, a redo pyeloplasty or ureterocalycostomy may need to be performed.

With long-term pyeloplasty success greater than 90 %, the follow-up for UPJO consists of office evaluations and imaging. In our practice, the patients have an office ultrasound performed 6 weeks and 6 months after their procedure. If there is clinical and radiographic improvement, yearly ultrasounds may or may not be recommended going forward. If the hydronephrosis worsens or the child remains symptomatic, radionuclide renography should be obtained for further evaluation.

## Conclusions

UPJO is the most common cause of significant hydronephrosis in newborns and young children. With a diverse presentation, it may manifest as a congenital abnormality or secondarily acquired later in life. The evolution of the management of UPJO in the pediatric population has shifted from early intervention to observational conservative management; however, the overall goal of treatment is to preserve renal function. Surgical options for treatment have remained the gold standard with high long-term success rates. There has been a recent push toward minimally invasive techniques to further decrease the morbidity of surgical treatment options.

## References

1. Hsu THS, Streem SB, Nakada SY. Management of upper urinary tract obstruction. In: Wein AJ, editor. Campbell-Walsh urology, vol. 4. 9th ed. Philadelphia: Saunders; 2007. p. 3359–82.
2. Hanna MK, Jeffs RD, Sturgess JM, Barkin M. Ureteral structure and ultrastructure: part II. Congenital ureteropelvic junction obstruction and primary obstructive megaureter. J Urol. 1976;116:725–30.
3. Sidhu G, Beyene J, Rosenblum ND. Outcome of isolated antenatal hydronephrosis: a systematic review and meta-analysis. Pediatr Nephrol. 2006;21:218–24.
4. Gonzalez R, Schimke CM. Ureteropelvic junction obstruction in infants and children. Pediatr Clin North Am. 2001;48:1505–18.
5. Tan BJ, Smith AD. Ureteropelvic junction repair: when, how what? Curr Opin Urol. 2004;14:55–9.
6. Lee RS, Borer JG. Robotic Surgery for ureteropelvic junction obstruction. Curr Opin Urol. 2006;16:291–4.

# Pediatric Renal Trauma

# 6

Bertram Yuh, Saul P. Greenfield, and Pierre E. Williot

## Impact

Urologic trauma is defined as injury to the kidneys, ureters, bladder, urethra, or external genitalia as a result of external force. Nearly half of childhood death between the ages of 1–14 in the United States can be attributed to traumatic incidents. The estimated cost of caring for these children is about 5–7 billion dollars per year in the United States. The social and economic ramifications are vast. After the central nervous system, the genitourinary system is the next most commonly affected by trauma. Fortunately, the majority of injuries are nonlethal and require no operative management. At least 90 % of genitourinary traumatic cases have associated injuries to other organs, complicating the clinical situation. Genitourinary trauma should thus be evaluated at centers experienced in complex trauma care. In trauma cases, time is of the essence, and therefore it is important to expediently and accurately identify urologic trauma so that it can be addressed within the whole scope of presentation and lead to the best outcomes.

B. Yuh, M.D. • S.P. Greenfield, M.D.
P.E. Williot, M.D. (✉)
Department of Pediatric Urology, Women and Children's Hospital of Buffalo, 219 Bryant Street, Buffalo, NY 14222, USA
e-mail: pwilliot@kaleidahealth.org

## Renal Trauma

At least 60 % of all pediatric urologic trauma affect the kidney. The pediatric kidney is more vulnerable to injury than the adult kidney for several anatomic reasons:

1. Size: The pediatric kidney is proportionally larger relative to body height.
2. Cushioning: The fat surrounding the kidney is less substantial.
3. Bony and muscular protection: The chest wall and rib cage are less mature and more flexible.
4. Location: The renal units are positioned lower in the abdomen.

Boys are more commonly affected by renal trauma than girls.

Congenital anomalies such as ureteropelvic junction (UPJ) obstruction or fused kidneys are more prone to significant injuries following minor impact.

## History and Presentation

Trauma to the kidneys can be subdivided into three groups based on mechanism:

- Blunt injuries
- Penetrating injuries
- Deceleration injuries

Some traumas involve a combination of mechanisms. The form of injury is important in regard to evaluation, management, and prognosis.

R. Rabinowitz et al. (eds.), *Pediatric Urology for the Primary Care Physician*, Current Clinical Urology,
DOI 10.1007/978-1-60327-243-8_6, © Springer Science+Business Media New York 2015

## Blunt Renal Injury

The vast majority of renal trauma, 80–90 %, is blunt. This is most commonly seen after motor vehicle accidents, sports injuries, assaults, and falls. Nearly all of these injuries are minor and require no surgery. The kidney has amazing recuperative properties and often will heal over time. Imaging is important to appropriately assess the extent of these injuries. Preexisting renal anomalies such as horseshoe kidney, UPJ obstruction, and tumor are more commonly found in trauma cases. These can present with gross hematuria out of proportion to the severity of the injury. Impressive symptoms after a minor injury should raise a flag for an underlying renal abnormality.

**Table 6.1** Examples of clinical presentations of blunt renal trauma

| |
|---|
| *Blunt injury* |
| A 10-year-old female is involved in a motor vehicle accident and presents with left-sided broken lower ribs, flank pain with bruising, and gross hematuria |
| *Blunt injury with underlying hydronephrosis* |
| A 16-year-old otherwise healthy male presents with visible blood in the urine (gross hematuria) and flank pain after getting punched lightly in the right side |
| *Penetrating injury* |
| A 12-year-old boy is found after being shot through and through below the right rib cage. In the emergency room, he is unstable and bleeding profusely |
| *Deceleration injury* |
| A 9-year-old boy sustains a fall onto his back from a height of 30 ft and presents with unconsciousness, hypotension, and transverse process fracture in the lumbar spine |

## Penetrating Renal Injury

Penetrating renal trauma from guns or knives is often more serious. 77–100 % of the penetrating trauma that affects the kidney also affects other organ systems. Commonly these children will be surgically explored for this reason. In these instances, the urologist will often work with the trauma surgeon in a collective surgical approach. The injuries may be more difficult to identify and control. Penetrating trauma is often more injurious than the initial survey may reveal. Blast effect from high-powered armaments may cause significant internal damage including extensive kidney and ureteral destruction.

## Deceleration Renal Injury

Deceleration renal injuries are most commonly seen with high-speed motor vehicle accidents and falls. Falls associated with these injuries are normally from a height greater than 20 ft. These children are often unstable and have many associated injuries, requiring operative management. While extreme deceleration can cause catastrophic damage to any individual, several injuries are more common in the pediatric population. A severe deceleration injury in a child should raise suspicion for two forms of serious renal injury:

### Ureteropelvic Junction (UPJ) Disruption

A traumatic separation between the kidney pelvis and the ureter interrupts the conduit for urine to flow into the bladder. As a result the renal unit becomes obstructed or spills urine into the retroperitoneum. The connection between the renal pelvis and the ureter can be torn by forces causing hyperextension of the spine or by extreme movements of the kidneys. This shearing is more common in children as the spine is more flexible and the kidney more mobile. A high index of suspicion for this type of injury is critical as the diagnosis of a UPJ disruption can be difficult and frequently delayed more than 36 h. Multiorgan trauma is the typical setting. The urine analysis is completely normal in 30 % of these cases.

### Arterial Intimal Tear

Children have less fat around their kidneys and their renal vessels are more mobile. Overstretching of the renal artery can lead to a tear of the innermost layer of the artery: the intima. This tear within the wall of the vessel will result in an endoluminal dissection of the intima with thrombosis and occlusion of the artery, leading to renal ischemia.

Deceleration injuries are not universally associated with rib fractures, lumbar bruising, or abdominal injuries. A fall from several stories onto one's feet can result in lower-limb fractures and ureteropelvic (UPJ) disruption. A child wearing a seat belt in a head-on vehicle collision could have whiplash with an arterial intimal tear and no other significant injuries. Examples of clinical presentations are shown in Table 6.1.

## Signs and Symptoms

The most common sign of renal injury after trauma is hematuria; however it is important to note that this is unreliable. In children, up to 70 % renal injuries may not have any gross hematuria or even blood on dipstick. Therefore a completely normal urine analysis does not rule out renal injury.

Other symptoms can include flank pain, nausea, and vomiting. There may be tachycardia or hypotension related to acute blood loss. Hypotension is also a variable sign as children often maintain their blood pressure even in cases where half of the circulating volume is lost.

## Physical Examination

Findings suggestive of renal injury:

1. Abdominal mass or tenderness
2. Abdominal distension
3. Flank bruising or tenderness
4. Lower rib or lumbar/thoracic vertebral body fracture

## Evaluation

First, immediate resuscitation must be initiated. The urologic workup is only part of the assessment and must not delay stabilization. Intravenous hydration should be started as soon as possible. Urinalysis and trauma labs (CBC, BUN, electrolytes, creatinine, liver enzymes, amylase, cross-match + red packed cells) should be obtained. Imaging will ultimately define the treatment plan for renal injuries but should be deferred in unstable patients. A Foley catheter SHOULD NOT be inserted if there is blood at the urethral meatus or vaginal introitus. This finding suggests urethral trauma and should lead to evaluation with a retrograde urethrogram.

In extreme cases, stabilization is not possible in the emergency/trauma room. In this circumstance, immediate surgical exploration can be lifesaving. The fascial layer around the kidney (Gerota) provides anatomic protection. As Gerota's fascia is a natural barrier frequently preventing exsanguination from a renal hemorrhage, it must not be opened unless (1) one faces a rapidly expanding retroperitoneal hematoma and (2) one can demonstrate contralateral renal function. Contralateral renal function can be rapidly demonstrated with a "one-shot IVP" on the operating table. This is performed with a single injection of 2 mL/kg of IV contrast material and a KUB (plain X-ray of the kidneys, ureters, and bladder) 10–15 min later. Confirmation of contralateral function allows exploration to proceed without risk of rendering the patient anephric. If the retroperitoneal hematoma is not expanding, it is better to complete the exploration without opening Gerota's fascia and perform a triple-phase CT scan (see technique below) in the postoperative period once the child is stable.

To accurately define the extent of renal injury and associated injuries, a CT scan is the gold standard. While ultrasonic investigations or intravenous pyelograms can be performed, the CT scan cannot be circumvented for definitive injury staging. CT provides information about associated injuries, fine anatomic detail, and possible differentiation between blood and urine.

The appropriate CT scan is a three-phase IV contrast abdomen/pelvis CT for complete visualization of the renal parenchyma, collecting system, and ureter. This three-phase CT scan includes:

1. A pre-contrast scan (fractures, stones, foreign body, calcifications, air, etc.).
2. An immediate post-contrast scan to delineate vascularization and perfusion.
3. A delayed scan (10–15 min) after contrast to evaluate the collecting system (renal pelvis + ureters + bladder) and to detect urine extravasation. Contrast in the urine at this point in time may be seen outside the kidney when the collecting system is violated. The evaluation of the bladder is also important and will be covered in the appropriate chapter.

These three phases are all imperative. A post-CT scan KUB is frequently very informative and can help highlight the extent of urinary extravasation, localization of fractures, and displacement of the bowel, air, and the bladder.

Renal outcome is correlated with the severity of injury, which is graded from one to five, in

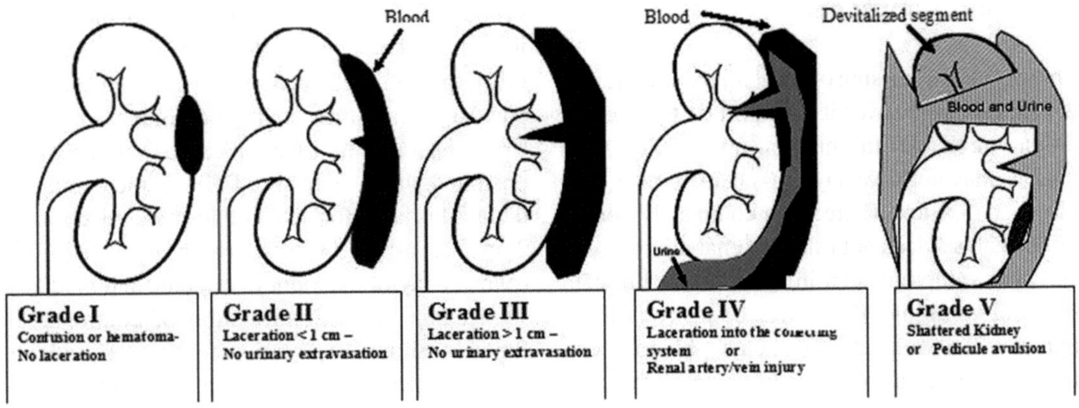


**Fig. 6.1** Grading system for renal injury severity

increasing degrees of severity (see Fig. 6.1). Higher-grade injuries are more likely to be complicated by urinary leakage, infection, and bleeding. The highest-grade injuries have a higher likelihood of requiring surgical intervention.

## Indications for Imaging

1. All penetrating trauma with microhematuria OR a mechanism suggestive of renal injury
2. Blunt trauma with one or more of the following:
   (a) Significant deceleration or high-velocity injury even without physical findings
   (b) Fractures of the spine and rib cage (suggestive clinical findings)
   (c) Gross hematuria
   (d) Microhematuria (>50 RBCs per high-powered field) with shock

The urologist should be involved if there is definite renal injury on CT scan or otherwise high index of suspicion for renal injury. While 99 % of these injuries require only observation, the rare few that need operative management are better served by being identified early. Imaging and clinical status provide the guidelines for management.

## Treatment

In the past, children with severe renal trauma were frequently explored. This leads to a high rate of nephrectomies. The main boundary limiting bleeding in severe renal injury is Gerota's fascia. By opening Gerota's fascia during an exploration, recurrence of a severe bleed can occur. This can convert a controlled bleed to an uncontrollable hemorrhage resulting ultimately in a lifesaving nephrectomy as the only option. Thus an "aggressive observation" approach dramatically improves renal preservation.

If the child is brought to the operating room for associated injuries, the urologist should maintain a conservative mindset and should avoid entering Gerota's fascia. If Gerota's fascia needs to be opened, it should be done only after the renal artery(s) and vein(s) are under control.

Facing an isolated UPJ disruption, an early primary repair should be performed. When the disruption is associated with significant renal trauma, the best management is a urinary diversion (percutaneous nephrostomy), followed by delayed repair.

Following the initial evaluation, a child with renal trauma should be observed closely and remain in bed. Aggressive fluid resuscitation should continue. Persistent or recurrent bleeding can occur, and thus close observation is desirable. In children, the blood pressure is normally the last parameter to drop. The blood pressure drops only when the blood losses are very significant or life-threatening. Close monitoring of the hemoglobin, hematocrit, and pulse is mandatory.

Radiographic monitoring of the renal injury can be undertaken in serial fashion several days after the insult with an ultrasound or CT scan. Strict bed rest is applied until there is gross hematuria as resolved and the child is stable. This may take several days. Once the urine clears, he or she is allowed to walk to his/her bathroom to urinate and defecate but should then return to his/her bed. When discharged from the hospital, the child must avoid any contact sports until the injury is completely healed and ideally should remain at home for 3–4 weeks.

Delayed bleeding occurs mainly within the first 10 days post injury but can occur up to 3 weeks later. Delayed retroperitoneal bleeding usually presents with pain, anemia, ecchymoses, and hemodynamic instability and can be life-threatening.

When there is urinary extravasation (grade IV and V injuries), a urologist must evaluate the need for the insertion of a double "J" ureteral stent, percutaneous nephrostomy, and/or percutaneous drainage of the urine collection.

Infection of the renal hematoma, urinoma, or development of an abscess may complicate matters. Broad-spectrum antibiotics and drainage of the infected fluid may be required.

## Follow-Up

Care for the patient beyond the acute traumatic episode is mainly radiographic. Follow-up triphasic CT scans of the abdomen and pelvis should be performed after 3 months in cases of severe renal injury. This helps elucidate the remaining anatomy and function after the insult. Other functional studies such as renal scans can be performed as well.

Long-term complications include hematuria, high blood pressure, and loss of renal function of the affected kidney. Delayed hematuria is suggestive of arteriovenous (AV) fistula. These are managed with selective embolization procedures. Hypertension secondary to trauma after a severe renal injury is seen in about 5 % of cases. This will usually manifest within 36 months of the injury. An AV fistula may also cause hypertension. Medication-resistant hypertension may require surgery or procedural intervention (embolization).

## Conclusions

Trauma is a significant cause of morbidity and mortality in children. Urologic injury is nearly always associated with trauma of other organ(s). Therefore, identification and treatment of urologic trauma must be undertaken within a larger scope of care. Patients should be swiftly assessed, stabilized, and managed by multidisciplinary teams. Most traumas to urologic organs will heal without surgical intervention. The key lies in the suspicion and identification of all degrees of injuries.

The mechanism of the injury can be as important as the objective findings. History of penetrating or blunt injury to the abdomen or deceleration injury provides information just as hematuria, flank pain, or flank bruising supply aids to diagnosis.

## Recommended Readings

Belman AB, King LR, Kramer SA. Clinical pediatric urology. 4th ed. Boca Raton: CRC; 2001.

Gillenwater JY, Grayhack JT, Howards SS, Mitchell ME. Adult and pediatric urology. 4th ed. Philadelphia: Lippincott Williams & Wilkins; 2002.

Ramchandani P, Buckler PM. Imaging of genitourinary trauma. Am J Roentgenology. 2009;192:1514–23.

Resnick MI, Novick AC. Urology secrets. 3rd ed. Philadelphia: Lippincott Williams & Wilkins; 2002.

Wein AJ, Kavoussi LR, Novick AC, Partin AW, Peters CA. Campbell-walsh urology. 9th ed. Philadelphia: Saunders; 2006.

# Renal Stones

# 7

Serdar Tekgül and H. Serkan Dogan

## Introduction

Namely, urolithiasis means the presence of calculi in any part of the urinary tract. It is one of the most important topics in urology. Pediatric and adult stone disease differs in both presentation and treatment which will be presented in this chapter.

## Epidemiology

In children, both sexes are affected equally, contrary to the adult population in which a male predominance is present. Stones are mostly located in the upper urinary tract whereas the bladder stones are mostly the problem of underdeveloped areas of the world. Although the stone disease in children is relatively rare in developed countries, it is seen more frequently in other parts of the world. Pediatric stone disease is considered to be endemic in Turkey, Pakistan, and some South Asian, African, and South American countries. In Germany, pediatric stones are 1–5 % of all urinary stones. However, for example, in Turkey 17 % of stone disease patients are in pediatric age group. Therefore, it is an important health problem in these particular areas of the world.

## History and Physical Examination

History and physical examination may not give clues about the disease especially in very young children. Presentation tends to be age dependent, with symptoms such as flank pain and hematuria being more common in older children. Nonspecific symptoms (e.g., irritability, vomiting) are common in very young children. There may be different patterns of clinical presentation. In patients who can verbalize the symptoms, intense pain that suddenly occurs in the back and radiates downward and centrally toward the lower abdomen or groin can be present. Hematuria may be present, usually gross, occurring with or without pain which is less common in children. Microscopic hematuria may be the sole indicator which is more common in children. Persistent microscopic hematuria, which consists of five or more red blood cells per high-power field in three of three consecutive centrifuged urine specimens obtained at least 1 week apart, should be further investigated for urinary stones. In some cases, stone can be identified during the radiologic imaging to evaluate the urinary tract infection. Additionally, in some asymptomatic cases, stones are diagnosed during abdominal imaging for another reason.

S. Tekgül, M.D. (✉)
Department of Urology, Pediatric Urology Division, Hacettepe University Faculty of Medicine, Ankara 06100, Turkey
e-mail: serdartekgul@gmail.com

H.S. Dogan, M.D.
Division of Pediatric Urology, Department of Urology, Uludag University Faculty of Medicine, Bursa, Turkey

R. Rabinowitz et al. (eds.), *Pediatric Urology for the Primary Care Physician*, Current Clinical Urology,
DOI 10.1007/978-1-60327-243-8_7, © Springer Science+Business Media New York 2015

# Evaluation

## Imaging Tests

A simple abdominal flat-plate X-ray and renal ultrasonography is very effective for identifying most of the stones in the kidney. However, abdominal gas can decrease the accuracy of these imaging tests. The most sensitive test for identifying stones in the urinary system is noncontrast helical CT scanning and is the first study obtained in many emergency departments. It is safe and rapid and has been shown to have 97 % sensitivity and 96 % specificity. Intravenous urography is rarely used in children but sometimes used to delineate the calyceal anatomy before percutaneous or open surgery.

## Metabolic Evaluation

Because of the high incidence of predisposing factors for urolithiasis in children and high recurrence rates, a complete metabolic evaluation of every child with urinary stones should be done. Metabolic evaluation includes: family and patient history of metabolic problems; analysis of stone composition; complete blood count; electrolytes; blood urea nitrogen; creatinine; calcium; phosphorus; alkaline phosphatase; uric acid; total protein; albumin; parathyroid hormone (if there is hypercalcemia); spot urinalysis and culture, including ratio of calcium, uric acid, oxalate, cystine, citrate, and magnesium to creatinine; and urine tests, including a 24-h urine collection for calcium, phosphorus, magnesium, oxalate, uric acid citrate, cystine, protein, and creatinine clearance.

Various metabolic problems can be determined after these studies. These problems may exist single or in combination. The most frequently detected metabolic problems in children are hypercalciuria, hyperoxaluria, hypocitraturia, hyperuricosuria, and cystinuria. The normal values in spot and 24-h collected urine are given in Tables 7.1 and 7.2 [1].

**Table 7.1** Normal spot values in urine

| | |
|---|---|
| Ca/Cr | |
| Child | <0.21 mg/mg |
| Infant | <0.6 mg/kg |
| Ox/Cr | |
| <6 months | <0.30 mg/mg |
| 6 months–4 years | <0.15 mg/mg |
| >4 years | <0.10 mg/mg |
| Uric acid | <0.53 mg/dL GFR |
| Citrate/Cr | >0.51 g/g |

**Table 7.2** Normal values in 24-h collected urine

| | |
|---|---|
| Calcium | <4 mg/kg/day |
| Oxalate | <40 mg/1.73 $m^2$/day |
| | <0.57 mg/kg/day |
| Citrate | >400 mg/g Cr |
| | >320 mg/1.73 $m^2$/day |
| Uric acid | <815 mg/1.73 $m^2$/day |
| | <10.7 mg/kg/day |
| Phosphorus | <15 mg/kg/day |
| Cystine | <75 mg/1.73 $m^2$/day |
| Mg | >1.2 mg/kg/day |
| Creatinine | 0.8–1.2 g/1.73 $m^2$/day |
| Volume | >20 mL/kg/day |

Besides these evaluations, stone analysis—if present—is very important to plan the medical treatment. Most of the stones (70–80 %) are composed of calcium (calcium oxalate or calcium phosphate). The other stone compositions are uric acid (4–8 %), cystine (2–6 %), and struvite (infection stones) (5 %).

## When to Refer?

Pediatric stone patient should be managed and treated with the cooperation of pediatric nephrologist and pediatric urologist. In acute episodes, in patients without hydronephrosis and fever, intravenous hydration and analgesics (oral, parenteral, or rectal route) are used to relieve the pain. In cases with hydronephrosis or fever or intractable pain, patient should be consulted to a pediatric urologist in order to decompress the obstruction via external or internal drainage. In elective cases, patient should be evaluated both by pediatric urologist and nephrologist.

**Table 7.3** Cause-specific medications for various conditions

| Medication | Dosage | Condition treated |
|---|---|---|
| Hydrochlorothiazide | 1–2 mg/kg/day | Hypercalciuria |
| Pyridoxine | 25–50 mg/kg | Primary hyperoxaluria |
| Orthophosphates | 25–50 mg/kg | Primary hyperoxaluria |
| Magnesium hydroxide | 5–10 mg/kg | Hypomagnesuria |
| Potassium citrate | 1–3 mEq/kg/day | dRTA and urinary alkalinization |
| Potassium citrate | 10 mg/kg | Hyperuricosuria |
| D-Penicillamine | 20–50 mg/kg/day | Cystinuria |
| Alpha-mercaptopropionylglycine | 10–15 mg/kg/day | Cystinuria |

## How to Manage?

The medical and interventional modalities are used to treat the pediatric stone patient. Most of the cause-specific medications are shown in Table 7.3.

The evaluation algorithm for pediatric stone disease patient is given in Fig. 7.1 [2].

The interventional treatment options are as follows:

### Extracorporeal Shock-Wave Lithotripsy (ESWL)

It means to disintegrate the urinary stone by focusing extracorporeally generated shock waves (electrohydraulic, electromagnetic, or piezoelectric) onto the stone located in the urinary tract. The disintegration success depends on the size, number, location, and composition of the stone. In children, it is performed under superficial anesthesia. SWL is not without complications; however, these complications are frequently self-limiting and transient. The most frequently observed complications are renal colic, transient hydronephrosis, dermal ecchymosis, urinary tract infection, formation of stone street, and very rarely hemoptysis and sepsis.

### Ureterorenoscopy (URS)

It means to reach, disintegrate, and extract the stone located in the ureter or kidney by semi-rigid or flexible endoscopic instruments. Energy sources to disintegrate the stone show variety, and these are electrohydraulic, pneumatic, ultrasonic, and laser (holmium:YAG). It is minimally invasive and patient comfort is at maximum. Complications occur in 0–7 % of cases and are generally minor, transient, and managed easily.

### Percutaneous Nephrolithotomy (PCNL)

It means to reach, disintegrate, and extract the kidney stone through an access developed via percutaneous route. It opened a new era in upper urinary tract stone management. Bleeding, postoperative fever or infection, and persistent urinary leakage are the most frequently reported complications of PCNL in children which are less frequent than in adults. This is attributed to fact that the surgeons gain a huge amount of experience before attempting such an operation in children.

### Open Surgery

Most of the stones in children can be managed by ESWL and endoscopic techniques. Yet, in some situations open surgery can be obviated. Very young children with large stones and/or a congenitally obstructed system, which also need surgical correction, are good candidates for open stone surgery. Severe orthopedic deformities may limit positioning for endoscopic procedures, and open surgery might also be required for such children. The recommendations for management of pediatric stone disease patient are given in Table 7.4 [2].

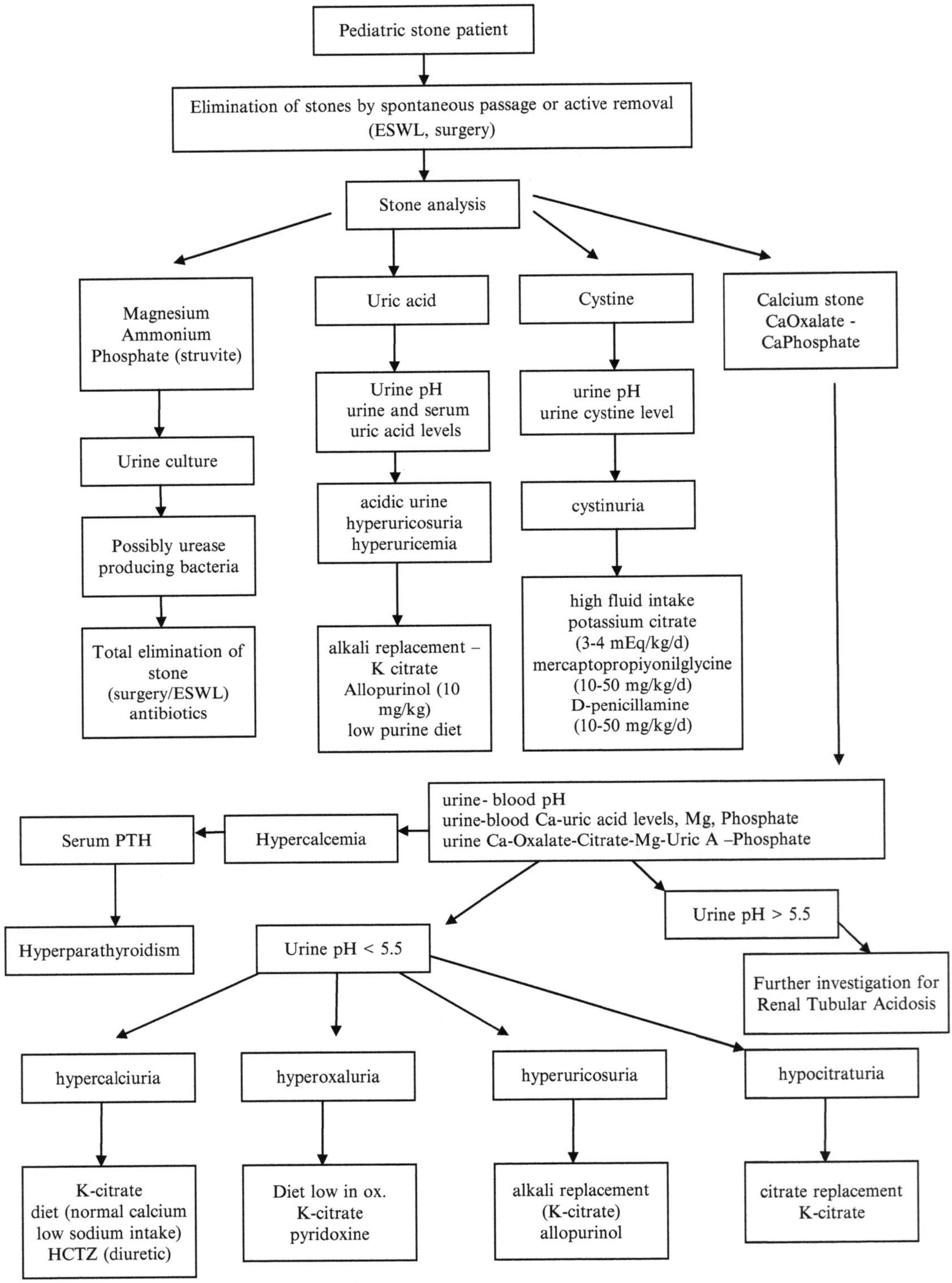


**Fig. 7.1** An algorithm providing information on performing metabolic investigations and planning medical treatment (HCTZ = hydrochlorothiazide; PTH = parathyroid hormone)

**Table 7.4** European Association of Urology (EAU) guideline recommendations for interventional management in pediatric stones

| Stone size and localization[a] | Primary treatment option | Level of evidence | Secondary treatment options | Comment |
|---|---|---|---|---|
| Staghorn cases | PCNL | 2B | Open, ESWL | Multiple sessions and accesses with PCNL may be needed. Combination with SWL may be useful |
| Pelvis <10 mm | ESWL | 1A | RIRS, PCNL | |
| Pelvis 10–20 mm | ESWL | 2B | PCNL, open | Multiple sessions with SWL may be needed. PCNL has similar recommendation grade |
| Pelvis >20 mm | PCNL | 2B | ESWL, open | Multiple sessions with SWL may be needed |
| Lower pole <10 mm | ESWL | 2C | RIRS, PCNL | Anatomical variations are important for complete clearance after SWL |
| Lower pole >10 mm | PCNL | 2B | ESWL | Anatomical variations are important for complete clearance after SWL |
| Upper ureter | ESWL | 2B | PCNL, URS, open | |
| Lower ureter | URS | 1A | ESWL, open | Additional intervention need is high with SWL |
| Bladder | Endoscopic | 2B | Open | Open is easier and with less operative time with large stones |

[a]Cystine and uric acid stones excluded

## References

1. Bartosh SM. Medical management of pediatric stone disease. Urol Clin North Am. 2004;31(3):575–87.
2. Tekgül S, Riedmiller H, Gerharz E, Hoebeke P, Kocvara R, Nijman R, Radmayr C, Stein R. EAU guidelines on Pediatric Urology, 2008.

## Recommended Reading

Docimo SG, Peters CA. Pediatric endourology and laparoscopy. In: Wein AJ et al., editors. Campbell-Walsh urology, vol. 4. 9th ed. Philadelphia: Saunders Elsevier; 2007. Chapter 131.

Dogan HS, Tekgül S. Management of pediatric stone disease. Curr Urol Rep. 2007;8(2):163–73.

# Pediatric Renal Tumors

# 8

Puneeta Ramachandra and Fernando A. Ferrer Jr.

## Introduction

Wilms tumors and non-Wilms renal malignancies constitute a significant portion of solid tumors diagnosed in children. Due to the efforts of large multicenter collaborative groups such as the Children's Oncology Group (COG) and the International Society of Paediatric Oncology (SIOP), significant progress has been made in the past 40 years in the treatment of these tumors. Using a multidisciplinary approach to treatment and developing a better understanding of the pathophysiology of pediatric renal tumors have resulted in improved survival and less treatment-related morbidity. In this chapter, our goal is to provide an overview of the most common pediatric renal tumors, concentrating largely on Wilms tumor, its diagnosis, and management. Oftentimes, the primary pediatrician is the first to make a diagnosis in children with renal masses. Appropriate treatment for these patients requires prompt referral to pediatric oncologists and pediatric surgeons skilled in the treatment of renal masses.

P. Ramachandra, M.D. (✉)
Division of Pediatric Urology, Children's Hospital Central California, Madera, CA, USA
e-mail: Puneeta.ramachandra@gmail.com

F.A. Ferrer Jr., M.D.
Department of Surgery, Division of Urology, University of Connecticut School of Medicine, Farmington, CT, USA

## Wilms Tumor

### Epidemiology

Wilms tumor is the most common primary malignant renal tumor of childhood. Also known as nephroblastoma, the incidence of Wilms tumor is approximately 7.6 cases per million children under age 15. The highest incidence of Wilms tumor is in the first 4 years of life, although children of any age and adults also may be affected. The median age at presentation is between 3 and 4 years of age [1]. More than 80 % of cases occur in children younger than 5 years of age. While solitary, unilateral lesions are most common, bilateral tumors occur in 7 % of patients, and about 12 % of patients will have multiple lesions within one kidney [2]. Bilateral tumors tend to present at an earlier age than unilateral tumors, and boys have a slightly younger mean age at diagnosis than girls. The incidence is nearly equal between boys and girls worldwide but demonstrates a slight predominance in girls in North America [3]. Based on the data from the Surveillance, Epidemiology, and End Results (SEER) Program, prognosis is excellent, with an overall 5-year survival of over 88 % for cases diagnosed between 1996 and 2004 [1].

Significant progress has been made in the treatment of Wilms tumor mainly as a result of large collaborative groups, such as the COG in the United States, the SIOP in Europe, and others,

R. Rabinowitz et al. (eds.), *Pediatric Urology for the Primary Care Physician*, Current Clinical Urology,
DOI 10.1007/978-1-60327-243-8_8, © Springer Science+Business Media New York 2015

which have helped develop a multidisciplinary approach to therapy. Newer research emphasizes reducing morbidity of treatment for low-risk patients and improving efficacy of treatment for the subset of high-risk patients with poor survival.

## Pathogenesis and Histology

Wilms tumor is an embryonal tumor that develops from remnants of immature kidney. This disease was once thought to occur as a result of the classic single-gene, two-hit model described in retinoblastoma, but now at least 10 different genes have been shown to be involved [4].

Wilms tumor has a great deal of histologic diversity. The classic triphasic pattern, which mimics the cell types in the developing kidney, is composed of varying amounts of three cell types: blastemal, epithelial, and stromal. Each of these components responds differently to therapy, and the proportions of different components may influence outcomes of therapy [5]. Tumors with unfavorable histologic features, also known as anaplasia, are associated with increased relapse and death rates [6].

## Presentation

Children with Wilms tumor may present in many ways. Most commonly, an asymptomatic abdominal mass is found. The parents may discover the mass while bathing the child, or a mass may be palpated by a pediatrician during a routine well-child physical examination. On occasion this mass may cross the midline. Other more rare signs and symptoms at presentation may include abdominal pain, gross hematuria, fever, or acute abdomen due to tumor rupture. In less than 10 % of patients, symptoms related to compression of adjacent structures may occur. These include varicocele, hepatomegaly, ascites, and congestive heart failure, all usually associated with extension of tumor into the inferior vena cava (IVC) or renal vein. The presence of a unilateral, right-sided varicocele should alert the physician to the possibility of a renal mass compressing or occluding the IVC. Unilateral, right-sided varicoceles are much less frequent than unilateral left-sided varicoceles, and when they are a result of an occlusion, will not collapse in a supine position. Hypertension secondary to renal ischemia has also been described in about 25 % of patients with Wilms tumor.

A palpable abdominal mass in a child should be considered malignant until proven otherwise. Initial workup will include a full physical examination and history, including family history of renal tumors or Wilms tumor-associated syndromes. During the full physical examination, it is important to note the presence or absence of commonly associated findings such as aniridia, genitourinary anomalies, or hemihypertrophy of body segments. Laboratory studies should include a complete blood count, liver and renal function tests, and possibly certain tumor markers. Acquired von Willebrand disease is found in almost 10 % of patients with newly diagnosed Wilms tumor. Patients with congenital mesoblastic nephroma or rhabdoid tumor of the kidney can have elevated serum calcium levels.

## Associated Syndromes

Other genitourinary abnormalities such as cryptorchidism, renal fusion abnormalities such as horseshoe kidney, and hypospadias are present in approximately 5 % of Wilms tumor patients. Because these other anomalies are much more common than Wilms tumor itself, a full evaluation for Wilms tumor is usually not warranted. A small minority of Wilms tumor cases are familial and associated with very specific mutations in some of these families.

Wilms tumor is associated with a number of syndromes. Generally, these syndromes can be divided into two types: those associated with overgrowth and those that lack overgrowth. Overgrowth syndromes include isolated hemihypertrophy, Beckwith–Wiedemann syndrome (BWS), Perlman syndrome, Simpson–Golabi–Behmel syndrome, and Soto syndrome. Syndromes not associated with overgrowth are Denys–Drash syndrome and WAGR syndrome

(Wilms tumor, aniridia, genital anomalies, and mental retardation). We will discuss a few of these syndromes in greater detail.

Hemihypertrophy, or overgrowth of a body segment, can occur as part of the BWS or an isolated entity. BWS is a rare disorder of developmental anomalies characterized by excessive growth at the organ or cellular levels. In addition to hemihypertrophy, features of this syndrome include macroglossia, nephromegaly, and hepatomegaly. The majority of cases of BWS arise sporadically, but as many as 15 % of patients exhibit apparent autosomal dominant heritability. BWS is caused by dysregulation of genes at chromosome 11p15, which control prenatal and childhood growth. The Wilms tumor 2 gene (*WT2*) has been identified at this site and is associated with BWS. Some mutations of the *WT2* gene result in an absolute increase of growth promoters, while others result in an absolute decrease in growth suppressors [6]. Several recent studies have looked at tumor risk in certain epigenetic subtypes of BWS. This data suggests that the risk of Wilms tumor is increased in those genetic subtypes that result in an increase in growth promoters, while those individuals whose subtype results in a decrease of growth suppressors may not be at increased risk of developing Wilms tumor. Over half of all individuals with BWS fall into this second category of patients; therefore, epigenotyping of the 11p15 helps to subclassify individuals with BWS into low-risk versus high-risk patients [6]. The overall incidence of tumors in patients with overgrowth syndromes is 10–20 %, including Wilms tumor, adrenocortical tumors, and hepatoblastoma. Patients with hemihypertrophy and BWS have a risk of developing Wilms tumor on the order of 4–10 %, with about 21 % of those patients presenting with bilateral disease. Patients with isolated hemihypertrophy have a 3 % risk of developing Wilms tumor. BWS patients who have kidneys in the 95th percentile of age-adjusted renal length are at the greatest risk for developing Wilms tumor.

Of the non-overgrowth syndromes related to Wilms tumor, the Denys–Drash syndrome (DDS) and WAGR syndrome are both associated with mutations of chromosome 11p13, the locus of the Wilms tumor 1 gene (*WT1*). *WT1* is thought to be a classic tumor suppressor gene which regulates many other genes known to be associated with cancer development [7]. Changes in only one of the two *WT1* alleles result in a spectrum of phenotypic variants with overlapping combinations of Wilms tumor, genitourinary abnormalities, and renal dysfunction. The WAGR syndrome was the first condition to be associated with a constitutional deletion of one allele of *WT1* and is found in 7–8/1,000 individuals with Wilms tumor [8]. The syndrome manifests with complete or partial aniridia, as a result of a mutation on chromosome 11p13 adjacent to *WT1*. Other features of the syndrome are ambiguous genitalia, cryptorchidism in boys, mental retardation, and an increased risk of renal failure (around 40 % of individuals by age 20). Rare patients may present without aniridia, depending on the location of their mutation. WAGR patients usually present at an earlier median age and are more likely to have bilateral tumors.

The Denys–Drash syndrome results from heterozygous germline mutations in *WT1* and manifests with a much more severe phenotype than WAGR syndrome. The classic triad of symptoms is Wilms tumor, nephropathy, and genitourinary abnormalities, ranging from mild hypospadias to male pseudohermaphroditism. Renal dysfunction, typically as a result of mesangial sclerosis, presents with hypertension and proteinuria. Eventually, renal failure results, requiring renal replacement by age 10.

Screening for Wilms tumor is recommended in patients with aniridia, BWS, or isolated hemihypertrophy. A renal ultrasound should be performed at approximately every 3 or 4 month intervals until past the high-risk age group. Tumors found on screening ultrasound are usually lower stage than those that are diagnosed after symptoms occur.

## Imaging

The role of imaging in pediatric renal masses is constantly evolving. Preoperative imaging is important in diagnosis as well as surgical planning. When a

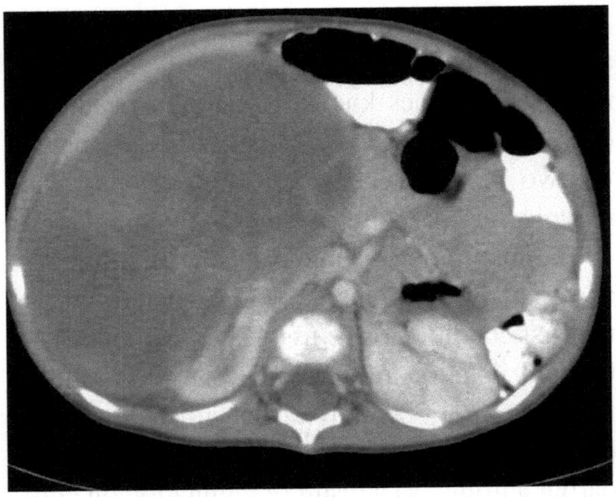

**Fig. 8.1** Contrast-enhanced computed tomography of the abdomen and pelvis demonstrating 7.6 × 12 × 13.6 cm right renal mass in a 1-year-old male. The contralateral kidney appears normal. The mass was first detected by the patient's parents during bathing

renal mass is suspected, ultrasound is usually the first study performed in children to determine if the lesion is solid or cystic. It is noninvasive and inexpensive and does not expose the child to ionizing radiation. CT or MRI of the abdomen is the next appropriate imaging study (Fig. 8.1), although no imaging modality can reliably distinguish between Wilms tumor and other solid renal tumors in childhood, as many of them have similar radiographic features. The goal of a CT or MRI is not to determine exact diagnosis, since the treatment of any solid renal tumors in children is likely to be eventual surgical excision. CT or MRI allows examination of the contralateral kidney and allows the surgeon to plan the appropriate operation for the lesion [9]. Patients noted to have bilateral renal tumors will most likely have bilateral Wilms tumors and should undergo preoperative chemotherapy before surgical excision. MRI and Doppler ultrasound can both detect tumor extension into the IVC, but Doppler ultrasound is much less expensive than MRI and does not require sedation. A CT of the chest should be performed to evaluate for lung metastases [10], while liver metastases can be seen on the abdominal CT. Regional lymphadenopathy seen on CT or MRI is a nonspecific finding in children and does not add any prognostic significance in patients with Wilms tumor or other renal tumors. These lymph nodes should be sampled at the time of surgery.

The presence of aniridia, hemihypertrophy, or other Wilms tumor-associated syndromes makes the diagnosis of Wilms tumor more likely when a renal mass is detected on imaging. Also, bilateral or multicentric tumors are much more likely to be Wilms tumors than other tumors. In the neonate with a renal mass, congenital mesoblastic nephroma (CMN) is the most likely diagnosis, even though familial Wilms tumor and rhabdoid tumor of the kidney (RTK) can also be diagnosed in the first few months of life. If the diagnosis based on surgical resection or biopsy is a lesion other than Wilms tumor, further metastatic workup is important. Bone scans and skeletal surveys may be performed after histological confirmation of the diagnosis as bone metastases are more common in clear cell sarcoma of the kidney (CCSK) and renal cell carcinoma (RCC). A CT or MRI of the head should be performed in RTK and CCSK to rule out brain metastases.

## Staging and Prognosis

Tumor stage is based on the anatomic extent of the tumor. The staging systems developed by the National Wilms Tumor Study Group (now known as the Children's Oncology Group Renal Tumors Committee) and the SIOP correlate well with outcomes and allow stratification of patients into various risk groups. The primary difference between these two staging systems is that the COG staging system assigns a stage based on prechemotherapy surgical findings while the SIOP staging system is based on the extent of the disease after chemotherapy.

Histology is a strong predictor of outcome. Anaplasia, defined by cells showing irregular mitosis, hyperchromasia, and enlarged nuclei, portends a much worse prognosis than favorable histology tumors. Furthermore, focal anaplasia, or anaplasia confined to only part of the tumor, offers a better prognosis than diffuse anaplasia [11]. Other than histology, certain biologic markers such as loss of heterozygosity of chromosomes 16q and 1p further stratify patients into risk groups for tailoring of therapy. Table 8.1 is a summary of the current COG staging system.

**Table 8.1** Stages of Wilms tumor

| Stages | |
|---|---|
| I | Tumor confined to the kidney, no intraoperative spillage, negative surgical margins |
| II | Tumor extends beyond kidney, surgical margins negative, no intraoperative spillage |
| III | Tumor spread outside of the kidney but confined to the abdomen, positive surgical margins, or intraoperative tumor spillage |
| IV | Hematogenous metastasis or distal lymph node spread |
| V | Bilateral disease |

## Treatment

The combination of stage, histology, and particular genetic abnormalities found in some tumors places the patient into a risk category which then determines which treatment regimen the patient will receive. Treatment philosophies differ between Europe, the United Kingdom, and North America. In all of these places, the vast majority of Wilms tumor patients are enrolled in ongoing study protocols and are treated based on currently defined risk groups. The goal in all of these trials is to improve overall and disease-specific survival, while diminishing treatment-related morbidity. A full discussion of these treatment protocols is beyond the scope of this chapter. In the most broad sense, the major difference between treatment strategies between the groups is timing of chemotherapy administration. Unlike the COG in North America, the SIOP in Europe administers preoperative chemotherapy to all patients without performing a biopsy. The advantage of this strategy is inducing tumor shrinkage and treating micrometastatic foci resulting in a greater number of "postchemotherapy stage I" tumors. The ultimate goal is to decrease the risk of tumor rupture and spillage at the time of surgery and reduce the morbidity associated with radiotherapy. The United Kingdom Children's Cancer Study Group (UKCCSG) also uses presurgical chemotherapy, but patients undergo biopsies of their lesions before treatment. The rationale behind this strategy is to avoid giving unnecessary chemotherapy to children with benign lesions and inappropriate chemotherapy to children with lesions other than Wilms tumor. Despite these considerable philosophical differences, all of the groups share the common goal of minimizing treatment for low-risk patients and identifying high-risk patients who might require more intense therapy.

As mentioned above, most patients treated in North America will undergo immediate nephrectomy, followed by adjuvant therapy based on pathological stage and other biological prognostic markers. Upfront chemotherapy is given to patients with bilateral tumors, tumors found to be inoperable at the time of surgery, or tumors with intracaval tumor extension above the hepatic veins. Importantly, as part of the current COG protocol, preoperative renal biopsy is no longer warranted in patients with bilateral renal tumors, based on evidence suggesting that in the vast majority of cases, bilateral pediatric renal tumors are in fact Wilms tumors.

## Other Renal Tumors

### Renal Cell Carcinoma

RCC accounts for about 5 % of malignant renal tumors in patients younger than age 20 and is the most common renal malignancy in the second decade of life. The mean age at diagnosis in pediatrics is between 8 and 11 years, but RCC has been found in children as young as 3 months old. Similar to Wilms tumor, a palpable abdominal mass is the most common finding at diagnosis, but hematuria is a relatively more common symptom in RCC than Wilms tumor. In contrast to adult RCC, there is no known association with any environmental factors such as cigarette smoking or dialysis. Papillary RCC occurs at a higher incidence in pediatric patients than adults and is associated with chromosomal translocations involving the *TFE* gene located at Xp11.2.

The treatment of pediatric RCC is similar to treatment in adults. The most important determinant of outcome in children is the ability to perform a complete tumor resection. Survival is excellent in patients who have stage I disease. Younger age at diagnosis is a favorable prognostic factor, and lymph node involvement does not necessarily portend a poor prognosis as it does in adults [12].

## Congenital Mesoblastic Nephroma

CMN is the most common renal tumor of infants. The mean age at diagnosis is 3.5 months. In this age group, a palpable abdominal mass is by the far the most common presentation. Outcomes after radical surgery are excellent in this group of patients. Adjuvant chemotherapy or radiation therapy is not routinely recommended for most patients. However, metastases and local recurrence can occur in certain histological variants of this disease.

## Clear Cell Sarcoma of the Kidney

CCSK accounts for about 3 % of pediatric renal tumors reported to the National Wilms Tumor Study Group and is the second most common renal tumor in children. Histologically, this tumor may mimic Wilms tumor, rhabdoid tumor of the kidney, and congenital mesoblastic nephroma. This disease is associated with a high risk of relapse after surgery, so most patients undergo postoperative irradiation. Thirty percent of relapses occur more than 3 years after initial diagnosis, thereby dictating long-term follow-up in these patients. Lower stage and younger age at diagnosis are associated with improved survival [12].

## Rhabdoid Tumor of the Kidney

RTK, which accounts for about 2 % of pediatric renal tumors, was originally considered a variant of Wilms tumor. It is now considered a sarcoma of the kidney and is the most aggressive and lethal of all pediatric renal tumors. Even patients with localized disease (stage I/II) have less than 50 % survival. Typically these patients are diagnosed at an early age and have advanced disease at the time of diagnosis. The disease often demonstrates resistance to chemotherapy and has a tendency to metastasize to the brain. RTK is also associated with second primary brain tumors in children. Both RTK and CCSK can occur at extrarenal sites [12].

## Multilocular Cysts and Cystic, Partially Differentiated Nephroblastoma

Multilocular cysts, or multilocular cystic nephroma, are rare, benign renal tumors usually found in young children, especially boys with a second peak incidence in young, adult women. The lesion is usually unilateral but some can be bilateral. Nephrectomy is often curative, and recurrence after incomplete resection via partial nephrectomy has been reported. Cystic, partially differentiated nephroblastoma is a similar entity usually diagnosed in the first 2 years of life. These may be considered part of the same disease spectrum. Surgical resection is also curative for this disease.

## References


1. National Cancer Institute. Surveillance epidemiology and end results. Online, 1975-2005. U.S. National Institutes of Health. http://seer.cancer.gov/statistics. Accessed 31 Dec 2008.
2. Breslow N, Beckwith JB, Ciol M, Sharples K. Age distribution of Wilms' tumor: report from the National Wilms' Tumor Study. Cancer Res. 1988;48:1653–7.
3. Breslow N, Olshan A, Beckwith JP, et al. Ethnic variation in the incidence, diagnosis, prognosis, and follow-up of children with Wilms' tumor. J Natl Cancer Inst. 1994;86:49–51.
4. Breslow N, Beckwith JB, Perlman EJ, Reeve AE. Age distributions, birth weights, nephrogenic rests, and heterogeneity in the pathogenesis of wilms tumor. Pediatr Blood Cancer. 2006;47:260–7.
5. Wierich A, Leuschner I, Harms D, et al. Clinical impact of histologic subtypes in localized non-anaplastic nephroblastoma treated according to the trial and study SIOP-9/GPOH. Ann Oncol. 2001;12:311–9.
6. Scott RH, Stiller CA, Walker L, Rahman N. Syndromes and constitutional chromosomal abnormalities associated with Wilms tumour. J Med Genet. 2006;43:705–15.
7. Lee SB, Haber DA. Wilms' tumor and the WT1 gene. Exp Cell Res. 2001;264:74–9.
8. Breslow NE, Norris R, Norkool PA, Kang T, Beckwith JB, Perlman EJ, Ritchey ML, Green DM, Nichols

KE. Characteristics and outcomes of children with the Wilms' tumor-aniridia syndrome: a report from the National Wilms' Tumor Study Group. J Clin Oncol. 2003;21:4579–85.

9. Ritchey ML, Kelalis PP, Breslow N, et al. Intracaval and atrial involvement with nephroblastoma: review of National Wilms' Tumor Study-3. J Urol. 1988;140: 1113–8.
10. Meisel JA, Guthrie KA, Breslow NE, Donaldson SS, Green DM. Significance and management of computed tomography detected pulmonary nodules: a report from the National Wilms Tumor Study Group. Int J Radiat Oncol Biol Phys. 1999;44:579–85.
11. Faria P, Beckwith JB, Mishra K, et al. Focal versus diffuse anaplasia in Wilms tumor—new definitions with prognostic significance: a report from the National Wilms Tumor Study Group. Am J Surg Pathol. 1996;20:909–20.
12. Ritchey ML, Shamberger RC. Ch. 130: Pediatric urologic oncology. In: Wein AJ et al., editors. Campbell-Walsh urology, vol. 4. 9th ed. Philadelphia: Elsevier; 2007.

# Ureteroceles

# 9

Pamela I. Ellsworth and Anthony A. Caldamone

## What Is a Ureterocele?

A ureterocele is a cystic dilatation of the terminal ureter. Ureteroceles occur most frequently in females (4:1 female/male) and almost exclusively in Caucasians. Ureteroceles are bilateral in 10 % of cases. The majority of ureteroceles (80 %) identified in children involve the upper pole ureter of a duplicated collecting system and are almost always associated with obstruction. Single-system ureteroceles do occur but are more commonly identified in adults. Unlike many congenital anomalies, the management of ureteroceles is individualized and does not lend itself to treatment algorithms.

## Classification

Ureteroceles are commonly described as intravesical (located entirely within the bladder) or ectopic. Ectopic ureteroceles are those that extend into the bladder neck or more distally into the proximal urethra.

Stephens described further classification of ureteroceles as follows:

A. Stenotic—the orifice is located within the bladder and is stenotic.
B. Sphincteric—the ureterocele orifice is located beyond the bladder neck.
C. Sphincterostenotic ureterocele—a sphincteric ureterocele with a stenotic orifice [1].

## Etiology of Ureteroceles

Several theories exist regarding the embryologic development of ureteroceles. It is known that at 37 weeks, Chwalla's membrane transiently divides the early ureteral bud from the urogenital sinus. One theory is that the stenotic orifice and ureteral dilatation are the result of incomplete dissolution of Chwalla's membrane [2]. Other theories regarding the etiology include abnormal muscular development or a developmental stimulus responsible for bladder expansion acting on the intravesical ureter [3, 4].

## Presentation

Today, ureteroceles are detected on prenatal ultrasonography. The fetal kidneys can be visualized as early as 16 weeks of gestation. Although the actual detection of a ureterocele may be difficult on prenatal ultrasound, the associated finding of prenatal hydronephrosis on prenatal

P.I. Ellsworth, M.D. (✉)
Division of Urology, UMassMemorial Medical Center, 55 Lake Avenue North, Worcester, MA 01655, USA
e-mail: pamelaellsworth@aol.com

A.A. Caldamone, M.D., F.A.A.P., F.A.C.S.
The Warren Alpert Medical School of Brown University, Providence, RI, USA

R. Rabinowitz et al. (eds.), *Pediatric Urology for the Primary Care Physician*, Current Clinical Urology, DOI 10.1007/978-1-60327-243-8_9, © Springer Science+Business Media New York 2015

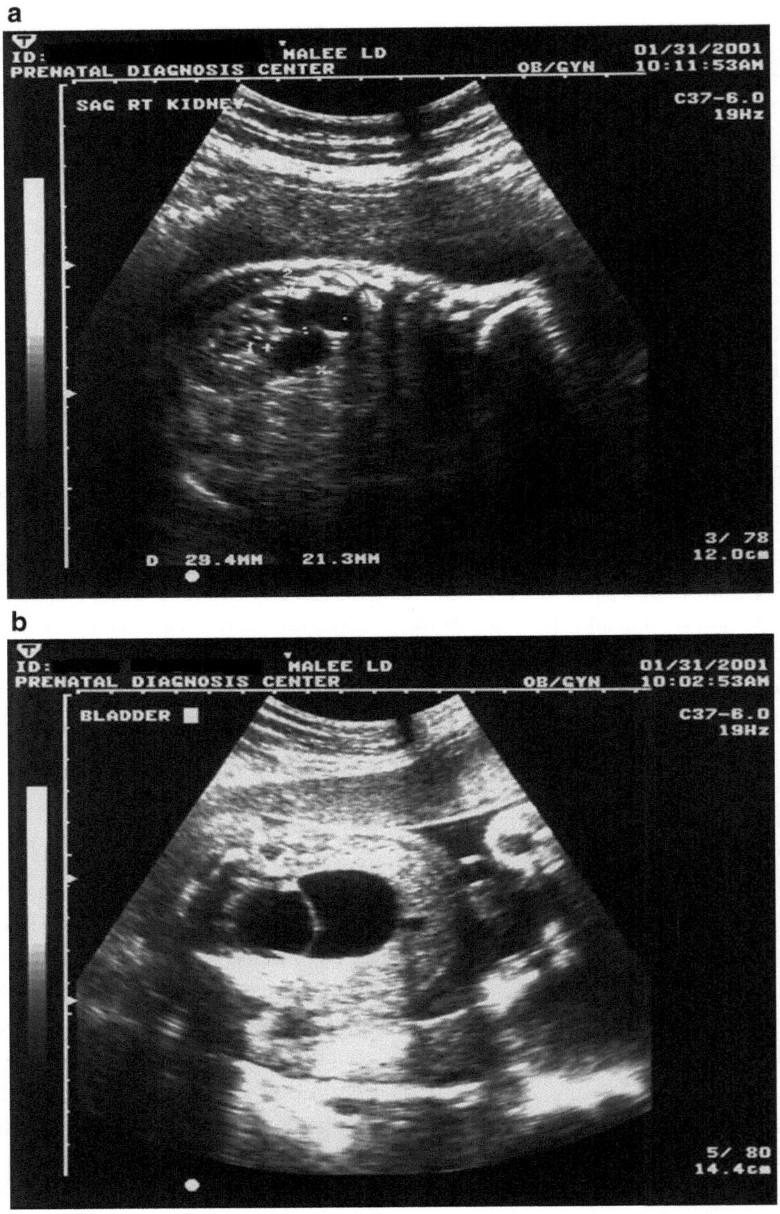


**Fig. 9.1** (**a**) Prenatal ultrasound demonstrating hydronephrosis. (**b**) Prenatal ultrasound demonstrating ureterocele in the bladder

ultrasound (Fig. 9.1a, b) should prompt further postnatal evaluation, which will lead to the confirmation of the diagnosis.

Not all ureteroceles are detected prenatally. Some ureteroceles are still diagnosed on clinical symptoms. The most common clinical presentation is an infant with a urinary tract infection or urosepsis. Rarely, an infant may present with a flank mass, representing the hydronephrotic kidney, failure to thrive, or with a vaginal mass secondary to a prolapsing ureterocele (Fig. 9.2). The differential diagnosis of a vaginal mass includes: urethral prolapse, sarcoma botryoides, paraurethral cyst, imperforate hymen, Gartner's

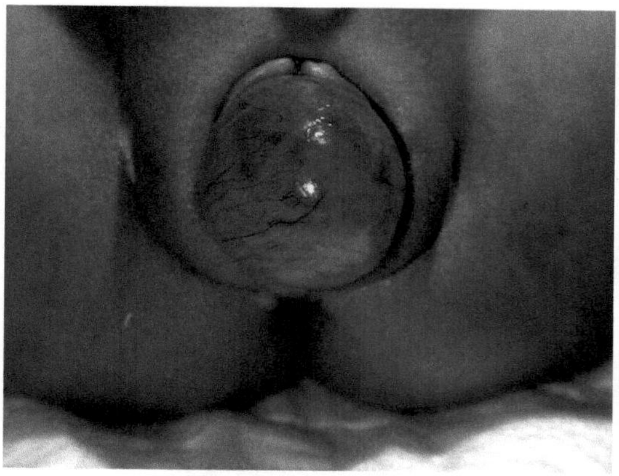

**Fig. 9.2** Prolapsing ureterocele

duct cyst, and a prolapsed ureterocele. The prolapsed ureterocele has a smooth round wall and usually slides down the posterior wall of the urethra; therefore, the urethra can be identified anterior to the mass and can be catheterized. Prolapse of the ureterocele may be intermittent and may cause bladder outlet obstruction. If the bladder outlet obstruction is significant, a distended bladder may be palpated on physical examination. Bladder outlet obstruction can lead to bilateral hydronephrosis.

## Physical Examination

The physical examination of a child with a history of prenatal hydronephrosis, prenatally detected ureterocele, or presenting with a urinary tract infection/urosepsis should include an abdominal, perineal, back, lower extremity, and focused neurologic examination. The abdominal examination should include examination of the upper abdomen to detect flank masses and the lower abdomen to assess for a distended bladder. The lower back and sacral area should be inspected for any abnormalities such as abnormal gluteal cleft, skin dimples, and hair patches which would be suggestive of an underlying neurologic abnormality. The genital examination should note whether or not there are any vaginal/introital masses, the urethral meatal position, and whether or not the hymen is patent. A focused neurologic examination should also be performed to rule out any neurologic abnormality. Ureteroceles may be associated with palpable flank masses, a distended bladder, or a vaginal mass in select cases.

## Radiological Evaluation

In newborns with a history of prenatal hydronephrosis or a ureterocele identified prenatally, a renal/bladder ultrasound should be obtained at approximately 48 h of life. The newborn should be started on antibiotic prophylaxis, amoxicillin 25 mg/kg per day as a single dosage, until the radiological evaluation is completed.

### Renal/Bladder Ultrasound

Clues to the presence of a ureterocele on ultrasound include the presence of a duplex system with hydronephrosis of the upper pole and a dilated upper pole ureter. The upper pole renal parenchyma may be of variable thickness and echogenicity. Severe upper pole parenchymal thinning or increased echogenicity of the parenchyma has been correlated with dysplasia [5]. Bladder ultrasound frequently shows a thin-walled cystic structure, the ureterocele, in the bladder and often extending through the bladder neck (ectopic ureterocele) (Fig. 9.3).

There are pitfalls of ultrasound which should be kept in mind. If the infant's bladder is distended, the ureterocele may be effaced and may not be detected. If the bladder is empty, it may be difficult to differentiate between the wall of the ureterocele and the wall of the bladder. Ectopic ureters may have similar findings on ultrasound as ureteroceles. Ectopic ureters are more commonly seen in duplex systems and affect the upper pole moiety. Ectopic ureters are most commonly obstructive and thus will be associated with hydronephrosis of the upper pole of the kidney and ureteral dilatation. Occasionally, the pelvic portion of a dilated ectopic ureter can be seen immediately posterior to the bladder and can impinge on the bladder mimicking a ureterocele (pseudoureterocele). The difference between

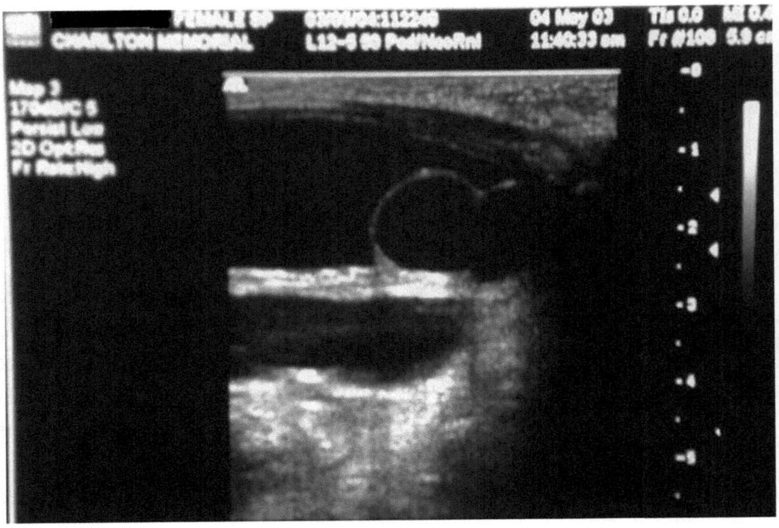

**Fig. 9.3** Ectopic ureterocele

a ureterocele and an ectopic ureter is that a ureterocele is separated from the bladder lumen by its thin wall, whereas an ectopic ureter is associated with a thicker bladder wall separating it from the intravesical space. Lastly, in some cases, the ureterocele may be associated with a normal caliber ureter and collecting system. The upper pole parenchyma may be atrophied and nonvisible, making the diagnosis of a duplicated system difficult.

## Voiding Cystourethrogram

Voiding cystourethrogram (VCUG) should be performed in any infant with a suspicious renal bladder ultrasound. The VCUG demonstrates the size and location of the ureterocele as well as the presence/absence of vesicoureteral reflux or bladder outlet obstruction. Reflux into the ipsilateral lower pole is common with reported rates of 44–63 % [6]. Reflux may also be seen into the contralateral kidney if the ureterocele is large enough to distort the trigone and the contralateral ureteral submucosal tunnel.

The appearance of a ureterocele on VCUG is that of a smooth, broad-based filling defect that is located near the trigone. It may be difficult to determine the side that the ureterocele actually arises from on VCUG, especially if the ureterocele is very large.

As with renal ultrasound, there are potential pitfalls with the VCUG. It is important to have images obtained early in the filling phase because some ureteroceles may efface later in filling and will not be visualized. When the bladder is full, the ureterocele may evert into the ureter and have the appearance of a diverticulum, due to poor detrusor backing. Periodic imaging during filling should prevent missing the ureterocele.

Renal/bladder ultrasound and VCUG are the initial radiologic studies performed for evaluation of hydronephrosis and a suspicion of a ureterocele. Further evaluation will depend on the ultrasound and VCUG findings.

## Cystoscopy

Diagnostic cystoscopy is rarely needed in the evaluation of a ureterocele. However, if the VCUG and ultrasound cannot adequately differentiate between an ectopic ureter and a ureterocele or if there remains a question as to the side of origin of the ureterocele, diagnostic cystoscopy may be useful.

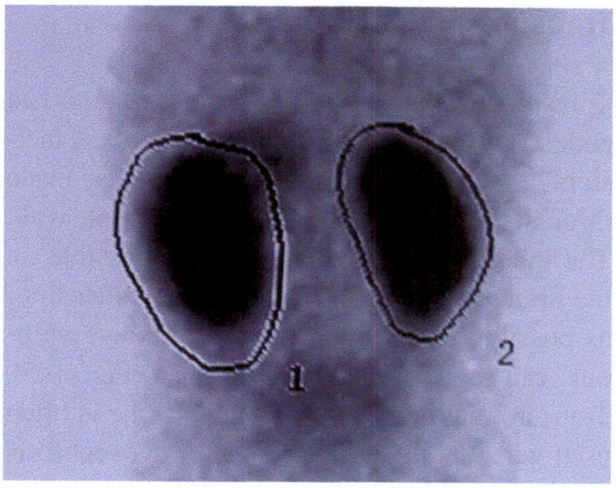


**Fig. 9.4** DMSA renal scan of ureteroceles; Fig. 9.5

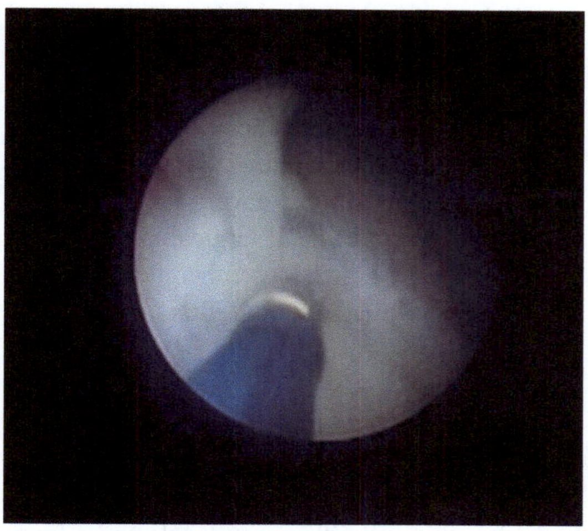

**Fig. 9.5** Transurethral incision of ureterocele

## Technetium-99m Dimercaptosuccinic Acid (DMSA) Renal Scan

The DMSA renal scan may prove useful in the management of the infant with a ureterocele. The DMSA renal scan may provide valuable information regarding the function of the upper pole, which will be useful in deciding the ultimate surgical management (Fig. 9.4).

## Diuretic Renography

Diuretic renography (furosemide mercaptoacetyl triglycerine renal scan, Lasix MAG3) can be useful in identifying the subgroup of patients with ureteroceles who are candidates for nonoperative management, including those children with ureteroceles with nonobstructed duplex system having relatively good upper pole function or those ureteroceles associated with a multicystic dysplastic nonfunctioning upper pole moiety.

## Management

Prophylactic antibiotics should be continued once the diagnosis of a ureterocele has been made. Early institution of antibiotic prophylaxis had led to a decrease in the rate of urinary tract infections in children with ureteroceles from 70–80 % to 3–15 % [6–8].

Prenatal detection of ureteroceles and the earlier institution of prophylaxis decrease morbidity and potential adverse outcomes related to urinary tract infections. Although this has not been demonstrated to have an effect on upper pole function, it is associated with a decrease rate of secondary procedures independent of the type of ureterocele.

In the vast majority of infants/children with ureteroceles, surgical intervention will be required. The goals of treatment are preservation of renal function, elimination of infection, relief of obstruction, management of vesicoureteral reflux if present, and preservation of urinary continence with minimal surgical morbidity. The decision regarding the type of surgical intervention depends on a variety of factors including whether or not prompt drainage is needed in the setting of pyonephrosis or urosepsis. The function of the upper pole moiety, the type of ureterocele (intravesical versus ectopic), and the presence of ipsilateral and contralateral reflux are all taken into account in the ultimate decision making.

In select cases, observation may have a role in the management of ureteroceles. Observation has been offered to children who had either no function to the upper pole or in whom there was function with adequate drainage as determined by an intravenous pyelogram (IVP) or diuretic renal scan, no evidence of contralateral renal or bladder outlet obstruction, and if reflux was present only low to moderate grade. With observation, prophylaxis is continued until toilet training or the vesicoureteral reflux is resolved. In an accumulation of reported cases, resolution of hydronephrosis has been seen in 43–67 %, improved in 0–43 %, and remained stable in 15–57 %. Only 1 child had increasing hydronephrosis requiring surgery. Vesicoureteral reflux resolved in 38–71 % of cases [9, 10]. It should be noted, however, this is only a select subpopulation, and these children must be followed carefully.

Options for surgical management include: transurethral incision of the ureterocele, upper pole nephroureterectomy, excision of the ureterocele, and common sheath reimplantation and ureteropyelostomy or ureteroureterostomy.

## Single-System Ureteroceles

The treatment of single-system ureteroceles is determined by the renal function. If the ipsilateral kidney has poor or no function, then a nephrectomy is indicated. If the affected kidney has satisfactory function and the ureterocele is intravesical, then transurethral incision of the ureterocele is successful in the majority of these patients.

## Duplex-System Ureteroceles

The management of ureteroceles in duplex systems is more complex than single systems and takes into account the location of the ureterocele (intravesical versus ectopic), the presence/absence of ipsilateral lower pole and contralateral reflux, as well as the function of the affected upper pole moiety. Controversy exists regarding the roles of each of the surgical therapies, and there is no single procedure that is effective for all cases of duplex-system ureteroceles; rather, the surgical approach must be individualized. The risk of requiring more than one surgical procedure is higher in individuals with ectopic ureteroceles.

## Transurethral Incision

Transurethral incision of a ureterocele is an endoscopic procedure in which a transverse incision or puncture using electrocautery is made through the full thickness of the ureterocele wall. The incision is made as distally as possible on the ureterocele and as close to the bladder floor as possible to provide effective drainage without causing vesicoureteral reflux (Fig. 9.5). Transurethral incision of the ureterocele is often used when an infant presents with pyonephrosis or urosepsis related to a ureterocele as it provides quick decompression of the ureterocele. In the elective management of ureteroceles, the success rate of transurethral incision as a definitive procedure is less with ectopic ureteroceles compared to intravesical ureteroceles. In the child with an intravesical ureterocele, 60 % or more of children will need no further procedures after endoscopic decompression of the ureterocele [11]. Children with ectopic ureteroceles have a greater chance of needing an additional surgical procedure(s) after transurethral incision, either for persistent obstruction or vesicoureteral reflux.

## Duplex System with Functioning Upper Pole

In duplex systems with a ureterocele and a functioning upper pole, ureteroureterostomy and ureteropyelostomy may be performed to salvage the upper pole (Fig. 9.6). These procedures are generally reserved for ureteroceles presenting without reflux into the ipsilateral lower pole ureter or contralateral ureters. The upper pole ureter is transected and anastomosed to either the renal pelvis of the lower pole of the duplex kidney or the lower pole ureter thereby diverting urine into the lower pole collecting system or lower pole ureter. The segment of upper pole ureter extending into the pelvis is excised, and the remaining stump of ureter is aspirated and allowed to collapse. This decompresses the ureterocele.

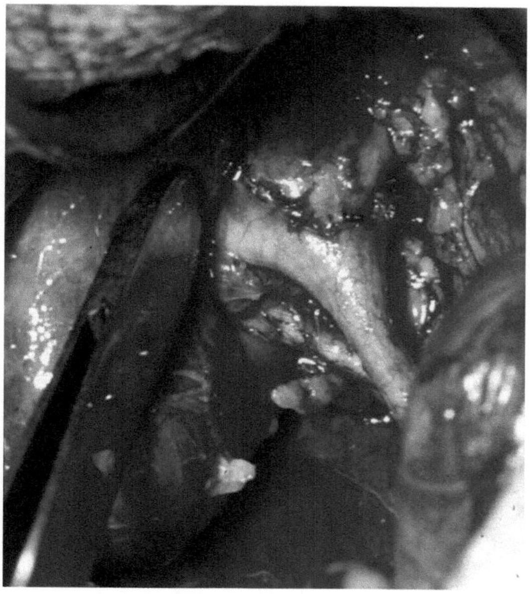

**Fig. 9.6** Ureteropyelostomy

Alternatively, if reflux is present to either the lower pole ureter or the contralateral ureter, then lower urinary tract reconstruction may be a more suitable alternative. In this approach, the ureterocele is excised, the floor of the bladder reconstructed, the duplex system ureters reimplanted via a common sheath approach, and if reflux is present on the contralateral side, ureteral reimplantation performed on that side also (Fig. 9.7).

## Duplex System with a Nonfunctioning Upper Pole

Upper pole nephroureterectomy, removal of the upper pole renal moiety and the upper pole ureter down to the level of the pelvis, is often successful in the setting of a ureterocele associated with a nonfunctioning upper pole moiety in the absence

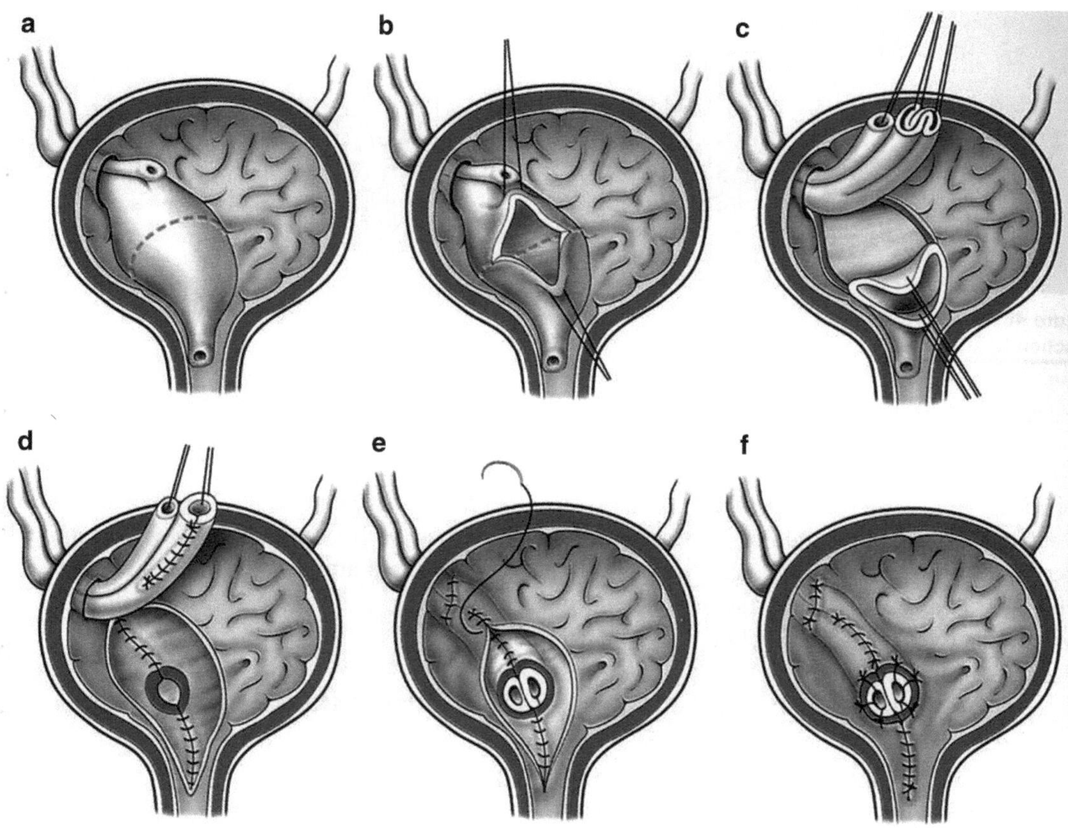


**Fig. 9.7** Excision of ureterocele and common sheath ureteral reimplantation (Reprinted with permission, Informa Healthcare from Clinical Pediatric Urology, 5th edition)

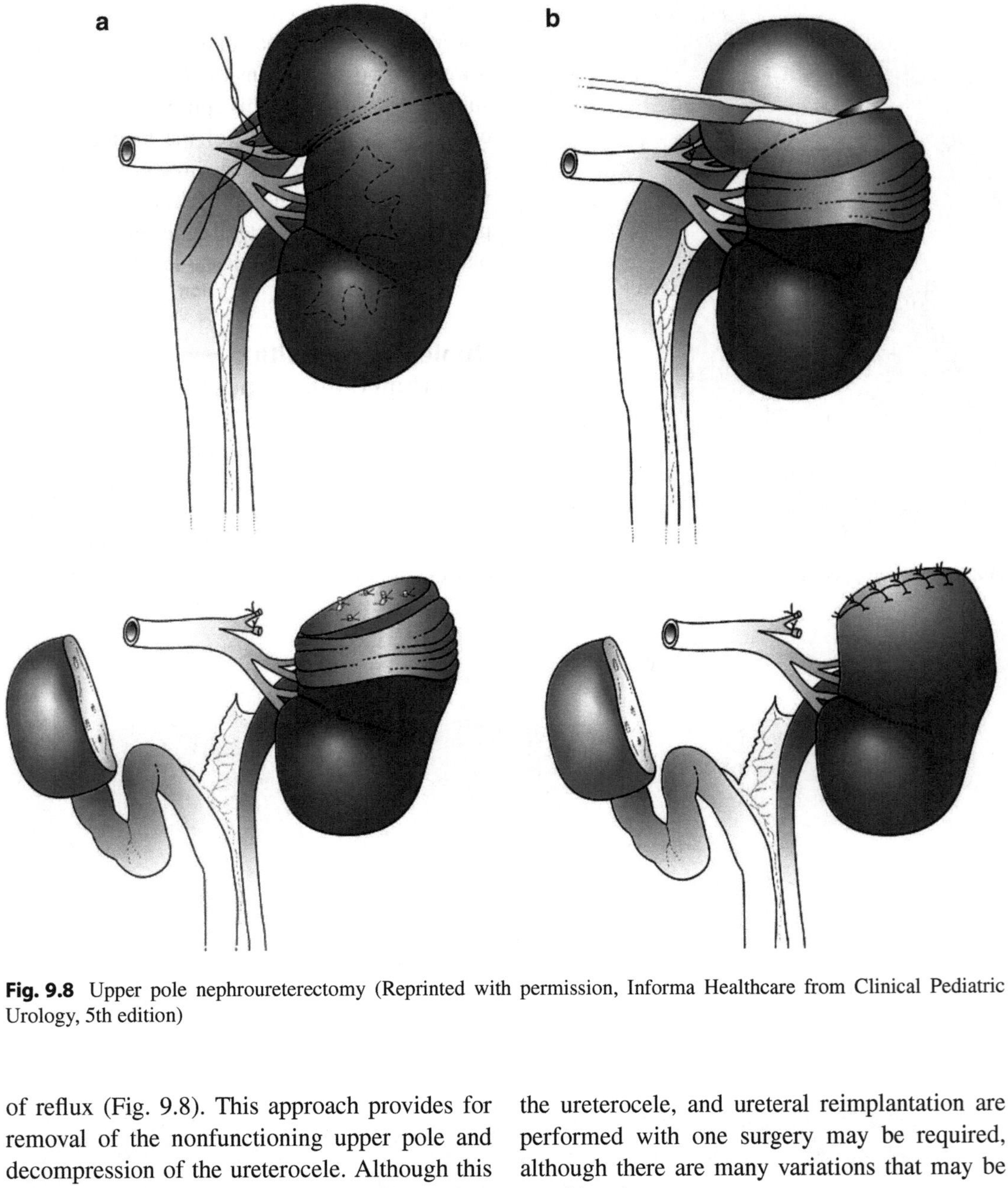


**Fig. 9.8** Upper pole nephroureterectomy (Reprinted with permission, Informa Healthcare from Clinical Pediatric Urology, 5th edition)

of reflux (Fig. 9.8). This approach provides for removal of the nonfunctioning upper pole and decompression of the ureterocele. Although this approach is associated with less morbidity than lower urinary tract reconstruction, a significant decrease in function in the remaining lower pole moiety has been noted in 8 % of children and a small decrease in function in 51 % [12]. Those children with reflux into the contralateral system and/or ipsilateral lower pole reflux and a non-functioning upper pole are the most challenging cases. In such children, a combined procedure whereby an upper pole nephrectomy, excision of the ureterocele, and ureteral reimplantation are performed with one surgery may be required, although there are many variations that may be considered.

## Long-Term Risks of Ureteroceles

### Hypertension

There does not appear to be an increased risk of hypertension related to the dysplastic upper pole moiety. Those children with associated reflux and urinary tract infections are at risk for hypertension similar to the reflux population.

## Incontinence

Children with extravesical ureteroceles with extension into the bladder neck and proximal urethra are at risk for urinary incontinence related to distortion of the bladder neck and proximal urethral anatomy from the ureterocele. In addition, these children often require excision of the ureterocele and ureteral reimplantation. Surgical dissection in the area of the bladder neck may further contribute to the risk of urinary incontinence.

## Altered Renal Function

Lower pole and contralateral renal function may be adversely affected in those children with bladder outlet obstruction related to the ureterocele. Bladder outlet obstruction should be suspected if the bladder is distended on ultrasound. The VCUG may demonstrate prolapse of the ureterocele into the bladder outlet during voiding.

The impact of early identification of ureteroceles on the function of the affected upper pole moiety is controversial. There are a few series that support improved upper pole function in those children with prenatally detected ureteroceles [7, 13].

## Conclusions

Prenatal detection of ureteroceles has allowed for prompt postnatal evaluation and institution of antibiotic prophylaxis. This has decreased the morbidity associated with ureteroceles; however, its effect on ipsilateral upper pole function remains controversial. In a child with a suspected ureterocele, a renal/bladder ultrasound and VCUG should be performed. These studies are important in confirming the presence of a ureterocele, identifying the anatomy and determining whether or not there is associated vesicoureteral reflux. DMSA renal scan is useful in assessing the upper pole renal function. The management of ureteroceles varies with the type of ureterocele, the function of the ipsilateral upper pole moiety, and the presence/absence of vesicoureteral reflux. The goals of treatment are preservation of renal function, elimination of infection, obstruction and reflux, and maintenance of urinary continence with minimal surgical morbidity.

## References

1. Stephens FD. Congenital malformations of the urinary tract. New York: Praeger; 1983. p. 320–2.
2. Chwalla R. The process of formation of cystic dilatations of the vesical end of the ureter and of diverticula at the ureteral ostium. Urol Cutan Rev. 1927;31:499.
3. Tokunaka S, Gotoh T, Oyanagi T, et al. Morphological study of the ureterocele: a possible clue to its embryogenesis as evidenced by a locally arrested myogenesis. J Urol. 1981;126:726.
4. Stephens D. Caecoureterocele and concepts on the embryology and aetiology of ureteroceles. Aust N Z J Surg. 1971;40:239.
5. Bolduc S, Upadhyay J, Restrepo R, Sherman C, et al. The predictive value of diagnostic imaging for histological lesions of the upper poles in duplex systems with ureteroceles. BJU Int. 2003;91:678–82.
6. Shekarriz B, Upadhyay J, Fleming P, Gonzalez R, Barthold JS. Long-term outcome based on the initial approach to ureterocele. J Urol. 1999;162(3 Pt 2):1072–6.
7. Van Savage JG, Mesrobian HG. The impact of prenatal ultrasonography on the morbidity and outcome of patients with renal duplication anomalies. J Urol. 1995;153:768.
8. Hulbert WC, Rabinowitz R. Prenatal diagnosis of duplex system hydronephrosis: effect on renal salvage. Urology. 1998;51(5A Suppl):23–6.
9. Han MY, Gibbbons D, Belman AB, Pohl HG, Majd M, Rushton HG. Indications for nonoperative management of ureteroceles. J Urol. 2005;174:1652–6.
10. Coplen DE, Austin PF. Outcome analysis of prenatally detected ureteroceles associated with multicystic dysplasia. J Urol. 2004;172:1637–9.
11. Hagg MJ, Mourachov PV, Snyder HM, et al. The modern endoscopic approach to ureterocele. J Urol. 2000;163(3):940–3.
12. Gundeti MS, Ransley PG, Duffy PG, et al. Renal outcome following heminephrectomy for duplex kidney. J Urol. 2005;173:1743–4.
13. Blyth B, Passerini-Glazel G, Camuffo C, et al. Endoscopic incision of ureteroceles: intravesical versus ectopic. J Urol. 1993;149:556.

# 10 Megaureter

Steve S. Kim, J. Christopher Austin, and Douglas A. Canning

## Introduction

A megaureter is in the broadest sense a purely descriptive term meant to indicate any ureter that is abnormally dilated. This label does not define a distinct pathologic entity per se, but rather encompasses a wide spectrum of both physiologic and pathophysiologic processes which culminate in a dilated ureter. Confusion arises when the terms megaureter, primary megaureter, and congenital megaureter are used interchangeably to specifically refer to a particular subset of all megaureters. In most instances, these labels are used to refer to those patients who present with either a primary non-refluxing obstructed megaureter or neonatal non-refluxing, non-obstructed megaureter. We hope to construct a framework for understanding the causes that lead to the development of a megaureter and to assist the primary care provider in formulating an appropriate and effective management strategy.

## Incidence and Epidemiology

Megaureter represents a relatively common anomaly of the newborn urinary tract. Overall, megaureters are thought to be the second leading cause of neonatal obstructive uropathy following only obstructions found at the ureteropelvic junction (UPJ). The vast majority of what constitute primary or congenital megaureters (meaning those found to be non-refluxing and either obstructed or unobstructed) were reportedly identified as the presumed cause for urinary tract dilation in 23 % of cases of all prenatal urinary dilation. With the increased utilization of fetal sonography, we expect megaureters to continue to be a prominent diagnosis found on neonatal evaluation.

With respect to gender differences, primary megaureters apparently occur roughly 2–4 times more often in boys than girls and are thought to occur slightly more often on the left side (1.6–4.5) than the right. Bilateral megaureters are thought to account for about 25 % of all cases. Of additional consideration is the reported association in 10–15 % of megaureters with a contralateral absent or dysplastic kidney which poses important management implications.

S.S. Kim, M.D.
USC Institute of Technology, 4650 Sunset Boulevard MS #114, Los Angeles, CA 90027, USA
e-mail: stkim@chla.usc.edu

J.C. Austin, M.D.
Division of Urology, Oregon Health & Science University, Portland, OR, USA

D.A. Canning, M.D., F.A.A.P., F.A.C.S. (✉)
Division of Urology, The Children's Hospital of Philadelphia, University of Pennsylvania School of Medicine, Philadelphia, PA, USA
e-mail: canning@email.chop.edu

R. Rabinowitz et al. (eds.), *Pediatric Urology for the Primary Care Physician*, Current Clinical Urology, DOI 10.1007/978-1-60327-243-8_10, 

## Definitions and Classification

By convention, any ureter that is larger in diameter than 7–8 mm is defined as a megaureter. Of crucial importance is the understanding of what processes give rise to the dilated ureter, moving beyond the simple descriptive nature of the term. The international classification for megaureters was established by Smith et al. in 1977. In this nomenclature, three major types of megaureters are emphasized based on the presence or absence of reflux and/or obstruction at the ureterovesical junction. The megaureters in this system are classified as either (1) *refluxing*, (2) *obstructed*, or (3) *non-refluxing* and *non-obstructed*. An additional category of *obstructed and refluxing* also deserves mention after its recognition as rare but distinct entity. Furthermore, each of these main categories is further subdivided into either an intrinsic primary ureteral etiology or a secondary non-ureteral etiology.

### Refluxing Megaureters

#### Primary Refluxing Megaureters

Primary refluxing megaureters encompass what we more traditionally have come to think of as dilating vesicoureteral reflux. In primary refluxing megaureters, the ureterovesical junction is presumed to be incompetent allowing for cyclical retrograde flow of urine into the ureter leading to progressive ureteral and upper urinary tract dilation. More regarding this particular subset of megaureters can be found elsewhere in the chapter on vesicoureteral reflux. Typically, the use of the term primary megaureter has not come to include this category which is more often thought of as simply vesicoureteral reflux.

#### Secondary Refluxing Megaureter

There are two types of secondary megaureters. Both syndromes require treatment of the underlying process, of which a megaureter is only one component. First, patients with the megacystis-megaureter syndrome are found to have bilateral high-grade vesicoureteral reflux along with a large thin-walled bladder created by a constant cycling of urine from a large-volume dilating reflux. The second possible systemic cause of secondary refluxing megaureter is the prune belly syndrome, also known as either Eagle-Barrett's syndrome or triad syndrome. Patients with prune belly syndrome may have ureterectasis as a part of a constellation of genitourinary findings. The ureteral dilation seen may be due to a variety of reasons including a secondary refluxing megaureter. These are only two specific examples of secondary refluxing megaureters, and the clinician must consider other causes as well.

### Obstructed Megaureters

#### Primary Obstructed Megaureters

Primary obstructive megaureters (POMs), along with the non-refluxing and non-obstructed megaureters, comprise what are typically referred to as primary or congenital megaureters. Primary obstructed megaureters are thought to be a result of an adynamic distal ureteral segment which creates a functional and/or true anatomic obstruction at the ureterovesical junction. Histologic studies of this distal aperistaltic segment have confirmed the presence of an abnormal collagen ultrastructure and altered ureteral concentrations of the neurotransmitter acetylcholinesterase. What was initially that to be a process analogous to Hirschsprung's disease was refuted by the identification of appropriate ureteral ganglia migration. Other than the presumed distal adynamic segment, other infrequent conditions that can cause a primary obstructed megaureter include congenital ureteral strictures and obstructing ureteral folds or valves.

It is at times difficult to distinguish primary obstructing megaureters from primary non-refluxing and non-obstructing megaureters as the definition of obstruction is subject to the vagaries of existing radiographic studies.

#### Secondary Obstructing Megaureter

The vast majority of secondary obstructed megaureters are related to functional obstructions associated with an elevated intravesical pressures and/or bladder outlet obstruction. In patients with neuropathic or non-neuropathic dysfunctional bladders, elevated intravesical pressures exceeding 40 cm $H_2O$ have been shown to generate enough resistance to impede flow of urine across a ureterovesical junction leading to ureteral dilatation and ultimately, renal deterioration. Patients with both spinal dysraphisms (tethered cord, myelomeningocele, etc.) and infravesical obstruction (posterior urethral valves, urethral atresia) are prime examples of secondary causes of ureteral obstruction. Aggressive management is imperative in these situations to avoid prolonged transmission of high pressure to the upper tracts that leads to renal deterioration.

## Non-obstructed and Non-refluxing Megaureters

### Primary Non-refluxing and Non-obstructed Megaureter

Primary non-refluxing and non-obstructed megaureters comprise the vast majority of neonatal megaureters encountered in practice. They are believed to be a clinically benign entity resulting from the polyuria of transitional nephrology. Fetal polyuria is marked by an immaturity of effective glomerular filtration, renovascular resistive indices, and overall concentrating ability creating a production of 4–6 times the normal amount of urine production seen later in infancy. High-volume urinary production leads to a state of transient ureteral dilation giving rise to a megaureter. Another potential contributing factor is the delayed maturation of distal ureteral architecture that transiently generates ureteral dilatation until full maturation occurs. Adding to this effect are the elevated voiding pressures of the infantile bladder resulting from a discoordinate urethrovesical unit. As previously mentioned, it becomes somewhat arbitrary as to what constitutes a non-obstructed system given the subjective nature of diuretic renal scans.

### Secondary Non-refluxing, Non-obstructed Megaureter

Secondary causes for a non-refluxing and non-obstructed megaureter include conditions that induce a state of polyuria including lithium toxicity, diabetes insipidus, and sickle cell nephropathy to name a few. Additionally, a transitory paralysis of normal ureteral peristalsis can be seen with bacterial endotoxin-mediated dilation in the context of an acute urinary tract infection. Just as in the other causes of secondary megaureters, the treatment lies in the treatment of the underlying condition.

## Refluxing and Obstructed Megaureter

The refluxing, obstructing megaureter represents a rare phenomenon that was not initially incorporated into the international classification system, but deserves mention as its own distinct category. Of the various categories, the refluxing and obstructing megaureter is the most difficult one to intuitively understand and conceptualize. Most of these rare cases occur in the context of ureteral ectopia, whereby a ureteral orifice aberrantly located in the bladder neck may be both incompetent causing reflux and become obstructed when the bladder neck musculature becomes contracted. Alternatively, a fixed, incompetent ureterovesical junction may lead to concomitant reflux and obstruction.

## History and Physical Exam

Increasingly, the diagnosis of a megaureter is being made on the basis of a prenatal screening ultrasound. Prior to the widespread utilization of fetal ultrasound, most megaureters presented with a constellation of clinical symptoms which subsequently lead to a diagnosis. This dichotomous presentation of the primary megaureter must be taken into consideration during the formulation of a management strategy given that it appears that they may represent differing phenotypic representations of a common set of circumstances.

For the most part, the antenatally detected megaureter represents a clinically asymptomatic process that appears to resolve spontaneously as the ureterovesical complex matures over time. A relative small group of these prenatally detected patients eventually manifest clinical symptoms and likely represent the subset of patients that in the past would have gone on to be diagnosed based on clinical symptoms.

Children with clinical symptoms leading to the diagnosis of a megaureter may have urinary tract infections, abdominal pain, gross and microscopic hematuria, and in extreme cases, renal insufficiency. There are no specific findings on the physical exam that direct the differential diagnosis toward a megaureter. Aside from a nonspecific finding of an abdominal or flank mass in severe cases, megaureters rarely demonstrate overt physical findings. Diagnosis is usually dependent on radiographic imaging.

## Evaluation

### Laboratory Evaluation

There are no specific laboratory tests required for the diagnosis of a megaureter. In the presence of a urinary tract infection, a urinalysis and urine culture are helpful to direct antibiotic therapy. Additional studies which may be useful include measurements of serum creatinine and estimated glomerular filtration rate to provide an assessment of overall renal function.

### Radiographic Evaluation

The diagnosis of a megaureter is usually based on radiographic findings. Accurate classification is paramount to the formulation of a therapeutic management plan. Radiographic investigations may provide both structural and functional information regarding the megaureter.

### Ultrasonography

The first step in the evaluation process begins with the clear identification of an abnormally dilated ureter on an imaging study. Currently, a vast majority of megaureters are detected by ultrasound (US), either as part of routine fetal screening or as the first-line imaging modality of choice in the clinically symptomatic pediatric patient. Ultrasound is the preferred initial imaging modality of choice for a variety of reasons. It affords the clinician not only structural detail of the entire urinary system (renal parenchyma, ureter, and bladder) but also is readily accessible and relatively inexpensive and, most importantly, presents no significant ionizing radiation and has minimal risks. It is for these reasons that we advocate ultrasonography (US) as the first imaging modality in the evaluation of the megaureter or of pediatric urinary symptoms.

### Intravenous Pyelography

Intravenous pyelography (IVP) provides structural detail of the affected ureter and distal ureterovesical junction as well as gives some idea regarding overall renal function. Limitations of IVP include the effect of renal immaturity on the ability to adequately visualize the urinary tract system and the level of ionizing radiation that is delivered to the pediatric patient. The use of IVP in the evaluation of megaureters is now largely historic but can occasionally be useful in helping to identify the location of the ureteral obstruction.

### Computed Tomography

Computed tomography (CT) provides excellent structural detail of the urinary tract. We do not advocate its use in the initial investigation of megaureters given its significant exposure to ionizing radiation and failure to provide any additional level of benefit. However, it is not unheard of for a pediatric patient with nonspecific abdominal or flank pain to undergo a CT scan as a diagnostic study, yielding a diagnosis of a megaureter.

### Magnetic Resonance Urography

Magnetic resonance urography (MRU) provides an excellent structural examination of the urinary tract. Additionally, the use of intravenous gadolinium enhancement affords the opportunity to assess functional information and may in the future become the study of choice in evaluating a host of urologic conditions. Currently, it remains an expensive and relatively inaccessible technology that often requires sedation. For these reasons, we do not advocate MRU as a first-line investigation at this time, but reserve it for cases involving more complex anatomical considerations (ureteral duplication, ureteral ectopia, etc.). We anticipate that as the image speed increases, sedation will become easier to manage even in the smaller babies, and MRU will become more widely utilized.

### Voiding Cystourethrogram

Voiding cystourethrograms (VCUG) are essential for identifying the presence of vesicoureteral reflux in the context of a diagnosis of a megaureter. Additionally, the VCUG provides structural insight into the urethra, bladder neck, and bladder to assess the presence of secondary causes of a megaureter. Its proper performance is relatively easy to achieve and, with the utilization of spot fluoroscopy, the amount of ionizing radiation can be kept to a reasonable level. Also, in the rare instance of refluxing and obstructing megaureters, the VCUG can provide information that would suggest an obstructive component which may not have otherwise been apparent.

### Diuretic Renal Scans

Diuretic renal scans (DRS) provide an important assessment of function by providing differential renal function and assessment of urinary tract obstruction. The renal scan is far from being an ideal examination and remains controversial in terms of how to interpret what constitutes urinary obstruction. Most diuretic renal scans are standardized to attempt to bring uniformity to the way the studies are performed. The radionuclide agents most often used are diethylenetriaminepentaacetic acid (99mTc-DTPA) or mercaptoacetyltriglycine (MAG3). An attempt to standardize hydration status, Lasix administration, and calculation of regions of interest is also made in an attempt to ensure reproducibility and accuracy. Despite these attempts, renal scans remain highly subjective and controversial in their ability to predict true urinary obstruction that would merit surgical interventions. Some have suggested that the drainage washout curves and t1/2 times are not accurate and that a detrimental change in overall differential renal function provides the best indication of obstruction. Another consideration in utilizing renal scans is the relative lack of tubular maturity in the neonatal kidney that may prevent an accurate assessment of function and obstruction. Some authors recommend delaying a renal scan until approximately 3 months of age when the kidneys have achieved maturity.

### Whitaker Perfusion Study

Alternatively, the Whitaker perfusion study can be performed to infer an obstructive uropathy based on differential pressure studies. This study has largely fallen out of favor due to its invasive nature (the requirement of percutaneous nephrostomy tubes) and relatively high margin of error in the face of a dilated, compliant collecting system. For these reasons, we do not recommend the Whitaker perfusion study, as we do not feel it offers any advantage over the renal scans except in cases where poor renal function results in poor concentration of radionuclide. In these cases, subjective assessment of drainage at the ureterovesical junction may help determine the need for surgery.

## Management

The management of primary or congenital megaureters has evolved over the past few decades as our understanding of the natural history of megaureters has grown. The principle philosophy behind therapeutic intervention in children with megaureter is preservation of renal function. Many children with primary megaureter improve the degree of dilation over time. It is reasonable to assume that a majority of these boys and girls spontaneously resolve or improve without the need for surgical intervention. With that in mind, the therapeutic strategy is therefore predicated on understanding the fundamental structural and functional etiologies that pertain to the megaureter. Additionally, the clinician must be able to recognize the potential for a secondary megaureter caused by another underlying disease process. The treatment of secondary causes of megaureter, regardless of the type of megaureter, is the aggressive treatment of the underlying etiology. Examples previously given of causes of secondary megaureters include neuropathic bladders, prune belly syndrome, and diabetes insipidus.

In the case of primary refluxing megaureters, the treatment recommendations consist largely of medical management with antibiotic prophylaxis and careful observation. Surgical interventions are reserved for those patients who persist with breakthrough urinary tract infections, pyelonephritis, and/or have documented renal scarring or deterioration. This topic is also somewhat controversial and is covered in more detail in the chapter addressing vesicoureteral reflux.

The primary non-refluxing, obstructed and non-refluxing, non-obstructed megaureters comprise two distinct categories of megaureters that likely lie on a continuous spectrum and present a therapeutic challenge in identifying which patients require intervention. In the clear case of an unambiguously obstructed ureter, few would disagree that surgical correction is warranted in order to prevent further renal deterioration. Unfortunately, the lack of an accurate and precise measurement of what truly constitutes an obstructed system leaves us unable to definitively answer which patients are clearly at risk, which patients are clearly obstructed, and which patients only require further observation. What was once uniformly treated with surgical reconstruction, the current knowledge that 70–87 % of these patients will either spontaneously resolve or improve has tempered our approach to the patient with the primary megaureter. Most pediatric urologists would now advocate a conservative course of expectant management consisting of antibiotic prophylaxis and serial radiographic surveillance. The development of recurrent febrile urinary tract infections or significant renal deterioration would prompt surgical intervention to mitigate further renal sequelae. Once again, the area of what constitutes significant renal deterioration is somewhat controversial and is subjective and largely based on clinical experience.

When initially confronted with a patient who is a diagnosed with a megaureter, one must take into consideration the circumstances of the diagnosis.

*Was the patient diagnosed based on clinical symptoms or detected incidentally on fetal imaging*? Presumably, a patient who presents with a clinical manifestation has transgressed into a clinically significant obstruction requiring a more timely evaluation. More frequently, the latter scenario is now what most clinicians encounter. Although it is reassuring to know that a vast majority of prenatally detected patients resolve spontaneously, one must be careful not to summarily discount the potential for these patients to later manifest significant disease. It is important to recognize that the clinical symptoms are preceded by a potentially lengthy preclinical period of ureteral dilation.

*Which patients with a megaureter should be referred to a pediatric urologist*? Given that it can be difficult for even pediatric urologist to discriminate which patients will require intervention on initial evaluation, we recommend that all patients who are diagnosed with a megaureter should be thoroughly evaluated by a pediatric urologist.

*Should patients be on antibiotic prophylaxis*? The protective effect of antibiotic prophylaxis remains one of the most controversial issues in pediatric urology. There is yet to be any conclusive evidence that antibiotic therapy confers a true benefit in the setting, but it is still a widely held belief that an obstructed and infected urinary system poses a serious threat to the safety of the child. This is an area that will require well-designed prospective randomized clinical trials to lend clarity to the issue. In the meantime, we still advocate the initial institution of daily low-dose prophylaxis (amoxicillin 25–50 mg/kg, trimethoprim 2 mg/kg) until a full risk assessment can be performed, including the exclusion of a refluxing megaureter.

## Conclusions

In conclusion, the term megaureter is a descriptive label that incorporates a wide spectrum of both physiologic and pathophysiologic causes. As we see a greater number of children diagnosed on ultrasound with a megaureter, it is important that the primary care provider be familiar with larger context of what processes give rise to a congenitally dilated ureter and have a working knowledge of the general categories of megaureter.

## Suggested Reading

Atala A, Keating MA. Vesicoureteral reflux and megaureter. In: Walsh PC, Retik AB, Vaughan ED, Wein AJ, editors. Campbell's urology. 7th ed. Philadelphia: WB Saunders Co; 1998. p. 1859.

Shokeir AA, Nijman RJ. Primary megaureter: current trends in diagnosis and treatment. BJU Int. 2000;86(7):861–8.

Shukla AR, Cooper J, Patel RP, et al. Prenatally detected primary megaureter: a role for extended followup. J Urol. 2005;173(4):1353–6.

# Ectopic Ureter

# 11

Armando J. Lorenzo and Antoine E. Khoury

## Definition

An ectopic ureter represents an anatomical variant in which the distal aspect abnormally inserts outside of its expected typical location within the bladder trigone. It can be seen in both single and duplicated system and can affect one or both renal units. Depending on the insertion point, two main problems may occur: abnormalities of urine flow and/or drainage past the continence mechanism. Therefore, ureteral ectopia is clinically relevant inasmuch as the anomalous insertion is associated with urinary incontinence, urinary obstruction, vesicoureteral reflux, or infections. There is an overlap between this diagnosis and other conditions such as megaureter and ureterocele, both covered in other chapters of this book.

## Incidence

Although the true incidence of ureteral ectopia is unknown, the condition is thought to be relatively rare (~1/2,000 children). It is more common in females, the majority of which have an associated duplication anomaly (80 %). In contrast, boys are more frequently found to have ectopic ureters that drain single systems [1, 2]. Rarely the process may present bilaterally (5–15 %) or involve a solitary kidney, situation that adds a sense of emergency to the work-up due to the potential compromise in renal function.

## Embryology and Pathophysiology

The ectopic ureteral insertion dates back to an abnormal takeoff of the ureteric bud during early embryogenesis. Depending on how far away from the normal point of origin, the insertion may be in close proximity or fairly distant to the bladder trigone (Fig. 11.1). Completely duplicated systems are of particular interest as two separate ureters enter at different points in the lower urinary tract. Drainage in such situations follows the Weigert-Meyer rule. Simply stated, this rule describes the rotation of ureters draining moieties of a duplicated system, whereby the upper part of the kidney drains medial and caudal to the lower pole one while the lower moiety drains more superiorly and lateral. Due to the more distal insertion of the upper pole ureter, this moiety is more commonly affected.

The location where the ureter ends has important *functional* implications. The more remote from the normal (expected) location, the greater the degree of renal dysplasia and the lower the likelihood of important functional parenchyma

A.J. Lorenzo, M.D., M.Sc., F.R.C.S.C., F.A.A.P., F.A.C.S.
Hospital for Sick Children, University of Toronto, Toronto, ON, Canada
e-mail: armando.lorenzo@sickkids.ca

A.E. Khoury, M.D., F.A.A.P., F.A.C.S. (✉)
Department of Urology, School of Medicine, University of California Irvine, Irvine, CA, USA
e-mail: aekhoury@uci.edu

R. Rabinowitz et al. (eds.), *Pediatric Urology for the Primary Care Physician*, Current Clinical Urology, DOI 10.1007/978-1-60327-243-8_11, © Springer Science+Business Media New York 2015 

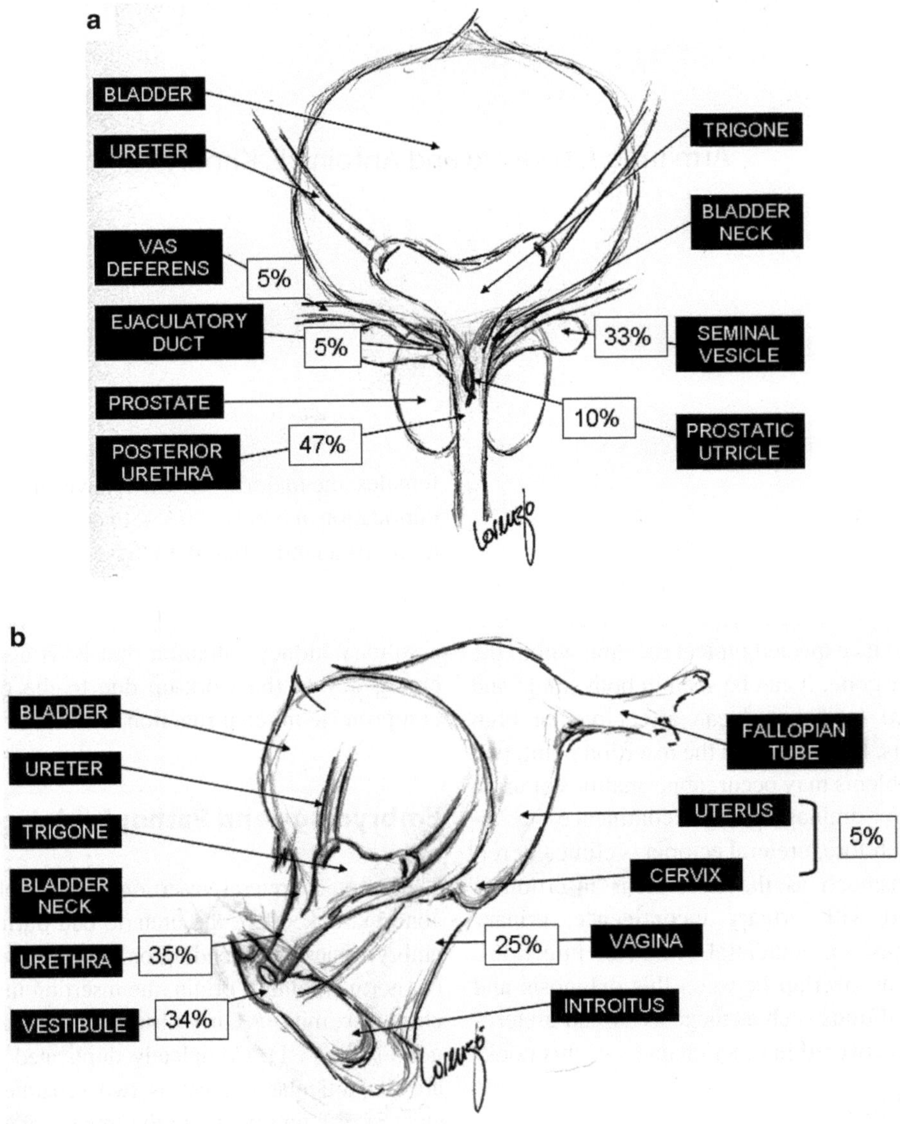


**Fig. 11.1** Location of ectopic ureteral opening in males (**a**) and females (**b**). Hydroureteronephrosis (panel (**a**)) and presence of a stone (panel (**b**), *white arrow*). Patient underwent ureteral reimplantation and stone removal soon after diagnosis

associated with such ureter. For practical purposes, this translates into congenital absence of normal parenchyma of the affected renal unit—or moiety, in a duplicated system—with little loss of overall renal function following resection. Furthermore, the location also has repercussions in regard to urinary continence. Importantly, this varies by patient gender (Fig. 11.1). In females, the ureter can drain in locations past the continence mechanism, situation that is not seen in males. Thus, continuous urinary leakage due to ureteral ectopia is clinically limited to female patients.

## Clinical Presentation

As is the case with several other pediatric genitourinary conditions, many otherwise asymptomatic children are detected by prenatal ultrasound or by abdominal ultrasonography carried out for an unrelated problem. Furthermore, children with

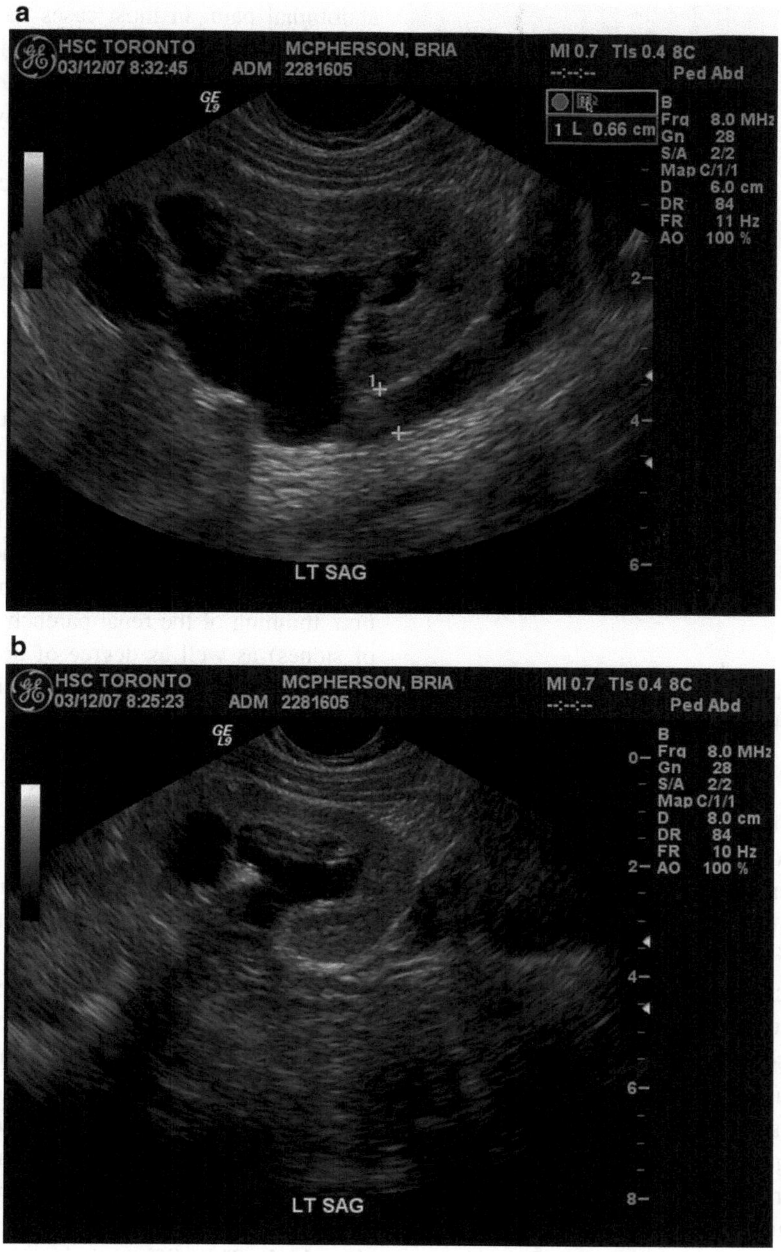


**Fig. 11.2** Solitary kidney with ectopic ureter and nephrolithiasis. Note hydroureteronephrosis (panel (**a**)) and presence of a stone (panel (**b**), *white arrow*). Patient underwent ureteral reimplantation and stone removal soon after diagnosis

other anomalies—such as imperforate anus and Mullerian abnormalities—are commonly found to have associated lower urinary tract problems. Considering the possibility of ureteral ectopia in the differential diagnosis of these patients helps accurately direct the initial management and prompt referral.

Children who escape incidental or prenatal diagnosis present with either clinical manifestations of obstruction (with or without infection) or urinary incontinence. The former may manifest itself as flank pain and recurrent pyelonephritis or lead to urinary stasis and stone formation (Fig. 11.2). Occasionally, symptoms are related

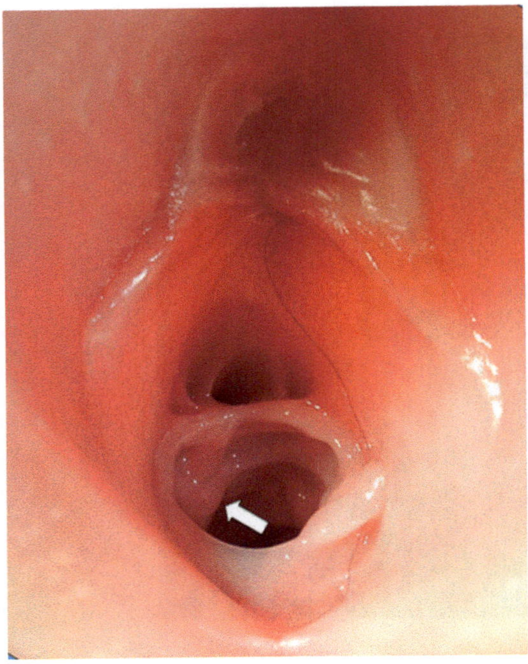

**Fig. 11.3** Physical exam of girl with continuous urinary incontinence. Ectopic ureteral orifice shown in figure (*white arrow*)

to drainage into structures derived from the mesonephric duct (such as vas deferens, seminal vesicles). Some of these boys manifest inflammatory changes of the scrotum due to bacterial or chemical irritation of the epididymis. A high level of suspicion is needed to correctly make this diagnosis. Therefore, children who present with recurrent episodes of epididymo-orchitis should undergo evaluation of the upper urinary tracts.

Continuous incontinence in a girl past the toilet training age should also raise concerns for an ectopic ureter. Not uncommonly these patients undergo evaluation by multiple healthcare providers prior to such consideration. Incontinence aside, recurrent episodes of vulvovaginitis and vaginal discharge are also commonly elicited on history. By exercising patience during physical exam, urine drainage in the area of the introitus may be detected, with the consequent pooling of urine in the vagina (Figs. 11.3 and 11.4).

Other rare presentations that should be kept in mind include a palpable abdominal mass secondary to upper tract dilation, hypertension due to renal scarring or dysplasia, and ill-defined abdominal pain. In most cases the diagnosis is not initially entertained, as ectopic ureters are relatively uncommon. However, keeping in mind that the source of the symptoms may be related to a congenital abnormality of the genitourinary tract will eventually lead to a correct diagnosis in most clinical scenarios.

## Initial Imaging Studies

Initial evaluation should include a renal/bladder ultrasound (RBUS), with subsequent selective voiding cystourethrogram (VCUG) for children in which the level of suspicion is heightened by the results of the ultrasound. The RBUS provides important information regarding the upper tracts (presence of hydronephrosis, evidence of duplication, thinning of the renal parenchyma, presence of stones) as well as degree of ureteral dilation and the relationship between ureter and bladder. The ease with ultrasonographic detection is related to the presence of obstruction, as the secondary hydroureteronephrosis is readily seen on RBUS. In the absence of dilation of the affected ureter, the ultrasound may appear normal or fail to show abnormalities of the affected renal unit.

Diagnosis is rarely confirmed by ultrasound alone, as other conditions may mimic the imaging findings, most notably primary megaureters and ureteroceles. An important distinction must be made between an ectopic ureter and ureterocele: The similarity in ultrasonographic presentations has led some to coin the term *pseudoureterocele* for dilated ectopic ureters that impinge on an otherwise normal bladder wall, thus creating a sonographic image similar to that of a ureterocele (Fig. 11.5). This differentiation is relevant when treatment is planned, as endoscopic puncture would be reasonable for some ureteroceles but ill advised in an ectopic ureter. Importantly, the sonographic appearance of an ectopic ureter and an obstructed or refluxing megaureter may be identical.

A VCUG is helpful in ruling out other pathologies (i.e., refluxing megaureter), detecting associated vesicoureteral reflux to other moieties, and – in some circumstances—showing

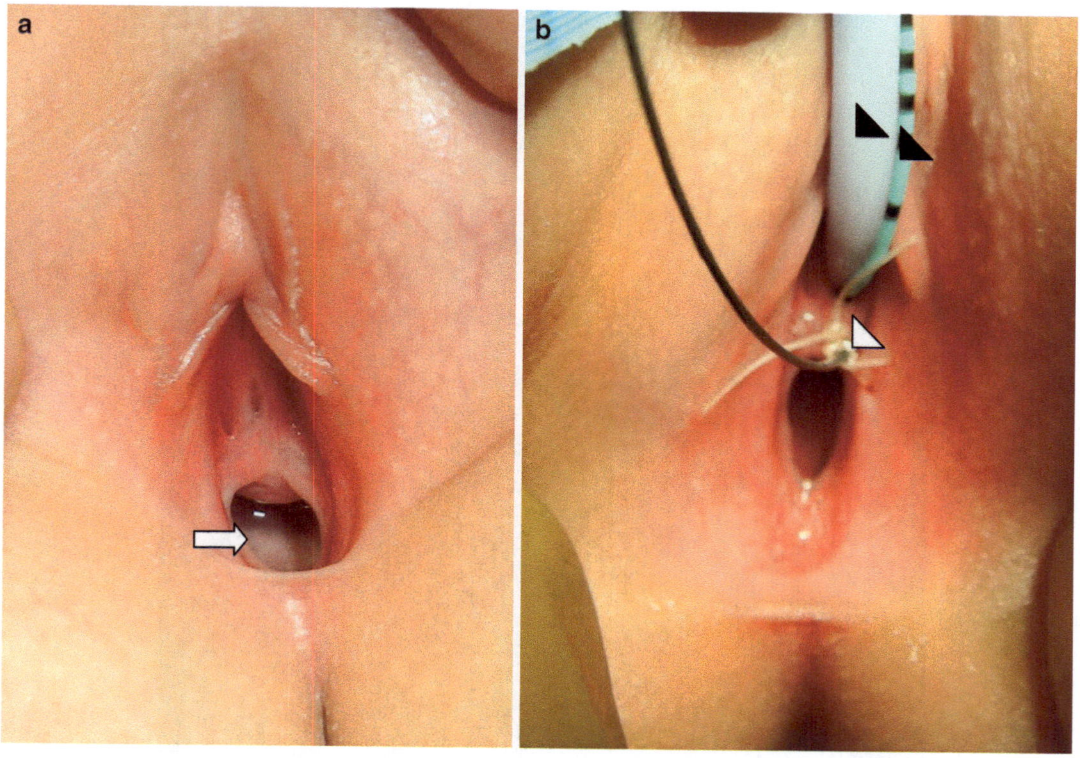


**Fig. 11.4** Exam under anesthesia of a girl with continuous urinary incontinence. The ectopic ureteral orifice could not be appreciated on physical exam in the office. Note pooling of urine in vagina (*white arrow*) and location of ectopic ureteral orifice (guide wire shown with *white arrowhead*). Note catheters going into bladder and normal ureter (*black arrowheads*) through the normal urethral meatus

the exact location of the ectopic ureteral orifice (Fig. 11.6). As catheterization and contrast injection are important for fluoroscopic visualization, ectopic ureters that are detected by VCUG generally enter the bladder neck or urethra. This study may also be of value in cases where the affected renal moiety has been removed and a residual stump predisposes the patient to recurrent infections. Due to the lack of anatomical detail, nuclear cystograms provide limited information and should not be employed during initial evaluation but reserved for the follow—up of vesicoureteral reflux.

## Treatment

Most patients with ectopic ureters that are referred to a pediatric urologist fall into three groups: a child who has urinary incontinence refractory to medications and/or behavioral treatment, a megaureter that fails to improve on serial evaluations, or hydroureteronephrosis discovered in a patient during the work-up of a febrile urinary tract infection or by antenatal ultrasound. During initial evaluation and while awaiting consultation, it is prudent to consider antibiotic prophylaxis and to aggressively evaluate any febrile illness to rule out an infectious process in a potentially obstructed system. Important considerations in the history, physical exam, and diagnostic work-up of these patients are presented in Table 11.1.

Indications for surgery include recurrent urinary tract infections, presence of symptoms (pain, urinary incontinence), nephrolithiasis, worsening degree of dilation, and loss of renal function. Many patients are followed over time with serial studies, particularly when asymptomatic. Some are managed conservatively based on the initial

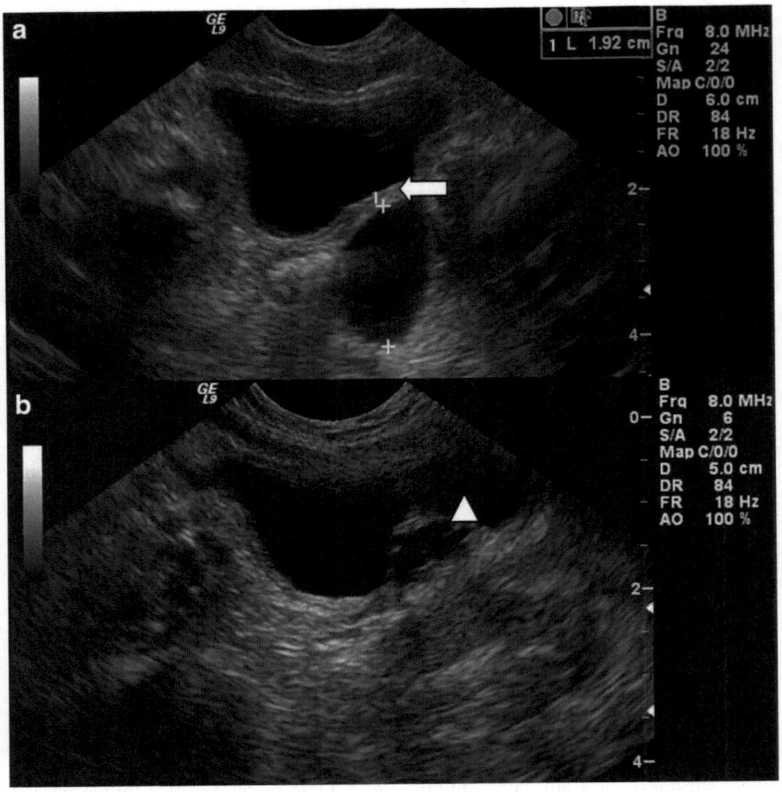


**Fig. 11.5** Ultrasound evaluation of the bladder showing a dilated ectopic ureter ("pseudoureterocele," panel (**a**)) and a "true" ureterocele (panel (**b**)). Note that the ectopic ureter is clearly extravesical, seen behind the bladder on its course to an abnormal insertion, with a thick septum of bladder wall between the ureteral and bladder lumens (*white arrow*). In contrast, the ureterocele is intravesical and has a thin wall inside the bladder lumen (*white arrowhead*)

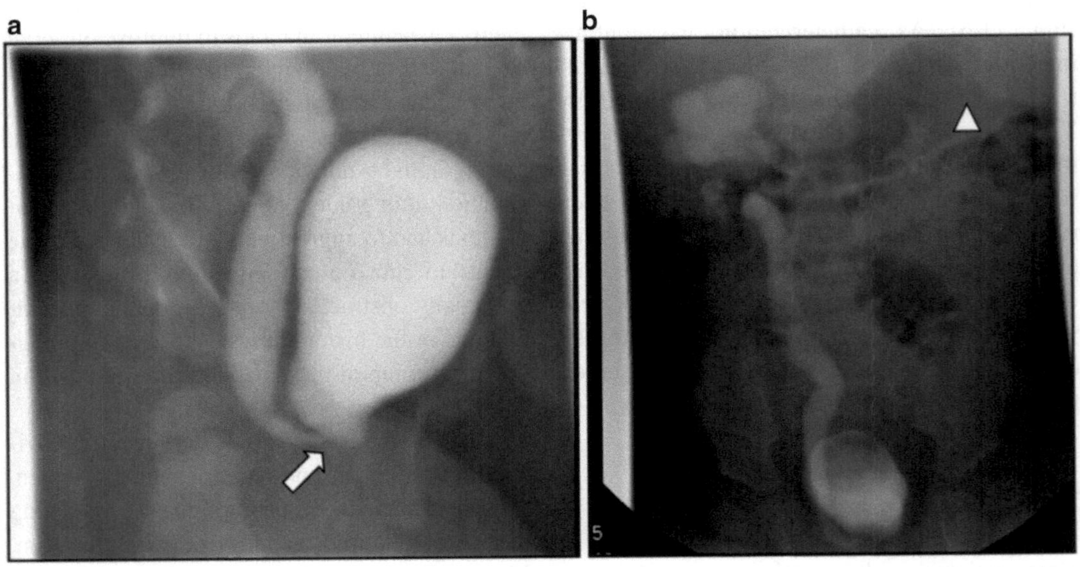


**Fig. 11.6** Voiding cystourethrogram in a girl with recurrent urinary tract infections. Note reflux detected into dilated system draining at the level of the bladder neck (*white arrow*, panel (**a**)) and the presence of contralateral vesicoureteral reflux (*white arrowhead*, panel (**b**))

**Table 11.1** Summary of important diagnostic points in ectopic ureters

| Ectopic ureter |
|---|
| *History* |
| Recurrent urinary tract infections |
| Continuous urinary incontinence |
| Recurrent episodes of epididymitis |
| Abdominal pain, nausea, vomiting |
| Hematuria |
| *Physical exam* |
| High blood pressure (rare) |
| Palpable abdominal mass (rare) |
| External genitalia with inflammatory changes |
| Epididymo-orchitis (scrotum and testicles) |
| Vulvovaginitis |
| Vaginal pooling with urine |
| Visualization of ectopic ureteral orifice |
| *Imaging studies* |
| Renal and bladder ultrasound |
| Voiding cystourethrogram |
| Renal scan (DMSA) |
| Magnetic resonance imaging (selected cases) |
| Retrograde pyelogram (selected cases) |
| Intravenous pyelogram (selected cases) |
| *Differential diagnosis* |
| Primary megaureter |
| Ureterocele |
| Vesicoureteral reflux |

evaluation thought to represent a primary megaureter. This condition tends to improve over time in many cases, therefore the diagnosis is not called into question until there is lack of improvement or the child develops symptoms. Since up to 15 % of orthotopic megaureters also fail to improve, the definitive diagnosis may not be firmly established until endoscopic evaluation is carried out, usually prior to surgical reconstruction.

Preoperative evaluation should include a functional assessment of the kidneys. This is achieved with renal nuclear scintigraphy (most commonly a 99mTc DMSA scan). The purpose is twofold: determine the differential function of the parenchyma associated with the ectopic ureter, and evaluate for abnormal renal locations (Fig. 11.7). In some circumstances the parenchyma may be so small and dysplastic that imaging studies (such as ultrasound and nuclear renal scan) may fail to identify it. Those selected children may then benefit from either exam under anesthesia with contrast injection in the ectopic orifice (retrograde pyelogram, Fig. 11.8) or more detailed evaluation with magnetic resonance imaging (MRI) of the abdomen and pelvis. The former study is usually performed at the time of planned surgical correction. The latter evaluation—although of exquisite anatomical detail and free of ionizing radiation—involves sedation or even general anesthesia depending on the age of the child; therefore, it is only used in cases where the diagnosis is in doubt and the findings are expected to change management.

Surgical management is tailored to the clinical presentation, the presence of an associated duplication anomaly, and the amount of renal function present in the affected moiety. Rarely, children who present with sepsis and fail to respond to antibiotics may benefit from temporary drainage, either percutaneously (percutaneous nephrostomy tube placement) or by creation of a urinary tract stoma (cutaneous ureterostomy). In selected cases where the obstructed ectopic ureter enters close to the bladder neck, balloon dilation may be attempted as a temporizing maneuver, although experience with this approach is limited. Definitive correction is achieved by either removal of the renal moiety associated with the ectopic ureter (if poorly or nonfunctioning) or by anastomosis to the bladder or ipsilateral ureter/renal pelvis (in duplicated systems). These options are summarized in Fig. 11.9. Either a laparoscopic [3] or open surgical approach may be employed depending on the age of the patient and the surgeon's experience with either technique. When a nephrectomy or heminephrectomy is performed, the child may later present with problems related to a residual ureteral stump, such as pain and recurrent infections (Fig. 11.10). Such patients should be considered candidates for surgical removal of the residual ureteral segment [4].

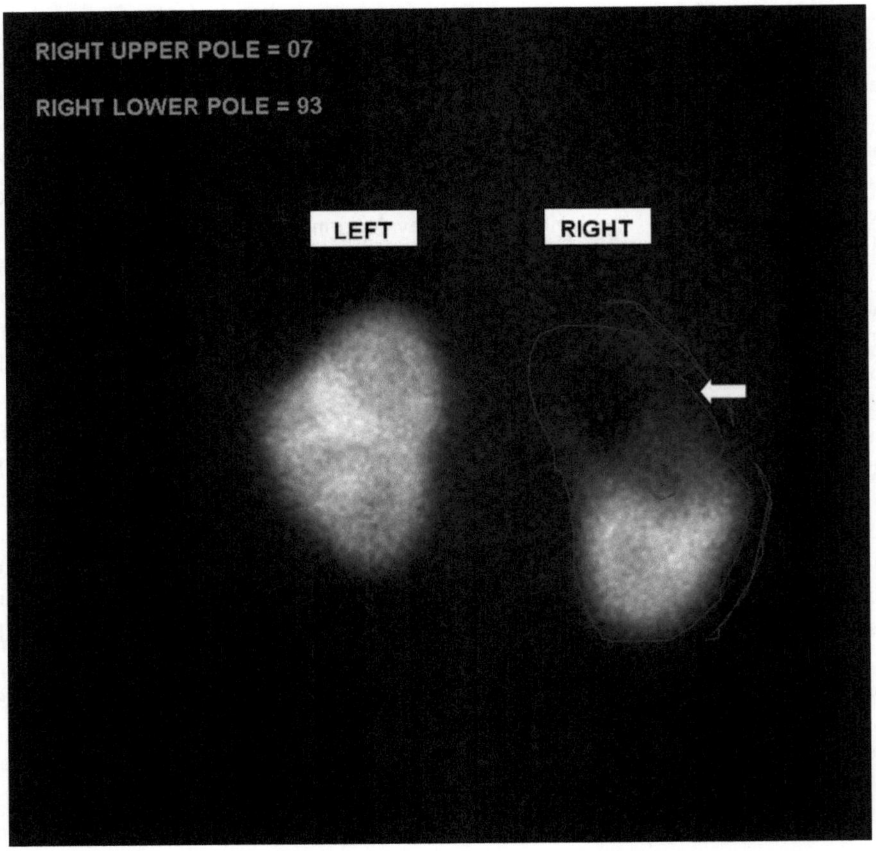


**Fig. 11.7** 99mTc-DMSA renal scan in patient with antenatal diagnosis of right hydronephrosis (*posterior view*). Postnatal evaluation demonstrated a right duplicated system with upper pole dilation and associated ureteronephrosis. Study demonstrates a poorly functioning upper pole (*white arrow*)

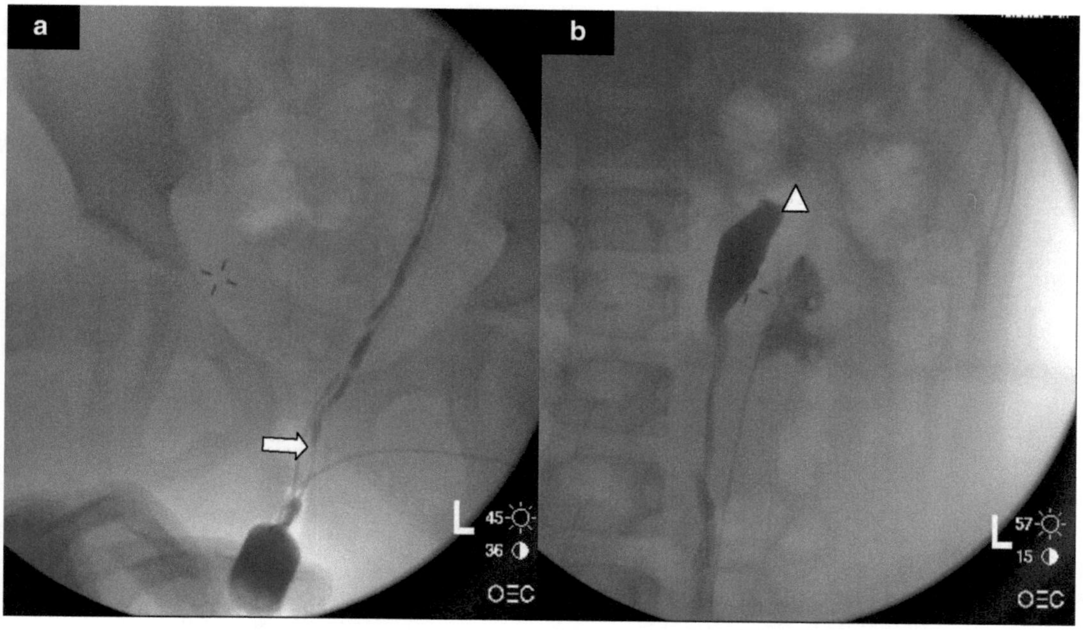


**Fig. 11.8** Retrograde pyelogram performed at time of upper pole heminephrectomy in patient with continuous urinary incontinence. DMSA renal scan (*not shown*) demonstrated lack of functional parenchyma. Panel A shows contrast injection in ectopic ureter (*white arrow*), with a guide wire in the lower pole ureter. Panel B shows the retrograde pyelogram for both moieties. Note the abnormal appearance of the upper pole moiety associated with the ectopic ureter. Urinary incontinence resolved after surgery

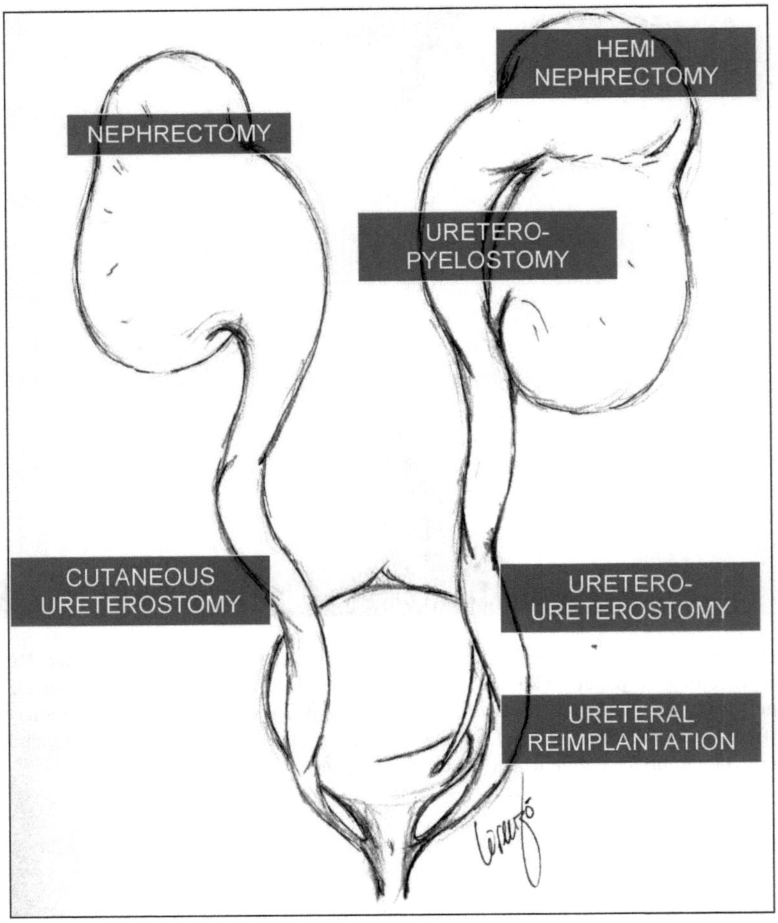


**Fig. 11.9** Surgical options for the management of ectopic ureters. Note *left side* corresponds to a single system and *right side* a duplicated one. Nephrectomy and heminephrectomy are reserved for situations with poorly functioning or nonfunctioning parenchyma. Cutaneous ureterostomy is a temporizing measure for patients with massively dilated or infected systems. Ureteropyelostomy, ureteroureterostomy, and ureteral reimplantation aim to direct unimpeded urine flow by anastomosis of the ectopic ureter to the normal renal pelvis, ureter, or bladder

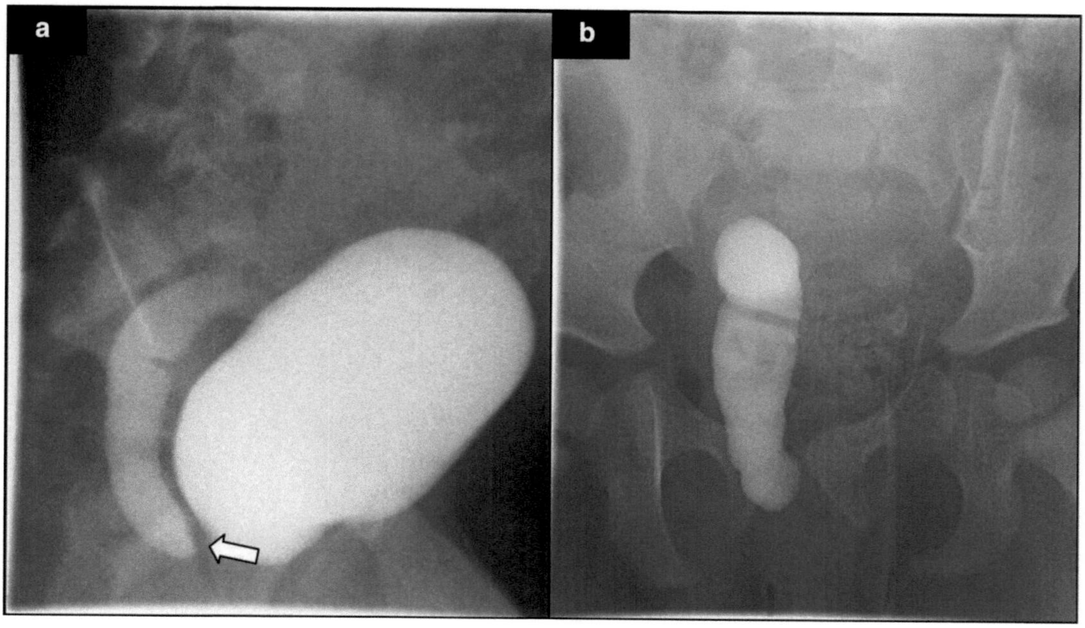


**Fig. 11.10** Voiding cystourethrogram in patient who had a previous laparoscopic heminephrectomy for an ectopic upper pole ureter and presented with recurrent urinary tract infections after surgery. Note ectopic ureter at the level of the bladder neck (panel (**a**), *white arrow*) and residual contrast in the ureteral stump after voiding (panel (**b**))

## References

1. Ahmed S, Barker A. Single-system ectopic ureters: a review of 12 cases. J Pediatr Surg. 1992;27(4):491–6.
2. Ahmed S, Morris LL, Byard RW. Ectopic ureter with complete ureteric duplication in the female child. J Pediatr Surg. 1992;27(11):1455–60.
3. Wang DS, Bird VG, Cooper CS, et al. Laparoscopic upper-pole heminephrectomy for ectopic ureter: surgical technique. J Endourol. 2003;17(7):469–73.
4. Plaire JC, Pope JC, Kropp BP, et al. Management of ectopic ureters: experience with the upper tract approach. J Urol. 1997;158(3 Pt 2):1245–7.

# Cystitis

# 12

Ilene Yi-Zhen Wong and Linda Dairiki Shortliffe

## Introduction

Cystitis, defined as inflammation of the bladder, is a common cause of pediatric office visits, second only to respiratory infection. Typically patients have a constellation of irritative voiding symptoms that include dysuria, frequency, incontinence, and urgency. Though the most frequent pathology leading to such symptoms is a bacterial infection of the bladder, one of the keys to understanding cystitis in children is an appreciation of the wide range of both infectious and noninfectious etiologies that can cause similar symptoms. These include viral cystitis, fungal infections, eosinophilic cystitis, interstitial cystitis, vulvovaginitis, and the extraordinary frequency syndrome.

## Epidemiology

Identification of an infectious cause of cystitis is paramount because of the potential complications of an untreated urinary tract infection (UTI), including progression to pyelonephritis and potential renal injury. Though it is difficult to determine the true incidence of UTI in the pediatric population, it is estimated that the cumulative childhood risk for UTIs is 2 % for boys and 8 % for girls, with greater than one million annual physician office visits [1]. The first 3 months of life are the only time in childhood when boys are at greater risk for UTIs than girls (1–4 % versus 0.5 %); data show that uncircumcised boys have a 12-fold increased risk for UTI compared to those who have been circumcised.

Children with an initial UTI are also at risk for recurrent UTI. Studies have shown recurrence rates in boys to be 18 % if first infection is discovered prior to age one and 32 % after the age of one. Recurrence rates for girls are even higher, being 26 % and 40 % respectively [2]. While these numbers refer primarily to symptomatic UTI, there are others who may have asymptomatic bacteriuria found on routine screening.

## History

In addition to localizing symptoms including dysuria, frequency, and urgency, cystitis may present with suprapubic tenderness or hematuria. A history of cloudy urine may be a pertinent positive, though foul-smelling urine has been shown to be an unreliable predictor of cystitis. In infants, nonspecific findings such as irritabil-

I.Y.-Z. Wong, M.D.
Academic Urology, 211 South Gulph Road, Suite 200, King of Prussia, PA 19406, USA

L.D. Shortliffe, M.D. (✉)
Pediatric Urology, Department of Urology, Stanford University Medical Center, 750 Welch Road, Suite 218, Stanford, CA 94305-5725, USA
e-mail: lindashortliffe@stanford.edu

R. Rabinowitz et al. (eds.), *Pediatric Urology for the Primary Care Physician*, Current Clinical Urology, DOI 10.1007/978-1-60327-243-8_12, © Springer Science+Business Media New York 2015

ity, poor feeding, and lethargy may be presenting factors.

Presence of fever, flank pain, and/or nausea/vomiting may be indications that the infection involves the upper urinary tracts, though a significant number (30–50 %) of febrile UTIs may be confined to the lower urinary tract if actually localized.

A standard medical history will identify immunocompromised patients (HIV positive, status post transplant, or chemotherapy) who may be at particular risk for viral or fungal cystitis. History of recent systemic viral illness (including varicella) in patients with competent immune systems may also point to a viral etiology for cystitis. Recent chemotherapy with cyclophosphamide can also cause hemorrhagic cystitis.

Sudden onset of urinary incontinence or bedwetting may be signs of cystitis. In general, a thorough history of the patient's elimination patterns (including constipation and the tendency to hold urine) should be elicited. A description of the patient's voiding pattern—namely, whether it is a smooth stream or is "staccato" with frequent stops and starts—may also help identify abnormal voiding patterns. Presence of an upward deflected stream suggests meatal stenosis.

It is important to obtain family history of vesicoureteral reflux (VUR) due to familial occurrence. If a first UTI occurs in an adolescent girl, one might be suspicious of sexual activity.

## Physical Exam

The physical exam of a child presenting with signs of cystitis should include a standard exam, with additional focus on abdominal and genital exams. Suprapubic tenderness, severe constipation, bladder distension, and renal or pelvic masses can all be detected on abdominal exam. Costovertebral angle tenderness should be assessed, though it is often absent in children with pyelonephritis.

Examination of the genitalia and perineum of girls can identify foreign bodies or general erythema consistent with vulvovaginitis, as well as labial adhesions. Placing the patient in a frog-legged position, gently grasping the labia majora, and spreading laterally and inferiorly to visualize the introitus best facilitates this exam. Careful examination of this area can also reveal signs of trauma consistent with sexual abuse, which can present with dysfunctional voiding and pain consistent with cystitis. Less commonly, a vaginal mass may represent a prolapsed ureterocele causing bladder outlet obstruction and predisposing to UTI.

The male genitalia should be examined for balanitis or severe phimosis, although practitioners should be aware that phimosis with adhesions are typically present in most infants. Meatal stenosis, often characterized by a pinpoint meatal opening lacking a slit-like appearance, may cause dysuria. Presence of a penile discharge suggests a urethritis. In a teenage boy, rectal prostatic palpation may be required to eliminate consideration of prostatitis.

Finally, in patients presenting with urinary complaints, the lower back should be examined for sacral dimples, sacral hairy patches, hemangiomas, or unusual creases that might suggest spinal dysraphism and possible neurogenic bladder. Such atypical dimples (those that are off center, deeper than 0.5 cm or more than 2.5 cm from the anal verge), subcutaneous lipomas, and dermal sinuses should be examined with either spinal ultrasonography (in infants younger than 3 months) or magnetic resonance imaging (MRI) looking for spina bifida or tethered cord.

## How to Evaluate

### Urine Collection

The initial evaluation for any child presenting with symptoms of cystitis is urine collection for urinalysis and culture and sensitivity. However, accurate sample acquisition is a challenge, particularly in infants and children who are not toilet trained.

#### Bagged Specimen Collection and Voided Urine Specimens

Placing a plastic bag over the perineum and waiting for the patient to void, or "bagged urine," is an attractive noninvasive method of urine collection for parents and clinicians. However, it is known that more than 60 % of such specimens will be contaminated with perineal flora. A bagged specimen may be of clinical utility if it shows a completely negative urinalysis/culture and eliminates suspicion of a UTI; false positives, though, may lead to delayed diagnosis and unnecessary tests and admissions [3].

In girls and in uncircumcised males, voided urine specimens have similar pitfalls to bagged specimens, namely, high contamination rates from periurethral and preputial flora.

### Catheterized Urine Specimens

Catheterized urine specimens via a sterile technique, while invasive, yield a significantly lower rate of contamination than bagged specimens (9 % versus 63 %). The initial portion of collected urine that may be contaminated by periurethral flora should be discarded to minimize contamination rates. Parents should be warned prior to urethral catheterization that there is a small risk of introducing periurethral bacteria into the bladder, causing de novo UTI. For this reason, antibiotic prophylaxis after catheterization may be prudent.

### Suprapubic Aspiration

Suprapubic aspiration is the "cleanest" method of urine collection and can be performed safely and with minimal patient discomfort with topical and injected local anesthesia. Using a 21 or 22 gauge needle, the bladder is identified 1–2 cm above the pubic symphysis and urine is aspirated. Occasionally (in approximately 20 % of attempts) the presence of an empty bladder can prevent obtaining an adequate sample of urine. If there is concern over localization of the bladder and/or bladder fullness, bedside ultrasonography can quickly assess the status and location of the bladder.

## Urinalysis

Overall, urinalysis has 82 % sensitivity for the detection of a UTI. Urine dipstick has become a standard initial step in the evaluation of UTI and has the advantage of being a cost-effective, rapid test. Traditional microscopic urinalysis offers both the quantification of white blood cells (WBC) and the ability to visualize bacteria, which may or may not be significant depending on the type of specimen obtained. The presence of the "triumvirate" of positive leukocyte esterase, positive nitrate, and positive identification of bacteria on microscopy approaches 100 % sensitivity for the detection of UTI. Similarly, when all three tests were negative, there is a close to 100 % negative predictive value [3].

The presence of pyuria (defined as >5 WBC per high-powered field in a centrifuged specimen) is a pertinent positive even in the absence of bacteria on microscopic exam, as it may represent viral or eosinophilic pathology. All this being true, the gold standard for detection of true UTI remains urine culture, which documents the precise organism involved and supplies vital information regarding antibiotic susceptibility patterns.

## Urine Culture

As noted above, diagnosis of a UTI cannot definitively be made without a positive urine culture. However, false positive cultures due to contamination occur frequently, depending on collection method. As outlined in Table 12.1, the number of colony forming units (cfu) of bacteria to diagnose a UTI depends largely on the type of specimen obtained. In 2011 the AAP recommended the presence of at least 50,000 colony-forming units (CFU) per mL of a uropathogen and urinalysis suggesting infection for establishing diagnosis [6].

Rarely, viral cultures are indicated for immunocompromised patients to differentiate between chemotherapy and radiation-induced cystitis and that caused by BK, cytomegalovirus, herpes simplex, or adenovirus.

## Laboratory Tests

The management of febrile infants and young children may benefit from the acquisition of a C-reactive protein (CRP) or complete blood count with differential. Children with CRP greater than 7 mg/dL and absolute neutrophil count greater than $10.6 \times 10^9$ are more likely to have a serious infection (i.e. pyelonephritis) requiring inpatient admission.

**Table 12.1** Criteria for the diagnosis of urinary tract infection

| Method of collection | Colony count (pure culture) | Probability of infection (%) |
|---|---|---|
| Suprapubic aspiration | Gram-negative bacilli: any number | >99 % |
| | Gram-positive cocci: more than a few thousand | |
| Transurethral catheterization | $>10^6$ | 95 % |
| | $10^4$–$10^6$ | Infection likely |
| | $10^3$–$10^4$ | Suspicious, repeat |
| | $<10^3$ | Infection unlikely |
| Clean void | | |
| Boy | $>10^4$ | Infection likely |
| Girl | 3 Specimens $\geq 10^6$ | 95 % |
| | 2 Specimens $\geq 10^6$ | 90 % |
| | 1 Specimen $\geq 10^6$ | 80 % |
| | $5 \times 10^4$–$10^6$ | Suspicious, repeat |
| | $10^4$–$5 \times 10^4$ | Symptomatic: suspicious, repeat |
| | | Asymptomatic: infection unlikely |
| | $<10^4$ | Infection unlikely |



## Imaging Studies

Imaging studies are rarely required for the acute management of cystitis. Exceptions to this generalization are instances in which the source of infection is unclear or the child has not responded to standard treatment. Imaging may also be beneficial when unusual infecting organisms (including fungi, *Mycobacterium*, or *Proteus*) are isolated or in children with a history of specific pathology of the urinary system including neurogenic bladder, papillary necrosis, or renal failure. In such cases, renal and bladder ultrasonography may be obtained to identify obstruction (characterized by hydronephrosis) or presence of a ureterocele, renal abscess, fungal ball, or urinary calculi. If uncertainty exists as to whether the infection has extended to the upper tracts, dimercaptosuccinic acid renal scans (DMSA) is a sensitive method for confirming acute pyelonephritis through the identification of focal changes in blood flow in acute infection [4], but computed tomography (CT) or MRI will show signs of upper tract inflammation and greater anatomic detail.

The goal of imaging in the majority of patients with cystitis is to rule out genitourinary abnormalities, which are more common in children with a documented UTI. Epidemiologic surveys show that 21–57 % of children who have bacteriuria have VUR upon evaluation, whereas an additional 5–10 % of children will have an obstructive lesion [3].

American Academy of Pediatrics (AAP) guidelines from 2011 recommend follow-up renal and bladder ultrasonography without routine voiding cystourethrograms (VCUG) for children between the age of 2 months and 2 years who have an initial documented febrile UTI. When the ultrasound reveals normal kidneys and bladder, the management benefit from VCUG findings are debatable [6, 8]. Notably, VCUG should be performed after a second infection or if initial ultrasound shows hydronephrosis, scarring or other a typical findings [6].

Children who present with gross hematuria should routinely undergo renal-bladder ultrasound to evaluate for retained bladder clots and assess for neoplasm.

## How to Manage

The acute management of cystitis typically hinges upon the results of urinalysis and urine culture. While waiting for urine culture results, it is appropriate to empirically treat children with moderate to severe symptoms who have confirmed pyuria and bacteriuria.

## Pyuria with Positive Urine Culture

### Bacterial Infections

Optimally, cystitis is treated with antibiotics that concentrate well within the urine. Clinicians should be aware of the local antibiotic resistance patterns of microorganisms. Though resistance rates for ampicillin, trimethoprim and cephalexin can range from 20 to 50 %, nitrofurantoin resistance is less frequent. Due to decreased tissue penetration, however, nitrofurantoin should not be used when pyelonephritis or urosepsis is suspected.

Duration of treatment has been under debate; while current AAP recommendations suggest 7 days of oral antibiotics for the treatment of uncomplicated cystitis, some data show that courses of 3–5 days are effective in the treatment of patients without urinary tract abnormalities. Current recommendations are to treat patients with febrile UTIs with culture-specific antibiotics for 7–10 days [3].

### Fungal Infections

Typically found in immunocompromised, recently hospitalized, or catheterized patients, fungal infections of the bladder can be a challenge due to frequent colonization and contamination. Generally, if pyuria is present and colony counts are greater than $10^4$ cfu/mL in a catheterized specimen, true infection is accepted. Due to the high incidence of renal pathology (renal fungus balls or fungal abscesses) in neonates with funguria, renal and bladder ultrasonography is recommended in premature infants.

Isolated funguria is typically treated with oral fluconazole (when sensitive) or, in the case of hospitalized and catheterized patients, with bladder irrigation with 5–15 mg amphotericin B for 60 min QID until negative cultures.

## Pyuria with Negative Urine Culture

### Viral Infection

Viral bladder infections are usually hemorrhagic in nature, leading one to suspect them in patients with pyuria, negative urine cultures, and hematuria. In immunocompetent children, viral cystitis is typically caused by adenovirus and is self-limiting. Supportive care with hydration leads to resolution in 2–3 weeks.

Immunocompromised patients are particularly susceptible to viral cystitis, with the BK polyomavirus, adenovirus 7, 11, 21, and 35, and herpes simplex viruses being the most commonly implicated strains. While recent literature has suggested that ribavirin may limit the course of adenoviral infections, treatment of such patients usually involves aggressive hydration (with or without diuresis) and management of the complications of ureteral and bladder clots as per below [3].

### Hemorrhagic Cystitis

Hemorrhagic cystitis may be bacterial or viral in etiology, as noted above, or may be secondary to chemotherapy (cyclophosphamide) or radiation therapy. Mild hemorrhagic cystitis can often be managed with continuous bladder irrigation, reversal of coagulopathies, and platelet replacement. If hematuria persists, prostaglandin E, formalin, or alum sclerotherapy may be administered, with operative intervention occasionally necessary in severe cases.

### Eosinophilic Cystitis

A poorly understood and rare inflammatory disorder, eosinophilic cystitis should be suspected in a child who presents with irritative voiding symptoms with pyuria, negative culture, and eosinophils in the urine. Diagnosis is confirmed by bladder biopsy, which reveals eosinophilic infiltration. The disease is more common in patients with a history of allergies and is thought to be caused by a reaction to antigenic stimuli. Evaluation consists of bladder ultrasound, which will typically identify bladder wall thickening, and the goal of management is removal of antigenic stimulus if found. Regardless of drug treatment, eosinophilic cystitis is self-limited and typically resolves in 7–12 weeks.

### Fastidious Organisms and Unusual Organisms

If cultures are negative despite pyuria and positive gram stain of bacteria, the presence of fastidious organisms (*Haemophilus*) should be suspected. Urine should be re-cultured with non-routine culture medium.

In addition, numerous other unusual organisms can affect the urinary tract, including schistosomiasis (detectable by the presence of eggs in the urine) and tuberculosis (diagnosed by culture for acid-fast bacteria). Clinical suspicion for these unusual disease processes may be engendered by a history of recent travel to endemic areas or the presence of systemic tuberculosis. If symptoms persist after appropriate medical treatment of these rare diseases, a specialist should evaluate patients.

## No Pyuria, Negative Urine Culture

Children who present with frequency and urgency in the face of negative urine culture and with a lack of pyuria pose a unique challenge. Physical exam is a key to rule out reversible etiologies including labial adhesions and meatal stenosis (diagnosed by observation of a deflected urinary stream). It is thought that hypercalciuria with urine calcium-to-creatinine ratio higher than 0.17/mg/dL may also cause urgency and frequency. Rarely, frequency and urgency symptoms can occur secondary to a prostatic, urethral, or bladder rhabdomyosarcoma, which typically presents with associated hematuria or bloody urethral discharge.

## Voiding Dysfunction

An often-abused term, voiding dysfunction is defined as a non-neurogenic incomplete relaxation or overactivity of the pelvic floor muscles during urination. It is characterized by interrupted voiding, incomplete bladder emptying, and the tendency to hold urine. It may be diagnosed via a combination of voiding diary and uroflowmetry or by more invasive urodynamics. Frequently it is associated with constipation, fecal impaction, and encopresis, forming a broadly defined "dysfunctional elimination syndrome." Treatment of dysfunctional voiding involves strict timed voiding, biofeedback, and a strict bowel regimen when indicated.

## Extraordinary Frequency Syndrome

Essentially a diagnosis of exclusion, extraordinary frequency syndrome has been described as a syndrome of excessive day and nighttime urinary frequency not attributable to other sources. It has been attributed to delayed maturation of the bladder and poor voiding habits. Unfortunately, it rarely responds to anticholinergics or fluid restriction but is a benign and self-limiting condition with a typical duration of 8 months in boys and 14 months in girls [7].

### Interstitial Cystitis

Characterized by urgency, frequency, and suprapubic pain relieved by bladder emptying, interstitial cystitis is a poorly understood disease that is ultimately diagnosed through cystoscopy, which reveals classic petechiae-like spots in the bladder known as "glomerulations." Fortunately this disease is rare in children and is primarily diagnosed in adult women. In children, conservative management with anticholinergics, antihistamines, and diet modification is typically recommended.

### Neurogenic Bladder

On rare occasions, patients with new spinal cord lesions leading to neurogenic bladder may present with urgency, frequency, and new onset incontinence. Post-void residual urine may be elevated, bladder may be palpable on physical exam, and a sacral dimple may be present. Workup includes a spinal ultrasound or MRI to rule out tethered cord or occult spina bifida. Patients in urinary retention may be catheterized or placed on clean intermittent catheterization until evaluation by a urologist.

## Management of Recurrent Cystitis

Approximately 20 % of patients with an initial bout of cystitis will recur, with the risk of recurrence increasing with each infection—a child with three previous infections has a 75 % risk of recurrence [2]. Recurrence can be classified into three categories based on etiology.

First, recurrence may be due to unresolved bacteriuria if the initial infection is inadequately treated due to bacterial resistance, poor adherence, subtherapeutic dosing, or poor renal concentration. This may be confirmed by follow-up culture and sensitivities, which are similar to the first infection and can be treated with culture-specific antibiotics at appropriate dosage levels.

Second, recurrence may be due to bacterial persistence due to an anatomic anomaly or infected foreign body. Diagnosis is typically made by careful history and imaging studies to evaluate for nephrolithiasis, urethral diverticulum, fistula, or other suspected anomalies.

Third, recurrence may occur due to reinfection after adequate treatment of the initial infection. Reinfection is the most common form of recurrent infection and often occurs in dysfunctional voiders and sexually active girls. As noted above, UTI may be a marker for sexual activity in adolescent girls [2, 8]. Sexually active girls may elect for post-intercourse antibiotic prophylaxis. Treatment of constipation and proper voiding hygiene may reduce risk of recurrence. Otherwise, high-risk patients may occasionally benefit from low-dose antibiotic prophylaxis (daily dosing at ¼ the full treatment dose of the antibiotic). The most common antibiotic agents used for prophylaxis due to their high urinary concentration are nitrofurantoin, trimethoprim-sulfamethoxazole, and cephalexin.

## When to Refer? What to Do with Abnormal Imaging Results?

The office pediatrician's challenge is to identify cystitis patients who are at risk of evolving into serious upper tract infections. Most uncomplicated febrile UTIs in children older than 1 month can be managed on an outpatient basis if the child is nontoxic, is able to tolerate orals, and has a reliable family. Referral to urology may be required based on either acute or follow-up imaging abnormalities, as well as recurrent symptoms or findings on physical exam.

### Acute Referral

As noted previously, acute imaging may be required for children with new onset azotemia, failure to respond to antibiotic therapy or clinical suspicion of a genitourinary abnormality. Such cases should be referred to a urologist, as there may be a need for acute surgical intervention depending on diagnosis. Identification of pyonephrosis or debris in the collecting system in patients with hydronephrosis or hydroureteronephrosis suggests an obstruction requiring intervention. Renal abscesses require surgical drainage if they do not respond to parenteral therapy within 48–72 h. Immunocompromised patients with hemorrhagic cystitis requiring blood transfusion may occasionally require operative clot evacuation and/or sclerotherapy.

### Urgent Referral

Expedited urology referral is indicated in patients with "complicated" UTIs, including those involving chronic catheterization, neurogenic bladder (due to spina bifida or cerebral palsy), or nephrolithiasis. If any signs of obstruction are associated with the UTI, acute urologic consultation should be sought.

### Elective Referral

Patients who are found on follow-up imaging to have VUR or hydronephrosis may have elective referral to urology after being placed on prophylactic antibiotics. Additionally, recurrent UTIs, extraordinary frequency syndrome, dysfunctional voiding, and interstitial cystitis can be managed by a referral to a urologist on an elective basis.

## References

1. Freedman AL. Urinary tract infection in children. In: Litwin MS, Saigal CS, editors. Urologic diseases in America. US Department of Health and Human Services, Public Health Service, National Institutes of

Health, National Institute of Diabetes and Digestive and Kidney Diseases. Washington, DC: US Government Printing Office; 2007; p. 441–57.
2. Marotte J, Lee K, Shortliffe L. Cystitis in infants and children. AUA Update Series, vol. 24, Lesson 19; 2005.
3. Shortliffe L. Infection and inflammation of the pediatric urinary tract. In: Wein A, editor. Campbell-Walsh urology. 9th ed. Philadelphia: Saunders; 2007. Chapter 112.
4. Rushton HG, Majd M. Dimercaptosuccinic acid renal scintigraphy for the evaluation of pyelonephritis and scarring: a review of experimental and clinical studies. J Urol. 1992;148:1726–32.
5. Hodson EM, et al. Interventions for primary vesicoureteral reflux. Cochrane Database Sys Rev. 2007;(3):CD001532.
6. American Academy of Pediatrics: Subcommittee on Urinary Tract Infection, Steering Committee on Quality Improvement and Management. Urinary Tract Infection: Clinical Practice Guideline for the diagnosis and management of the initial UTI in febrile infants and children 2 to 24 months. Pediatrics. 2011;128(3):595–610. doi:10.1542/peds.2011-1330.
7. Zoubek J, Bloom DA, Sedman AB. Extraordinary urinary frequency. Pediatrics. 1990;85:1112.
8. Weir M, Brien J. Adolescent urinary tract infections. Adoles Med. 2000;11:293–313.

# Vesicoureteral Reflux

# 13

Marco Castagnetti, Waifro Rigamonti, and Gianantonio Manzoni

## Introduction: What Is the Entity?

Vesicoureteral reflux (VUR) refers to a retrograde flow of urine from the bladder into the upper urinary tract. It can be uni- or bilateral and occur in single or duplex systems, usually affecting the lower moiety.

VUR is defined primary when it is due to an intrinsic defect of the vesicoureteral junction; instead, secondary when it is due to another cause such as bladder outlet obstruction, neurogenic bladder, or bladder dysfunction. Only primary VUR will be addressed in this chapter.

VUR is not a pathological condition per se but because of its possible consequences on renal function. Two kinds of renal damage can be associated with VUR, the congenital renal dysplasia and the pyelonephritic renal scar(s). Neither necessarily affects all the children found with VUR.

Renal dysplasia is congenital and seems increasingly to be associated with rather than be due to VUR. In some patients, VUR (usually high grade) and renal dysplasia would be two aspects of a maldevelopment involving all the urinary tract. Patients presenting with sever bilateral renal dysplasia will develop chronic renal failure early on in life. At present, no treatment can improve a dysplastic damage of the kidney.

Renal scars, instead, follow an infection of the kidney, namely, a pyelonephritis. In this case, VUR is considered to be a risk factor for the ascent of the bacteria and thereby the renal infection. As the risk of developing chronic renal failure and hypertension in the long run is proportional to the number of scars, administration of treatment in order to prevent the recurrence of renal infections is generally considered worthwhile. Nevertheless, the major issue is that not all the patients diagnosed with an acute febrile urinary tract infection (UTI) have in fact a pyelonephritis, and not all the cases diagnosed with a pyelonephritis will necessarily develop a scar. Moreover, acute pyelonephritis can occur even in the absence of VUR, and other factors than the VUR are important for the development of scars eventually including factors related to the child and the environment. Among the former, it is apparent that children developing a more severe immune reaction are at increasing risk of developing renal scars. Among the environmental factors, it has been suggested that some bacterial strains might be more virulent than others.

Prevention of the renal damage is essential to avoid the long-term sequelae of VUR-related

M. Castagnetti, M.D.
Section of Paediatric Urology, Urology Unit, University Hospital of Padova, Padua, Italy

W. Rigamonti, M.D.
Paediatric Surgery and Urology Unit, Burlo Garofalo Hospital, Trieste, Italy

G. Manzoni, M.D., F.E.A.P.U., F.R.C.S. (✉)
Department of Pediatric Urology, Fondazione IRCCS Cà Granda, Ospedale Maggiore Policlinico, Via della Commenda, 10, 20122 Milan, Italy
e-mail: gianantonio.manzoni@policlinico.mi.it

R. Rabinowitz et al. (eds.), *Pediatric Urology for the Primary Care Physician*, Current Clinical Urology, DOI 10.1007/978-1-60327-243-8_13, © Springer Science+Business Media New York 2015

renal damage, therefore the key points for the management of patients with VUR are the differentiation of congenital dysplasia and acquired scars and the selection of the cases at higher risk of developing recurrent UTIs and progressive renal scaring. Indeed, recurrent UTIs occur in less than one-third of patients with VUR diagnosed after a febrile UTI, and progressive renal scaring is estimated to occur in less than 10 % of cases. Therefore the follow-up and treatment of all the patients with VUR would involve an unacceptable cost for both the patients and the medical system. In patients requiring treatment, instead, the latter should be the most effective to prevent recurrent UTIs and progressive renal scaring, and the major issue at present is to determine which treatment among continuous antibiotic prophylaxis, endoscopic treatment, and open surgery is the best to achieve this goal also in comparison to no treatment at all.

## Why Is the Entity Relevant to a Primary Care Provider?

VUR is one of the most common urological anomalies in children. The incidence in the general population is less than 1 % and varies in different races, Asian and African children having a lower incidence than Caucasian ones. Up to 40 % of patients diagnosed with a prenatal hydronephrosis have a primary VUR. Up to 50 % of patients diagnosed with a UTI have VUR, with prevalence inversely proportional to age. VUR has been reported to occur in 1/3 of sibling of indexed cases, and about 30 % of these cases have been reported to present renal scars. Female to male ratio is 3:1 considering VUR, but males are predominant among patients presenting with a febrile UTI (more than 80 %). Females are instead predominant among patients presenting with lower urinary tract symptoms due to voiding dysfunction.

VUR is a condition of medical interest because of its relation to the development of renal damage, hypertension, and chronic renal failure. Approximately 30–50 % of patients with VUR develop renal scarring. VUR is one of the most common causes of paediatric hypertension accounting for up to 10 % of cases. The prevalence of hypertension in patients with VUR is about 15 %, which is twice the expected in the normal Caucasian population. VUR is also responsible for up to 30 % of paediatric end-stage renal disease cases and 20 % of cases of renal failure before the age of 50 years.

## History and Presentation

Patients with VUR usually can present in one of two ways, either with an asymptomatic urinary tract dilatation or with a UTI. Asymptomatic cases can also be diagnosed during the screening of siblings of indexed children. Several factors should be considered in the evaluation of asymptomatic patients diagnosed antenatally with a urinary tract dilatation including the appearance of the urinary tract dilatation, the status of the renal parenchyma, and the amount of the amniotic fluid on the antenatal ultrasound scan (US). In most of the cases, a definitive differentiation between a refluxing or obstructive dilatation can only be made postnatally. However, several factors can suggest the presence of a VUR rather than an obstruction based on the antenatal history. VUR is usually diagnosed earlier than obstructive dilatations. VUR more often presents as a dilatation involving both the renal pelvis and the ureter, and the dilatation fluctuates over subsequent scans or during the same scan in relation to the degree of bladder filling. The amount of amniotic fluid is usually normal in patients with VUR unless the presence of two small, nonfunctioning, dysplastic kidneys. Conversely, the presence of oligohydroamnios and bilateral hydro-ureteronephrosis should always elicit the suspicion of obstruction, especially in male foetuses.

UTIs are the second major presenting modality of VUR. UTIs should be differentiated in febrile and non-febrile. The presence of fever usually corresponds to a renal localization of the infection; non-febrile UTIs instead are infections usually confined to the lower urinary tract.

Febrile UTIs are more often the presentation of infants in whom the infection tends to quickly

**Table 13.1** Features of children with primary vs. VUR with dysfunctional voiding

| | Primary | DYSF voiding |
|---|---|---|
| Age at diagnosis | Newborn-infant | Child |
| Sex preference | Male | Female |
| Presentation | Prenatal diagnosis – febrile UTI | UTI, constipation, urinary incontinence |
| Grading | High | Low |
| Behaviour | Persistent | Intermittent |
| Vesicoureteral junction | Abnormal | Normal |
| Risk of associated renal damage | +++ (Dysplasia) | + |
| DMSA | Often abnormal | Usually normal |

develop in urosepsis. In some infants, however, the diagnosis can be difficult as the fever is a very non-specific symptom; moreover the history of UTIs cannot be clear-cut and rather appear as a failure to thrive.

Non-febrile UTIs usually cause symptoms such as urgency or frequency. This presentation is more common in older children, especially females 3–5 years old. In these patients, it is quite common a tendency to postpone voiding and to present urgency, minor degrees of diurnal incontinence, or nocturnal enuresis. In most of these cases, VUR is actually secondary to a voiding dysfunction. An abnormal bowel habit can also be present, and the distended rectum compressing the urethra can further exacerbate the voiding difficulties and increase perineal bacterial colonization and the risk of UTIs. The common sphincteric mechanism shred by the bowel and urinary tract can account for the association of bladder and bowel habit abnormalities, also called "dysfunctional elimination syndrome (DES)". A comparison of main features in patients with primary VUR and patients with VUR and voiding dysfunction is given in Table 13.1.

## Physical Examination

In children with primary VUR, general physical examination is usually normal. Examination of the genitalia is always important. In the male, it is essential to rule out a tight phimosis, meatal stenosis, and any congenital penile anomalies (hypo or epispadias). Therefore, it may be relevant to observe the urinary stream, the presence of voiding in a preputial reservoir, or the presence of straining during micturition. In females, both labial fusion and major anatomical abnormalities (urogenital sinus, epispadias) potentially causing a vaginal voiding should be ruled out.

Observation of the buttock and sacral region is always mandatory to detect potential malformations of the region, which could be associated with an occult spinal dysraphism.

## How to Evaluate

Irrespective of the initial suspicion of VUR whether suggested by a prenatal dilatation or a UTI, the final diagnosis of VUR relays upon the imaging of the retrograde flow of urine from the bladder into the upper urinary tract.

"Traditional" imaging of reflux usually requires a trans-urethral catheterization for the intra-vesical injection of a contrast agent. Catheterization requires to be performed under sterile conditions.

Any imaging of reflux should be performed at least 2 weeks after an acute UTI, as any infection of the bladder can cause a bladder hyperactivity leading to false positives.

Three main techniques are available for the diagnosis of VUR: the fluoroscopic *voiding cystourethrography* (*VCUG*), the isotopic voiding urosonography (VUS), and the voiding cystoscintigraphy (VCS). Any of these techniques should be performed with a cycling method, which means that ideally three subsequent cycles of filling/voiding should be performed in each case.

The VCUG is in fact the only technique allowing for a proper evaluation of the morphology of the bladder outlet and of the urethra. For this reason it should be considered the investigation of choice in males at first evaluation. In order to properly see the urethral profile, an oblique view during micturition is mandatory (Fig. 13.1). Moreover, VCUG has been considered the only imaging modality

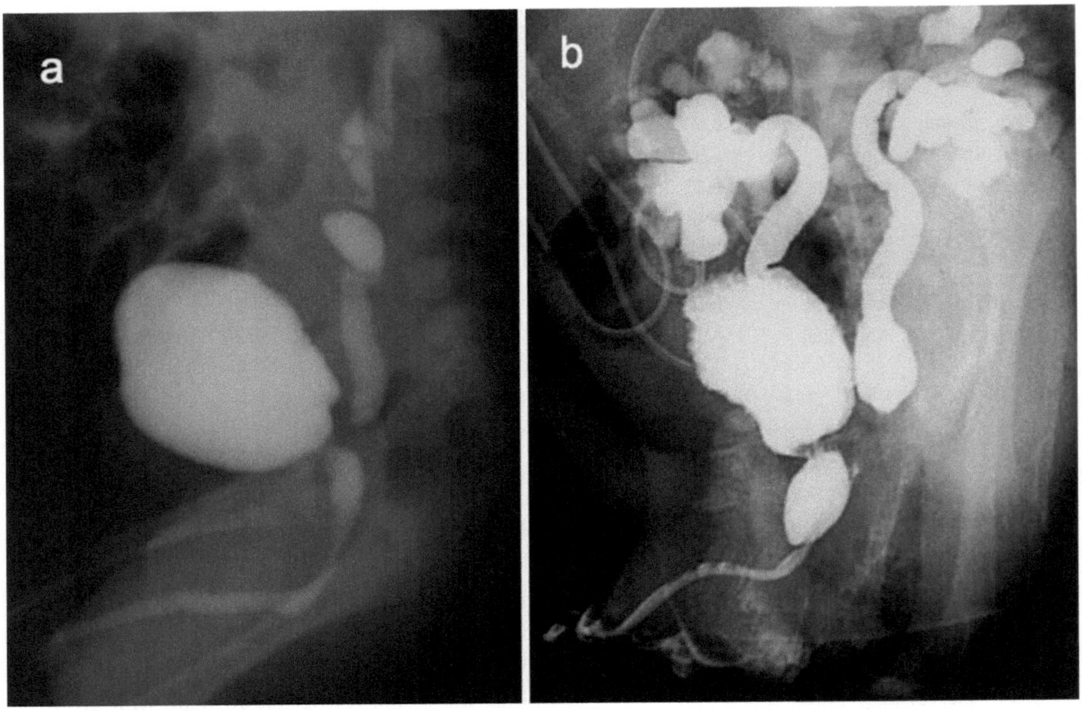


**Fig. 13.1** Oblique view during micturition on a voiding cysto-urethrography: (**a**) normal urethral profile and (**b**) dilated posterior urethra

allowing for an accurate grading of reflux, with five grades being described (international classification) (Fig. 13.2). Nevertheless, the critical importance of VUR grading on the management of reflux is nowadays widely questioned, and multiple cycles can lead to discrepancy in the presence, laterality, and grading of VUR inasmuch as 40 % of cases.

Since reflux is an intermittent phenomenon for the clinical management, it may practically suffice to differentiate between high- and low-grade refluxes, i.e. refluxes occurring in a dilated or non-dilated system (Fig. 13.2). Among the major disadvantages of VCUG are its invasiveness and the radiation exposure. The latter vary widely in relation to the technique and the equipment used for the investigation. It has been calculated a lifetime risk of fatal cancer per examination of 1 in 10,000.

Radiation exposure is completely avoided in the VUS. This might theoretically combine the assessment of the morphology of the urinary tract and the imaging of reflux. The major disadvantage is that, as for the standard US, it is highly operator dependent. Moreover it does not allow simultaneous visualization of the lower and upper urinary tract as usual with VCUG (Fig. 13.3) and does not allow for an easy and reproducible evaluation of the posterior urethra. VUS therefore has so far gained acceptance only in centres where there are competent radiologists devoted to this technique with a tight collaboration between the physician who perform the investigation and the paediatric urologist. The direct voiding cystoscintigraphy is the most sensitive test in the detection of reflux (Fig. 13.4). In the everyday use, it is probably the most reproducible test for the first evaluation in females and for the follow-up in both sexes. Finally an indirect voiding cystoscintigraphy can also be performed, avoiding an unpleasant trans-urethral catheterization, but only in the older toilet-trained patient. The indirect voiding cystoscintigraphy, as the terminal part of a dynamic scan, after the upper tract has emptied allows combining the study of reflux to an evaluation of renal function, but the main disadvantage is its lower sensitivity with regard to both the detection of reflux and of renal scars.

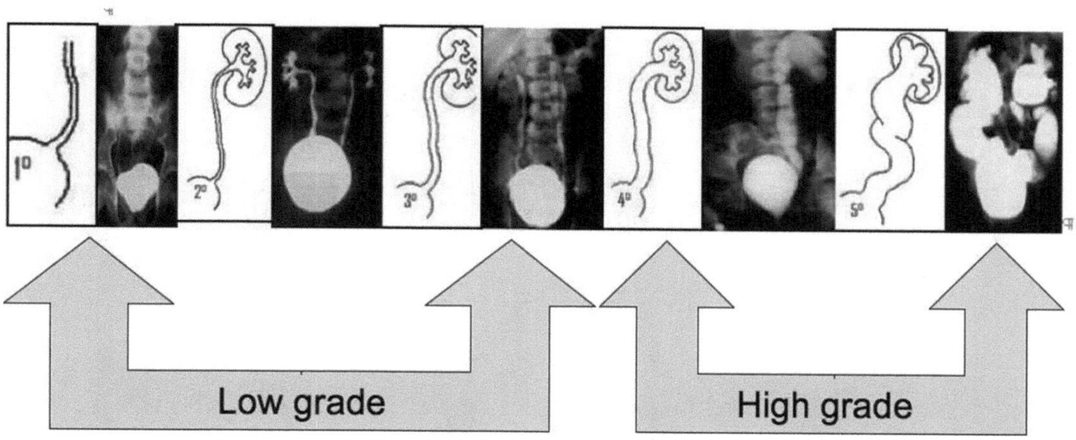


**Fig. 13.2** Grading of reflux

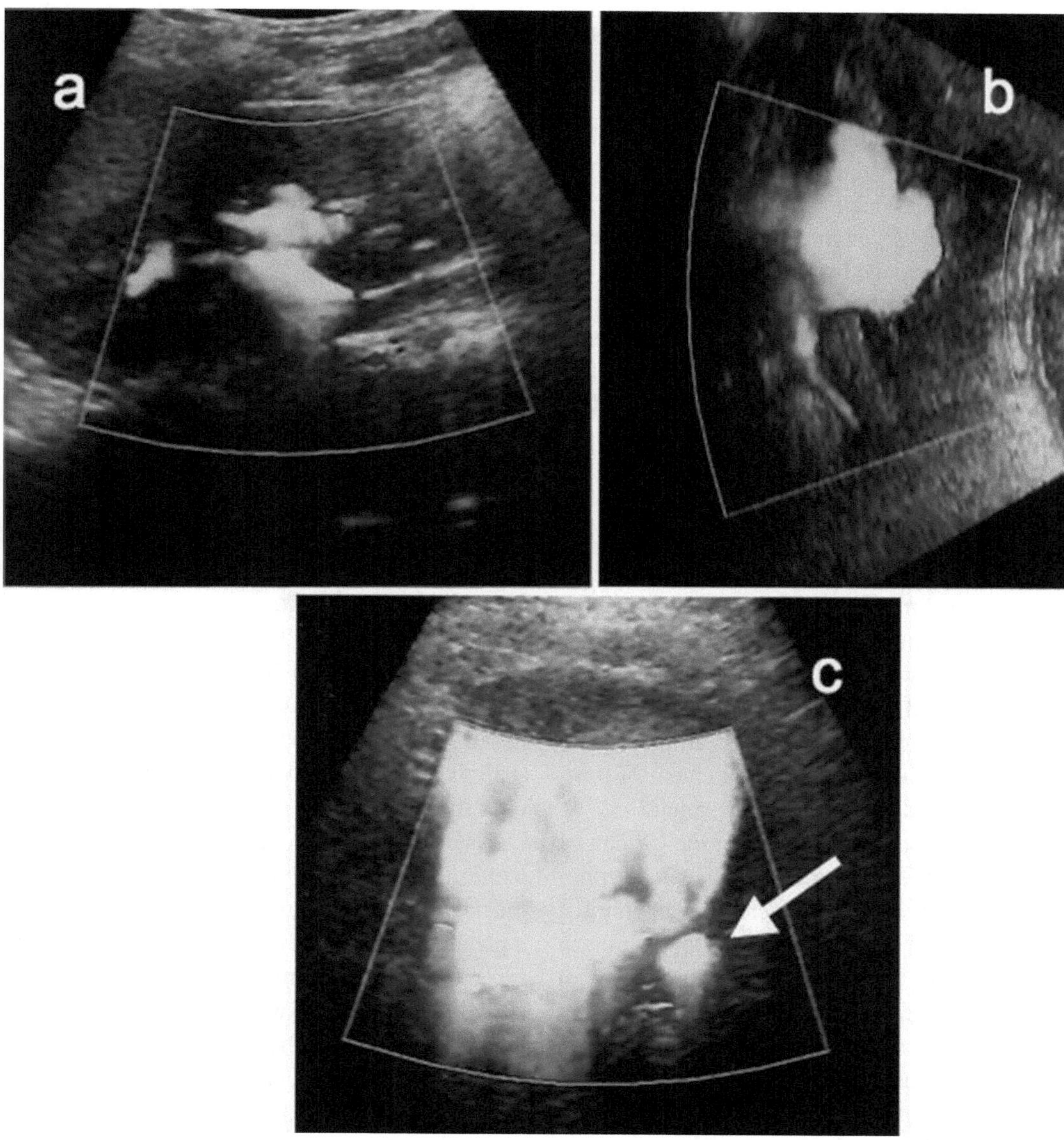


**Fig. 13.3** Imaging of reflux on voiding cysto-sonography: (**a**) right reflux, (**b**) left reflux, and (**c**) bladder with left ureter (*arrow*)

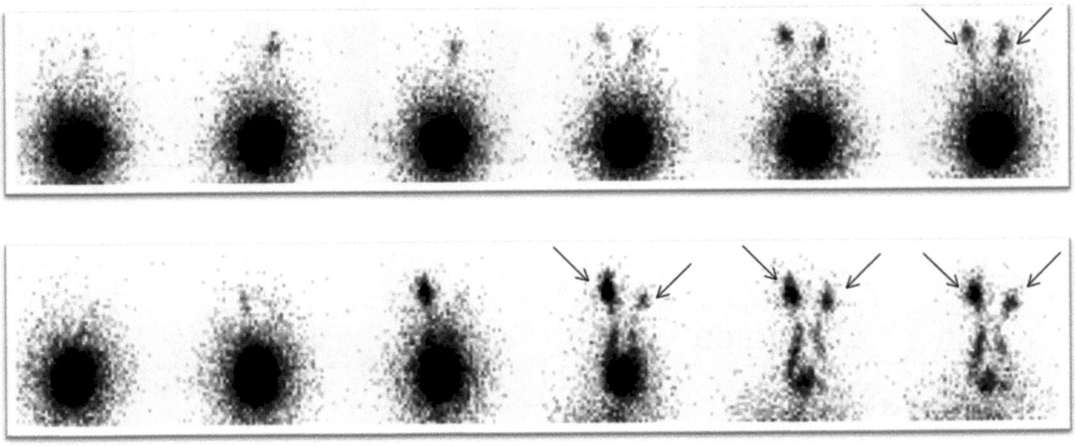

**Fig. 13.4** Bilateral reflux (*arrows*) on a direct voiding cystoscintigraphy

Besides the imaging of VUR, the classical algorithm for the evaluation of patients with VUR includes the assessment of the morphology of the urinary tract by US and the evaluation of the kidney function/damage by DMSA scan.

US is a noninvasive investigation widely used in the diagnosis and assessment of patients with VUR. It is an operator-dependent procedure and even in experienced hands has sensitivity of less than 85 % and a very low specificity. It allows for the evaluation of multiple morphological features of the kidneys, ureters, and bladder. To begin with, it allows for an evaluation of the characteristics of the renal parenchyma and the measurement of the dimensions of the kidney(s), renal pelvis, and ureter. The urinary tract should be evaluated both with a full bladder and after voiding. Bladder wall thickness before and after voiding should also be assessed. Particularly in toilet-trained children, the measurement of post-micturition residue should be determined.

It is questionable as to whether the US can be of use during the acute phase or if it can corroborate the diagnosis of a suspected pyelonephritis. Particularly with the use of colour Doppler, it can provide useful additional information, but it remains an operator-dependent test with quite a low specificity.

The static renal 99m-dimercaptosuccinic acid (DMSA) scintigraphy, otherwise, has classically been used for the evaluation of kidney function and to rule out the presence of renal damage, which appears with a defect in the distribution of the tracer within the kidney. The DMSA scan can be differentiated between the acute and non-acute phase. The former is performed within 7 days from a febrile UTI. This is the most accurate test for the diagnosis of an acute pyelonephritis as it allows for a localization of the infection into the affected kidney. The non-acute DMSA, instead, is performed at least 6 months after the last UTI, as this is the minimum period required for acute lesions to mature into irreversible parenchymal scar.

## How to Investigate

The above-mentioned investigations have to be used differently in asymptomatic patients diagnosed with a urinary tract dilatation on a prenatal scan than in patients with a non-febrile infection or in those presenting with a febrile UTI.

Asymptomatic patients should be subjected to a different diagnostic protocol in accordance with the degree of the prenatal dilatation. Patients with a prenatal antero-posterior pelvic diameter on the transverse plane <10 mm should only undergo a US within a couple of weeks after birth and more invasive tests only if the US shows a progression in the urinary tract dilatation or other abnormalities of the urinary tract (i.e. dilated ureter(s) and/or an abnormal bladder). Those with a prenatal dilatation >10 mm should undergo a US scan 3–5 days after birth and an imaging investigation for the reflux within the first month, but in males with bilateral hydro-ureteronephrosis and/or an abnormal bladder on the US, this evaluation should be performed sooner. First imaging modality in males should be the VCUG in order to achieve a clear definition of the anatomy of the urethra. VUS or VCS could be the imaging of choice in females. A VCUG may be preferable also in a female with evidence of a duplex system or in other anatomical abnormalities on the US, namely, whenever a greater anatomical detail is considered necessary for the choice of treatment.

If the test is positive for VUR, a baseline DMSA should be performed within the first months of life.

Patients with a non-febrile UTI should undergo a US only, and if it is strictly normal, do not undergo any more invasive investigations unless the UTI recur. If non-febrile UTI presents in toilet-trained children, especially females, a voiding dysfunction should always be suspected and bladder and bowel habit carefully assessed.

Patients presenting with a febrile UTI represent a very controversial group with regard to their assessment. The first issue regards the diagnosis of acute pyelonephritis. The condition should be suspected in every child with fever and without any reasonable source of infection. The first controversial issue regards the modality of urine sample collection. The three main alternative methods include external collection, catheterization, or suprapubic puncture. The latter is the most invasive way but it avoids any risk of contamination. If it is deemed unsuitable, and the sample is collected by spontaneous voiding, the diagnosis should be corroborated by at least two samples collected apart from each other, and the mid-urine stream should be collected to reduce the risk of contamination. The latter is clearly not possible in infants, and a reasonable approach in these patients could be to get the first sample by an external bag and a second by catheterization if the first is positive for UTI.

Irrespective of the method used for collection of the urine sample, if the diagnosis of febrile UTI is confirmed, the following step is to ascertain as to whether the infection involves the kidney or not. Pyelonephritis is always associated with a rise in the markers of infection. The procalcitonin seems to be the most specific marker of renal infection, but the ideal cut-off is still to be found, and the test is not always available and bares elevated costs.

As previously mentioned, the acute DMSA is the most accurate investigation for the diagnosis of acute pyelonephritis, allowing for a specific and definitive localization of the infection to the kidney.

Interest in acute DMSA has recently increased, as it seems to be able to allow for a more precise selection of cases deserving further evaluation. Indeed, among the patients with a febrile UTI, only those with an acute pyelonephritis would deserve imaging of reflux; the latter could instead be spared in patients with a febrile UTI without renal involvement. In this way, more invasive imaging could be avoided in up to 40 % of cases diagnosed with a febrile UTI. According to such a protocol, the imaging of reflux (VCUG, VUS, or VCS) should be postponed to the initial acute DMSA and be performed only in the presence of a positive DMSA finding (Fig. 13.5).

The limit of this approach is that since not all the lesions found on an acute DMSA give rise to a scar, a second DMSA theoretically should be performed 6 months later. Therefore, an alternative option to further simplify the management of these patients could be to skip the acute DMSA, accepting a diagnosis of pyelonephritis based only on the clinical picture and the laboratory findings, and wait for the 6-month DMSA than carry on with the imaging of reflux only in the patients with evidence of a scar on such DMSA.

## How to Manage

The main acute problem in patients with VUR is pyelonephritis/urosepsis.

The ideal treatment in patients with an acute pyelonephritis includes basic support, antibiotic treatment, and a temporary urinary diversion. Empirical antibiotic treatment should be started soon after collection of a urine sample

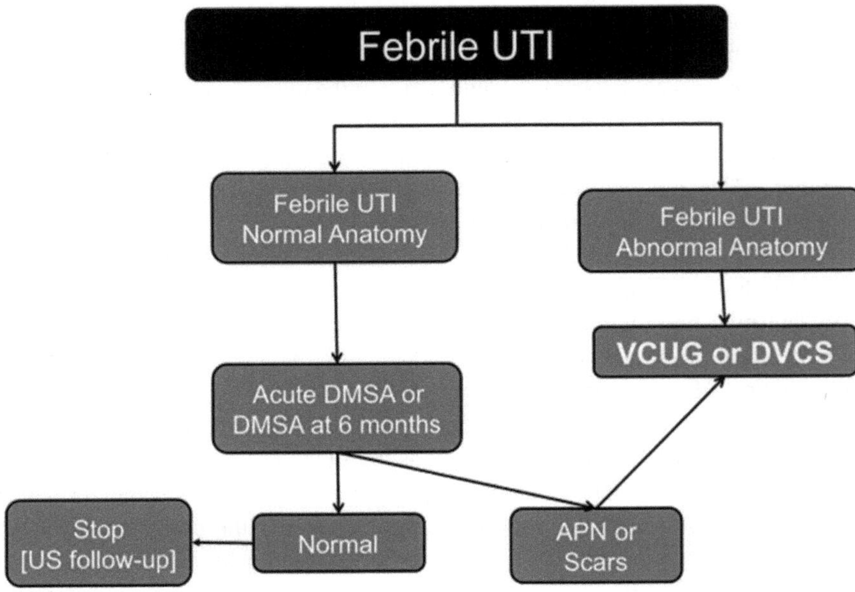


**Fig. 13.5** Algorithm for the diagnosis in children at first febrile urinary tract infection

for urinalysis. Therefore, antibiotic treatment should be tailored to each case based on the results of the urine culture. It is controversial which antibiotic scheme should be used in patients with an acute pyelonephritis, whether the antibiotic should be administered intravenously or orally, how long for, if treatment could be administered at home or the child should be kept as an inpatient. Only as a practical rule, patients <1 year, patients with systemic signs or vomit, and those at risk of low compliance should be admitted and receive at least initially a parenteral treatment. If domiciliary treatment is elected daily, follow-up should be ensured.

With regard to urine diversion during an acute infection, insertion of trans-urethral catheter is the best method to keep the system decompressed and obtains a temporary suppression of VUR. Placement of an indwelling catheter should be considered in all the patients with systemic signs related to the infection and be maintained until a complete clinical response is achieved.

After an acute pyelonephritis, if further investigations are deemed necessary, the patient should always be kept on prophylaxis until such investigations are undertaken.

Elective treatment modalities in children with VUR include observation, antibiotic prophylaxis, endoscopic or surgical treatment, and more rarely a urinary diversion.

From a historical perspective in the 1950s, all VURs were considered to be secondary to a bladder outlet obstruction, and treatment options aimed at reducing bladder outlet resistances or widening the outlet. During the 1960s and 1970s, several studies showed that VUR can be due to a primary abnormality of the vesicoureteral junction and that it was associated to renal damage; therefore this prompted early surgical treatment of all cases found with VUR. Several techniques were devised, all relying upon the principle that lengthening of the intramural ureteral segment was necessary to prevent VUR. Between the 1970s and 1980s, the correlation among reflux, UTIs, and renal damage became clearer. Several studies showed that sterile reflux did not lead to the development of any renal damage. Antibiotic prophylaxis was therefore introduced in the management of patients with VUR. Moreover, following up patients on prophylaxis, it became also clear that the VUR could improve or resolve spontaneously. Thereafter during the 1980s and 1990s, the comparison of surgical vs. prophylactic treatment became the subject of international, multicentric, and randomized trials. These studies showed that the benefit of surgery over antibiotics is questionable. Finally, three main changes have characterized the last decade in terms of treatment of VUR. Firstly, the minimally invasive endoscopic treatment has become increasingly popular. Secondly, even the need for an antibiotic prophylaxis has been questioned, and ongoing studies are currently comparing the prophylaxis vs. observational treatment alone with use of antibiotics only in case of acute UTIs. Thirdly, genetic studies have shown that in some patients the renal damage can be associated rather than be due to reflux, and therefore in such cases progression of damage is independent form treatment. Indeed, the evidence coming from these studies has found clinical confirmation in the observation that all the above-mentioned improvements in treatment have not changed the number of patients developing chronic renal failure and eventually requiring a renal transplant.

It seems therefore possible to conclude that, in patients with high-grade VUR and small dysplastic kidneys bilaterally at birth, the final outcome does not improve even despite successful surgical treatment of VUR. Continuous antibiotic prophylaxis is recommended in patients with high-grade reflux since no data are available on patients with high-grade VUR followed up off prophylaxis. Patients with low-grade reflux and otherwise normal kidneys have a low risk of developing recurrent febrile UTIs and progressive renal scarring, and, therefore, observation off prophylaxis might be reasonable.

Endoscopic treatment can be offered to the patient developing recurrent febrile UTIs or progressive renal scarring. Endoscopic treatment consists of a submucosal injection of bulking agents. This produces a combined partial elevation of the meatus while lengthening the intramural segment of the ureter. The original technique included only the injection of a small amount of the agent at 6 o'clock position, just below the ureteral orifice. With this technique, the procedure proved effective only in case of low-grade reflux. The amount of injected material has progressively been increased, improving the effectiveness of treatment without any apparent increase in the risk of obstruction. Moreover, in order to treat also high-grade VURs, a technical modification has been recently introduced including hydro-distension of the orifice and intra-ureteral injection of the substance. With regard to the injected substance, the cross-linked bovine collagen was initially used; it was then switched to polytetrafluoroethylene. Nowadays, dextranomer/hyaluronic acid copolymer (Deflux®, Oceana Therapeutics Ltd, Dublin, Ireland) is the bulking agent of choice in most European and North American centres. The above-mentioned modifications have been made possible to extend the use of the endoscopic treatment to almost any degrees of VUR with an average success rate as high as 80 %, including refluxes in duplex systems. The procedure is also safe being associated with a less than 1 % complication rate. The major complication of endoscopic treatment is a transient ureteral obstruction. This is usually asymptomatic and self-limiting. If symptomatic, insertion of a ureteral catheter should be considered. Therefore the need for a formal ureteral reimplantation is quite exceptional.

The high effectiveness and the low morbidity of the endoscopic treatment have led some groups to suggest it as a better option than prophylaxis in patients deemed to require treatment in order to avoid any issue related to the long-term administration of antibiotics, especially in terms of compliance with treatment. It should be emphasized, however, that the effectiveness of endoscopic treatment in preventing recurrent febrile UTIs and progressive renal scarring is currently unknown.

Based on present knowledge, our preferred approach is to keep patients on prophylaxis until 6 months of age and to wait for the achievement of full urinary and bowel continence and to offer an endoscopic treatment only to those cases that develop recurrent infections in spite of prophylaxis or after its discontinuation. This is consistent with a policy focusing more on renal damage than on the VUR itself, and this is based on the principle that only the renal damage due to infections can be affected by treatment, and therefore only patients keen to develop infections need for treatment.

Also our follow-up protocol has been tailored to this principle, and we have progressively reduced the number of follow-up controls required to rule out the persistence/disappearance of reflux. Checking for VUR means to commit ourselves to take same action if it persists, which is probably not necessary if it does not affect renal damage. Nowadays, we do not recommend any imaging of reflux before discontinuation of the prophylaxis or even after endoscopic treatment unless symptoms develop. A follow-up DMSA scan can instead be considered a few years after the baseline one, even in the absence of symptoms in the meanwhile, to rule out the development of new scars, as the latter can occur even in the absence of clear-cut pyelonephritic episodes. Eventually, a final DMSA assessment is, in our opinion, mandatory at puberty to assess renal function and scarring as the patients enters adult life.

Finally, urinary diversion can be considered as a reasonable option, but only in infants with recurrent breakthrough febrile UTIs or with borderline chronic renal failure. If a urinary diversion is considered appropriate, we favour the use of either a vesicostomy or preferably a low unilateral "refluxing" cutaneous ureterostomy, which is not interfering with the bladder.

Treatment of VUR secondary to voiding dysfunction goes beyond the scope of this chapter, but it should be mentioned that in cases in which signs of bladder dysfunction are present, the latter should be addressed primarily. In these cases, the use of anticholinergic drugs, bladder training with time-voiding scheme, and resolution of constipation, if present, represent the cornerstones of treatment.

## Suggested Reading

Ardissino G, Avolio L, Dacco V, Testa S, Marra G, Viganò S, Loi S, Caione P, De Castro R, De Pascale S, Marras E, Riccipetitoni G, Selvaggio G, Pedotti P, Claris-Appiani A, Ciofani A, Dello Strologo L, Lama G, Montini G, Verrina E, ItalKid Project. Long-term outcome of vesicoureteral reflux associated chronic renal failure in children. Data from the ItalKid Project. J Urol. 2004;172:305–10.

Brandström P, Jodal U, Sillén U, Hansson S. The Swedish reflux trial: review of a randomized, controlled trial in children with dilating vesicoureteral reflux. J Pediatr Urol. 2011;7(6):594–600.

Elder JS, Diaz M, Caldamone AA, Cendron M, Greenfield S, Hurwitz R, Kirsch A, Koyle MA, Pope J, Shapiro E. Endoscopic therapy for vesicoureteral reflux: a meta-analysis. I. Reflux resolution and urinary tract infection. J Urol. 2006;175:716–22.

Hansson S, Dhamey M, Sigstrom O, Sixt R, Stokland E, Wennerstrom M, Jodal U. Dimercapto-succinic acid scintigraphy instead of voiding cystourethrography for infants with urinary tract infections. J Urol. 2004; 172:1071–4.

Hoberman A, Charron M, Hickey RW, Baskin M, Kearney DH, Wald ER. Imaging studies after a first febrile urinary tract infection in young children. N Engl J Med. 2003;348(3):195–202.

Kirsch AJ, Perez-Brayfield M, Smith EA, Scherz HC. The modified sting procedure to correct vesicoureteral reflux: improved results with submucosal implantation within the intramural ureter. J Urol. 2004;171(6 Pt 1): 2413–6.

Roussey-Kesler G, Gadjos V, Idres N, Horen B, Ichay L, Leclair MD, Raymond F, Grellier A, Hazart I, de Parscau L, Salomon R, Champion G, Leroy V, Guigonis V, Siret D, Palcoux JB, Taque S, Lemoigne A, Nguyen JM, Guyot C. Antibiotic prophylaxis for the prevention of recurrent urinary tract infection in children with low grade vesicoureteral reflux: results from a prospective randomized study. J Urol. 2008; 179:674–9.

Routh JC, Bogaert GA, Kaefer M, Manzoni G, Park JM, Retik AB, Rushton HG, Snodgrass WT, Wilcox DT. Vesicoureteral reflux: current trends in diagnosis, screening, and treatment. Eur Urol. 2012;61:773–82.

# Posterior Urethral Valves

# 14

Erica J. Traxel and Curtis A. Sheldon

## Introduction

Posterior urethral valves (PUVs) are a congenital obstruction of the male posterior urethra. They represent the most common form of urinary tract obstruction in children. The incidence of this condition is between 1:3000 and 1:8000, with 400–500 new cases each year in the United States. The spectrum of this disease is wide in its age of presentation, ranging from antenatal to adolescent, and in its degree of disease severity, including minor voiding dysfunction as well as renal failure. Understanding of this condition has progressed over the last several decades, and subsequently treatment approaches have evolved.

PUVs were first identified and classified by Hugh Hampton Young in 1919 [1]. He differentiated PUVs into three types. Type I valves, which account for over 90 % of all PUVs, begin distal to the verumontanum and extend distally in an anterolateral direction, joining at the 12 o'clock position. Type II valves are mucosal folds that run between the bladder neck and verumontanum. Type II valves are nonobstructive and thus generally asymptomatic, making their true incidence unknown, such that some urologists even doubt their existence. Type III valves, which make up less than 10 % of all PUVs, are a concentric annulus located just distal to the verumontanum, resembling a stricture.

PUVs have significant implication for males with this disease. The resulting bladder outlet obstruction leads to elevated voiding pressures, triggering bladder wall hypertrophy in order to generate sufficiently high pressures to overcome the obstruction. Eventually, the bladder is unable to compensate and post-void residuals (PVR) gradually increase. Subsequently resting/filling bladder pressures rise as well. This increase in pressure is transmitted to the upper tracts, leading in time to renal damage. Even after intervention to relieve the bladder outlet obstruction, there can be already irrevocable alterations in bladder and renal histology, leading to permanent modifications in bladder and renal function. These changes can affect a patient's lifestyle, relating to a high incidence of urinary incontinence. They can also have very morbid consequences, including recurrent urinary tract infections (UTIs), end-stage renal disease (ESRD), and even death. Due to improvements in hemodialysis, antibiotics, and neonatal intensive care units, the mortality related to PUVs has decreased from a traditional level of 50 % down to 5 % [2]. Despite advances in the care of children with PUVs and earlier detection via prenatal ultrasonography, the incidence of chronic renal insufficiency in this population is still high, ranging from 34 % at 10 years of age to 51 % at age 20 years [3]. Such potentially severe long-term effects point to the importance of early diagnosis and intervention.

E.J. Traxel, M.D. (✉) • C.A. Sheldon, M.D.
Cincinnati Children's Hospital Medical Center,
3333 Burnet Avenue, Cincinnati, OH 45229, USA
e-mail: erica.traxel@cchmc.org

R. Rabinowitz et al. (eds.), *Pediatric Urology for the Primary Care Physician*, Current Clinical Urology,
DOI 10.1007/978-1-60327-243-8_14, © Springer Science+Business Media New York 2015

## History and Physical Examination

The signs and symptoms associated with PUVs are varied and depend upon the age at which they present and the severity of underlying renal dysplasia. Careful history taking is paramount to the diagnosis of PUVs, as no outward physical sign of PUVs will manifest itself, at least not until the sequelae of ESRD are present. Quite often today, the diagnosis of PUVs may be entertained even while in utero. Such is the case when routine prenatal ultrasonography reveals findings that suggest PUVs, as will be discussed further in the section on imaging studies.

In an infant or child with PUVs for whom prenatal care was lacking or failed to show any clue as to the presence of PUVs, one of the first demonstrations of PUVs may be a UTI, urinary retention, urinary incontinence, hematuria, dribbling, or a weak urine stream. Any male who has a UTI should undergo a screening renal/bladder ultrasound to evaluate for anatomic abnormalities, such as hydronephrosis or a thick-walled bladder. The patient should also undergo a voiding cystourethrogram (VCUG). Additionally, any male with a febrile UTI should prompt a referral to a pediatric urologist.

Some boys after the expected age of toilet training may experience nocturnal enuresis along with occasional daytime accidents related to delays in voiding. While these behaviors are not inherently worrisome, the boy in whom consistent day- and nighttime wetting persists should make the medical practitioner wary of the potential for PUVs. Such a patient should undergo a screening renal/bladder ultrasound as well as uroflow studies and determination of a PVR. As most general pediatric clinics are not outfitted with the equipment necessary to perform these studies, such patients should likely be referred to a pediatric urologist. It can be exceedingly difficult to discern children who are merely "dysfunctional eliminators" from those with underlying pathology such as PUVs. For this reason it is important to preserve a high index of suspicion for a possible diagnosis such as PUVs.

Physical examination of the patient with undiagnosed PUVs is perhaps most helpful at identifying other pathologies that could contribute to overlapping signs and symptoms. A child with "prune belly" or Eagle-Barrett syndrome has congenital dilation of the urinary tract leading to stasis and infection. These children will have a characteristic lack of abdominal musculature and bilaterally undescended testes. A child with a neurogenic bladder related to spinal cord abnormalities leading to voiding dysfunction and UTIs may have a characteristic sacral dimple or tuft of hair in the lumbosacral area. A child with anterior urethral valves (AUVs) can sometimes have a ballooning or outpouching of the anterior urethra evident on the ventrum of the penis. A child who has been circumcised and developed urethral meatal stenosis can have voiding symptoms of urinary urgency, frequency, and dysuria. Such a patient will have a small-appearing meatus. However, not all children with a small meatus have urinary symptoms.

## Evaluation

### Imaging

Ultrasonography is the initial screening imaging modality for all patients with PUVs. This may be done as a standard prenatal ultrasound. Significant obstructive uropathy can be seen as early as 18–19 weeks of gestation. Infants with PUVs can have bilateral hydroureteronephrosis, renal parenchymal thinning, thickened bladder wall, and oligohydramnios (Fig. 14.1). Certainly these findings are not inherently indicative of PUVs, as they can also be seen in Eagle-Barrett syndrome, but they raise suspicion of PUVs. The addition of fetal MRI in cases of suspected PUVs can better delineate anatomy, including fetal lung volumes, in order to aid prenatal practitioners and parents in decision-making during the pregnancy as well as prepare neonatologists and parents for a potentially complicated neonatal course.

Other possible ultrasound findings include unilateral hydroureteronephrosis associated with

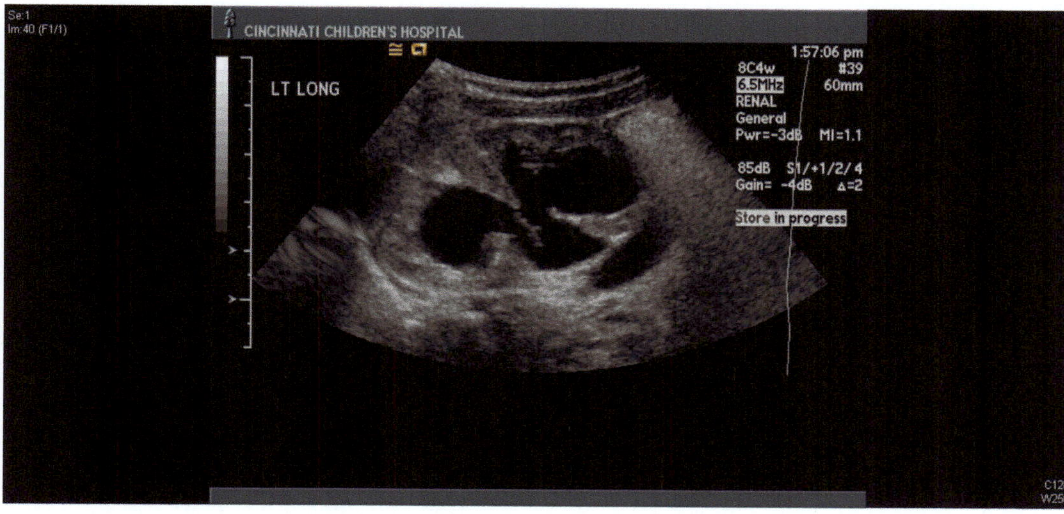


**Fig. 14.1** Renal ultrasound in a male with PUVs demonstrating significant hydronephrosis with lower pole parenchymal cortical thinning as well as a dilated proximal ureter

a cystic or dysplastic kidney. In these instances, the child may have VURD syndrome, that is PUVs, unilateral vesicoureteral reflux (VUR), and renal dysplasia. This finding actually may portend well for overall future renal function, as essentially one renal unit has been sacrificed while the other has been preserved and often has become hypertrophied. Other findings that portend a better long-term prognosis include urinary ascites and bladder diverticulum, as each of these provides a mechanism whereby high pressures in the obstructed bladder may be relieved without compromising renal function.

Another important finding on ultrasound can be the degree of echogenicity within the renal parenchyma and the differentiation between renal cortex and medulla. Patients with normal renal echogenicity and normal corticomedullary differentiation will usually go on to have adequate to normal long-term renal function. However, those in whom ultrasonography demonstrates increased echogenicity and loss of corticomedullary differentiation do not always end up with renal insufficiency [4].

The VCUG is the definitive radiologic test in diagnosing PUVs and has the benefit of providing real-time documentation of voiding with fluoroscopy. Of note, it can sometimes be difficult to pass a catheter retrograde into the bladder, as it may encounter resistance at the hypertrophied bladder neck and then coil within the capacious posterior urethra. In this instance, a coude tip catheter may better bypass the bladder neck. Typical VCUG findings in PUVs include a dilated posterior urethra terminating at the level of visible valve leaflets just distal to the verumontanum. Other findings may include a trabeculated bladder, bladder diverticuli, unilateral or bilateral VUR, and an elevated PVR (Figs. 14.2 and 14.3).

Nuclear renal scans are also used in patients with PUVs to quantify renal function. Mercaptoacetyltriglycine (MAG3) and dimercaptosuccinic acid (DMSA) scans are used to determine differential renal function, particularly in cases of VURD syndrome. These scans are also used to quantify glomerular filtration rate (GFR) when renal dysplasia and insufficiency is anticipated.

## Laboratory Assessment

Certainly in any instance when a child displays symptoms of a UTI, a urinalysis with macroscopic and microscopic analysis along with urine culture should be obtained. In the case of a child with

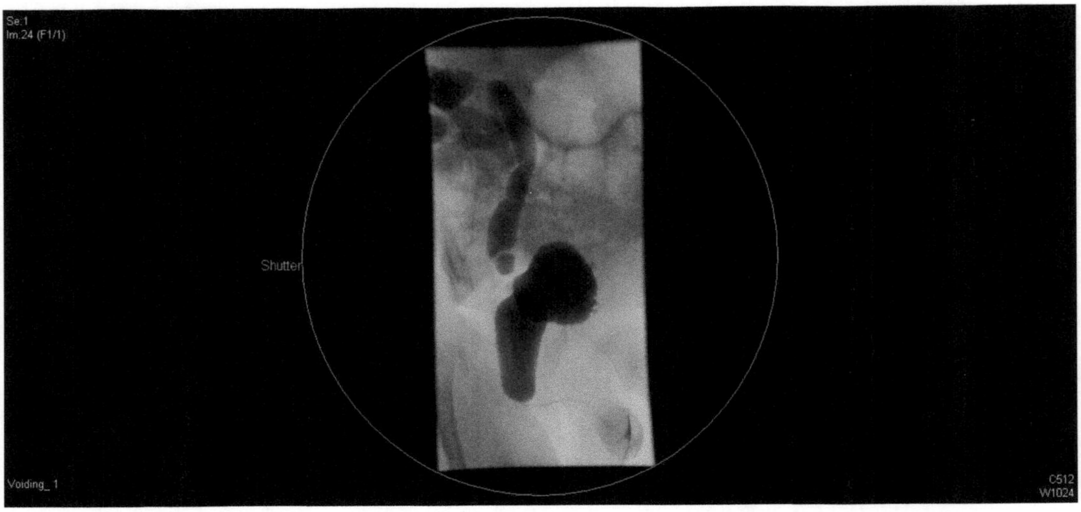


**Fig. 14.2** VCUG showing a dilated posterior urethra, trabeculated bladder, and right-sided grade V VUR

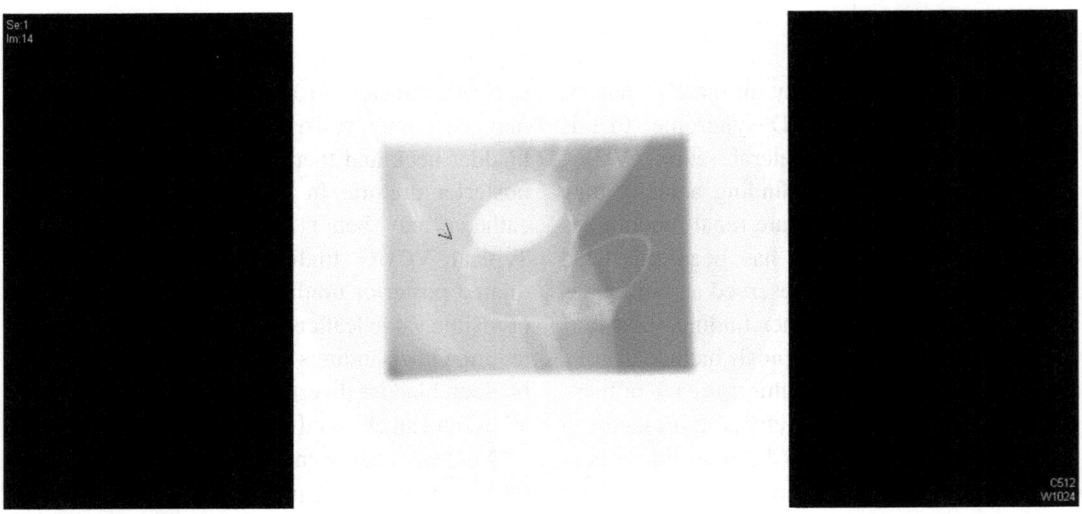


**Fig. 14.3** VCUG demonstrating a lucency in the posterior urethra representing the location of the PUVs. Also the arrow points to contrast entering into the utricle

known PUVs, this is especially important as they are at higher risk of pyelonephritis if they have concomitant VUR. Moreover, a child with known PUVs who experiences a fever of unknown origin, even without urinary tract symptoms, should have a urinalysis and urine culture performed.

The other key lab test to acquire in PUVs is a renal profile including serum creatinine. When an infant is first born, his serum creatinine will reflect that of the mother. Within about 72 h, the serum creatinine will reflect the infant's renal function, which typically should nadir around 0.2 or 0.3 mg/dL. The level at which the serum creatinine nadirs has prognostic importance, as it is believed that a serum creatinine of 0.8 mg/dL or less at age 12 months predicts lifelong adequate renal function, while a higher level suggests eventual renal insufficiency [5]. As the boy ages and grows, his renal function will only worsen in terms of his GFR, in that a finite number of nephrons will have to provide renal function for an increasing amount of body mass.

## Urodynamics

Urodynamics play an integral role in the physiologic assessment of the valve bladder. While not all boys with a diagnosis of PUVs must undergo urodynamic testing, it is essential in understanding the underlying bladder functioning in patients with voiding symptoms. Certainly a boy with voiding symptoms but normal urodynamic findings can be treated with behavioral modification, such as timed voiding. Also, urodynamic testing is important to ensure stable bladder dynamics in those patients requiring renal transplantation so as to protect the allograft and optimize its function.

Urodynamics testing usually encompasses uroflowmetry, cystometry, urethral pressure profilometry, and sphincter electromyography. While it is possible for a child with a history of PUVs to have an entirely normal voiding pattern and normal urodynamic findings, those patients with voiding dysfunction will typically fall into one of three urodynamic patterns of voiding, as supported by several studies [6]. These categories include myogenic bladder failure, bladder hyperreflexia, and bladder hypertonia with small capacity. Myogenic failure describes the inability of the bladder to generate a sustained bladder contraction sufficient to initiate voiding and to empty the bladder. These patients often void by Valsalva with a low flow rate and an elevated PVR. Incontinence in this group is attributed to overflow. A hyperreflexic bladder shows uninhibited detrusor contractions occurring early in filling. These patients usually have a normal bladder capacity and empty to completion but experience incontinence due to the urgency associated with the uninhibited contractions. A hypertonic small-capacity bladder has high filling pressures with a capacity that is smaller than that expected for age. There is usually no instability associated with filling, and emptying is to completion in this group. Incontinence in this category is related to a small functional capacity with bladder pressures greater than sphincteric pressures. There can be overlap among these three categories, and it is therefore important to tailor therapy to the individual urodynamic findings in each case.

## Management

### Preoperative Intervention

In the case of neonatal diagnosis or suspicion of PUVs, the child is first assessed for adequate pulmonary function. If stable, evaluation proceeds with ultrasound and placement of a urethral catheter (typically a feeding tube) in anticipation of a VCUG. It is important to start the child on antibiotic prophylaxis with amoxicillin. If the diagnosis of PUVs has been confirmed or has not been ruled out by imaging, the child can then proceed to the operating room within a few days of life. In a child with pulmonary hypoplasia or who is otherwise too ill or too premature for endoscopic intervention, the bladder outlet obstruction can be temporized with placement of a urethral catheter and surgery deferred until a later date.

### Surgical Intervention

The goal of surgical intervention is to relieve obstruction within the urinary tract. There are several options for surgical treatment, including primary endoscopic valve ablation, vesicostomy and delayed valve ablation, and primary valve ablation with upper tract diversion. Generally primary valve ablation is preferred. Fiberoptic technology is now sufficiently advanced that cystoscopes are small enough to use on neonates in all but the smallest of infants. When performing cystourethroscopy in an effort to diagnose PUVs, the scope is positioned just distal to the verumontanum while the surgeon applies suprapubic pressure to a full bladder so that the valves, if present, will balloon up toward the scope. The valves are then incised at the 5, 7, and sometimes 12 o'clock positions. This can be done either with a cold knife or a cutting electric current. The incidence of complications following endoscopic intervention ranges from 5 to 25 % and include urinary incontinence and stricture [7]. These complications can be minimized by avoiding incision of the bladder neck.

Cutaneous vesicostomy is a surgical alternative used in infants too small to permit endoscopic intervention. It then serves as a temporizing measure while waiting for the child to grow enough to undergo endoscopic valve ablation. It is also used in children in whom renal function does not improve despite bladder decompression with transurethral catheterization or even after transurethral incision of PUVs.

If a child's renal function fails to improve despite transurethral ablation of valves and even cutaneous vesicostomy, some practitioners progress to higher diversions, such as cutaneous ureterostomy and pyelostomy. It is known that in some children, the hypertrophied detrusor leads to obstruction at the ureterovesicular junction (UVJ). In such instances, higher diversion may be beneficial. Options like percutaneous nephrostomy tube placement are viable in the short term, but long term are associated with an increased risk of infection. Many would argue against higher urinary diversion, believing that it will defunctionalize the bladder as it prevents bladder cycling. It appears in studies that the different forms of surgical intervention do not have a benefit in terms of progression to ESRD or time to continence, but patients who have undergone higher diversion require a significantly larger number of surgeries [3].

In the neonate with PUVs, most urologists would recommend circumcision, as it has been shown that uncircumcised males under the age of 6 months are at increased risk of febrile UTI.

## Medical Management

Even after successful surgical relief of obstruction, it is crucial to follow these patients for a prolonged period of time in order to ascertain the presence of voiding dysfunction and possible renal insufficiency. In patients who do develop voiding problems, a thorough evaluation is necessary, including repeat imaging studies to ensure that no residual valve tissue is obstructing the urethra. Also urodynamic testing should be done to assess bladder physiology.

Depending upon the results of further testing, therapies to alleviate voiding dysfunction can include timed voiding, double- or triple-voiding, fluid restriction, clean intermittent catheterization, overnight indwelling catheter drainage, and anticholinergic medication. Patients who go on to develop renal insufficiency should be followed not only by a pediatric urologist but also a nephrologist. These patients often develop hypertension requiring medication as well as acidosis requiring bicarbonate supplementation. Those with significant renal insufficiency can also require growth hormone. In those who progress to ESRD, the urologist and nephrologist must coordinate care, to ensure that the patient has a functional bladder that can store adequate volumes of urine at low pressures in preparation for transplantation.

## References

1. Young HH, Frontz WA, Baldwin JC. Congenital obstruction of the posterior urethra. J Urol. 1919;3:289–307.
2. Connor JP, Burbige KA. Long-term urinary continence and renal function in neonates with posterior urethral valves. J Urol. 1990;144:1209–11.
3. Smith GHH, Canning DA, Schulman SL, Snyder HM, Duckett JW. The long-term outcome of posterior urethral valves treated with primary valve ablation and observation. J Urol. 1996;155:1730–4.
4. Duel BP, Mogbo K, Barthold JS, Gonzalez R. Prognostic value of initial renal ultrasound in patients with posterior urethral valves. J Urol. 1998;160:1198–200.
5. Duckett JW. Are "valve bladders" congenital or iatrogenic? Br J Urol. 1997;79:271–5.
6. Peters CA, Bolkier M, Bauer SB, Hendren WH, Colodny AH, Mandell J, Retik AB. The urodynamic consequences of posterior urethral valves. J Urol. 1990;144:122–6.
7. Nijman RJM, Scholtmeijer RJ. Complications of transurethral electro-incision of posterior urethral valves. Br J Urol. 1991;67:324–6.

# Bladder Exstrophy

# 15

Thomas E. Novak and Yegappan Lakshmanan

## Introduction

### Definitions

Bladder exstrophy and epispadias are a spectrum of uncommon, severe congenital defects that involve the genitourinary and pelvic musculoskeletal systems. The complex embryology and genetics of this disease are not well understood. A number of theories have been proposed which include premature rupture of the cloacal membrane, arrested mesenchymal ingrowth, and failure of cranial yolk sac progression during development [1]. In its classic form, bladder exstrophy describes the condition in which an exteriorized bladder template develops in association with a diastasis of the pubic symphysis. This pubic separation results in the characteristic genital and pelvic abnormalities which are described below. Epispadias can be viewed as the least severe form of exstrophy in which the bladder is closed and covered by a normal abdominal wall, but the pubic separation and genital abnormalities persist. Isolated epispadias is described in detail elsewhere and comments will be limited to its relevance in the patient with bladder exstrophy.

T.E. Novak, M.D.
Division of Urology, San Antonio Military Medical Center, San Antonio, TX, USA
e-mail: thomas.e.novak.mil@mail.mil

Y. Lakshmanan, M.D., F.A.A.P. (✉)
Children's Hospital of Michigan, Detroit, MI, USA
e-mail: ylaksh@dmc.org

## Relevance

### Epidemiology

Bladder exstrophy is rare, with a reported incidence of 1 in every 10,000–50,000 live births with males affected approximately twice as often as females. The incidence of isolated epispadias is more rare (1 in 100,000) and even less common in females. In its classic form, associated chromosomal abnormalities or defects of the central nervous system, heart, and digestive tract are extremely uncommon. Thus, bladder exstrophy is usually an isolated defect of the genitourinary system. Furthermore, surgical techniques have been developed and refined such that reconstruction is now performed with the expectation that these children will enjoy an excellent quality of life. This is an extremely important consideration in the modern era of prenatal diagnosis in which concerned parents will likely seek consultation regarding the impact of this defect on their child's future.

### Evidence

From a scientific standpoint, studies regarding bladder exstrophy and epispadias are limited by the extreme rarity of the condition. The overwhelming majority of literature on this subject

R. Rabinowitz et al. (eds.), *Pediatric Urology for the Primary Care Physician*, Current Clinical Urology,
DOI 10.1007/978-1-60327-243-8_15, © Springer Science+Business Media New York 2015

exists as small, single institution series which are often retrospective and span several decades. There has been recent interest in the regionalization of the management of complex surgical problems such as this, with the potential for a benefit on outcomes research. Indirectly, however, we can glean the importance of treating this condition from several studies which have investigated the profound negative impact of urinary incontinence and sexual dysfunction on quality of life and social and psychological well-being.

Children with bladder exstrophy can survive without surgical reconstruction. The earliest descriptions of treatment focused on the development of an apparatus that could suitably fit over the exposed bladder to absorb the urine and keep the clothes dry. Beyond the social implications, however, left untreated, the chronic exposure of the bladder mucosa to the environment is harmful and over time may lead to painful ulcerations and even malignant changes. Excision of the bladder template and urinary diversion in the form of ureterosigmoidostomy were popularized as the first continence procedure for bladder exstrophy. Although this procedure was successful in some cases and is still used in some parts of the world today, long-term outcomes have been disappointing, and the risk of rectal cancer at the ureteral anastomotic site has been a cause for this approach to be largely abandoned in regions where modern closure techniques are available.

## Diagnosis

### Prenatal

Diagnosis by prenatal ultrasound (US) is possible and becoming more common with advances in sonographic techniques. An absence of bladder filling is the most common characteristic fetal finding. Other suggestive findings include: an anterior abdominal mass, low-set umbilicus, abnormal widening of the iliac crests, and an anteriorly displaced scrotum with a small phallus in male fetuses [2]. The differential diagnoses include cloacal exstrophy, omphalocele, and gastroschisis. The use of maternal magnetic resonance imaging (MRI) in the antenatal evaluation of severe congenital defects is being investigated.

## History

Historical information contributes minimally to the diagnoses. Routine questions regarding the prenatal course, maternal health, and family medical history are warranted.

## Physical Exam

In the absence of prenatal diagnosis, bladder exstrophy/epispadias is readily diagnosed by physical examination at birth.

### General

Because these are typically isolated defects, children with exstrophy and epispadias are most often born at term and in no particular distress. The face, neck, thorax, lung, and heart exams are expected to be normal.

### Abdomen

The umbilicus is lower than normal and is involved in the defect. Below the umbilicus and starting from it, the exstrophic bladder template is visible as a circular patch of reddened mucosa from which the ureteral orifices will actively drain urine (Figs. 15.1 and 15.2). Polyps may develop on the template over time secondary to exposure of the fragile urine-soaked mucosa to the environment. The pubic symphysis is variably separated, and the diastasis between the two sides is palpable. In children with isolated epispadias, the bladder is not exposed, but pubic separation may still be present.

### Genitalia

The appearance of the genitalia varies depending on the sex. In males, the urethra lies as an open plate on the dorsal surface of the corporal bodies with the penis splayed open (Fig. 15.1). The pubic separation gives the corpora a shorter length and upward deflection. The corpora are, however, wider than normal. The testes are usually descended, but inguinal hernias are extremely common (especially in males). In females, the pubic diastasis results in an absence of a mons pubis with a bifid clitoris and lateral displace-

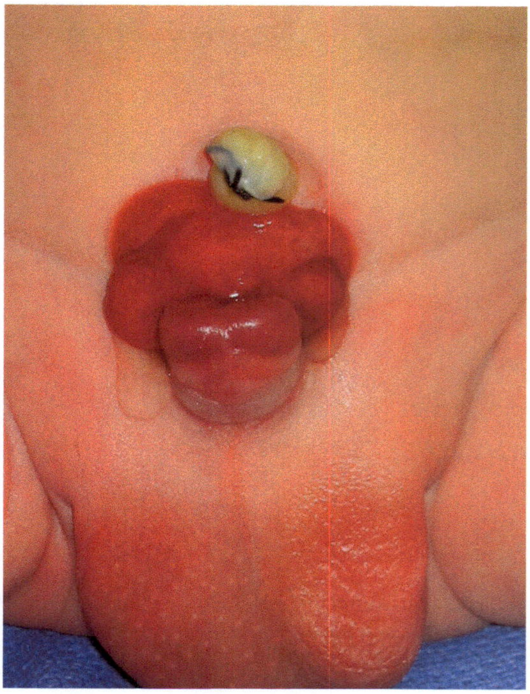

**Fig. 15.1** Newborn male with bladder exstrophy and epispadias. Note the silk suture on the umbilical stump

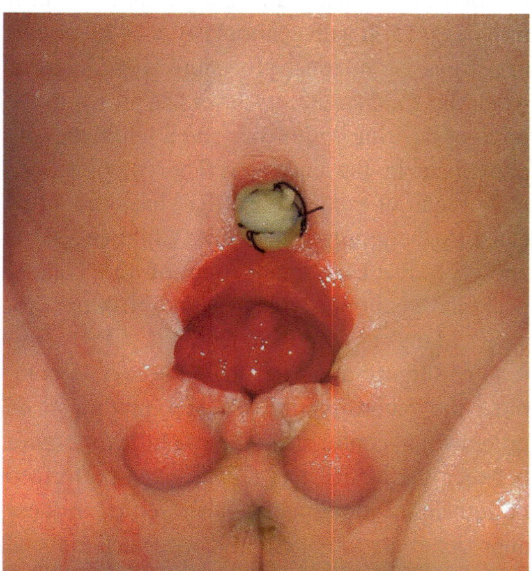

**Fig. 15.2** Newborn female with bladder exstrophy. Note the anterior displacement of the anus. The female genitalia are repaired during the time of primary closure

ment of the labia (Fig. 15.2). The anus is typically patent with normal sphincter innervation, but the location is displaced anteriorly when compared to controls.

## Evaluation

### Laboratory

No immediate laboratory information is required. However, in children who will undergo immediate closure, type and screen with baseline CBC, serum electrolytes, and coagulation studies will assist in preparation for surgery.

### Imaging

#### KUB

A plain abdominal radiograph allows for precise measurement of the pubic diastasis. This factor is considered in the surgical approach as described below.

#### Renal US

A baseline renal sonogram should be obtained.

### Cross-Sectional Imaging

The use of computed tomography (CT) and MRI in the presurgical planning is investigational. Comparison studies of pelvic anatomy before and after closure have provided useful insights that allow for ongoing modification of surgical technique.

### Procedures

The umbilical cord should be ligated with a heavy silk suture (Fig. 15.1). If a plastic cord clamp is used initially, this should be changed in order to prevent it from irritating the bladder mucosa. Likewise, the bladder template should be kept moist with periodic saline irrigation and covered with either a hydrated gel or Saran-type dressing. Petroleum-based gauze dressings are discouraged as they may dry and denude the mucosa when removed.

## Consultation

Consultation with a pediatric urologist with experience in exstrophy management should be made at the time of diagnosis. As mentioned previously, prenatal diagnoses and counseling are becoming more common. In the event that the diagnosis is made at delivery, immediate urologic consultation is appropriate. This consultation is urgent as the timing of initial closure may have an impact on management (as detailed below). Orthopedic consultation may be necessary depending on the need for osteotomy.

## Management

### Role of Primary Care in Initial Management

One advantage of prenatal diagnosis is that it allows time for movement to a center with the proper anesthetic, surgical, critical care, and nursing resources. Full-term delivery by cesarean section is recommended. The bladder template should be maintained, covered, and moistened with saline as needed until closed. If delayed closure is necessary, pediatricians should be aware of the high incidence of indirect inguinal hernia and the potential for incarceration while awaiting surgery. Latex precautions should be universally used because of the high incidence of latex sensitivity developing in these children after numerous surgical procedures.

## Initial Closure

The details of surgical closure are provided elsewhere and are beyond the scope of this text [3]. With respect to technique, there are two approaches to anatomic closure which are most commonly used in North America. The modern staged reconstruction of exstrophy (MSRE) has been popularized by the group at Johns Hopkins. This approach involves initial closure of the bladder, abdominal wall, and pelvis at or near birth (Fig. 15.3) with genitoplasty at 6–12 months of age and a continence procedure after 5 years or when the child's maturity level has grown to the point of desiring continence and a willingness to participate in the endeavor. The complete primary repair of exstrophy (CPRE) has been advocated by the group from Seattle Children's. This approach involves remodeling of the bladder neck and genitoplasty at the time of initial closure. Many children undergoing CPRE still require surgery at a later time in order to complete the reconstruction of their urethra or in order to gain continence. There is little difference between the MSRE and CPRE when performed on females. The ultimate goals of either of these approaches are to obtain the same functional and cosmetic results. A direct comparison of the two methods has not been performed.

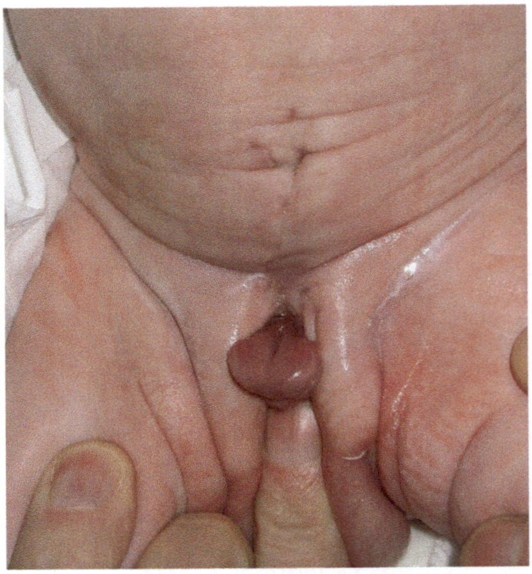

**Fig. 15.3** Male from Fig. 15.1 following primary closure in the MSRE approach. Note that this leaves the child with epispadias which is repaired during the first year of life

The timing of initial closure requires consideration for the child's age and size of the bladder template. The bladder template size can be initially evaluated in the nursery by the pediatric urologist using a pair of sterile gloves. Examination is subsequently performed under anesthesia by the surgeon. In children with a suitable bladder template, closure within the first 72 h of life is preferable if all necessary resources are available. Within these first 3 days, the infant's pelvis is usually malleable enough such that closure is possible without osteotomy (cutting of the pubic bones). Osteotomy is performed in conjunction with closure in the following circumstances: (1) outside of the initial 72-h window in primary closures (i.e., delayed closure), (2) primary closures associated with an extremely wide pubic diastasis, and (3) repeat closure after failure of the primary closure (i.e., secondary closure). Postoperatively, the children are placed in traction and immobilized for 4–6 weeks depending on the type of closure and use of osteotomy. This state of immobilization presents a number of unique challenges (feeding, pain control, parental bonding) and potential complications (skin breakdown, neurovascular injury). It takes a team of dedicated physicians, nurses, and social workers to help the patient and family get through this time.

## Genitoplasty

The genital defect was described above. Female genitoplasty is performed at the time of bladder closure regardless of the approach. In males, the alternate approaches have been outlined with respect to timing. In boys whom genitoplasty is delayed until 6–12 months of age, the intramuscular injection of testosterone enanthate (2 mg/kg) 5 and 2 weeks prior to surgery helps to promote phallic growth [4]. The pediatric urologist might ask the pediatrician to assist with this task. The goals of genitoplasty are to relocate the urethra to the ventral side of the corporal bodies while producing a phallus that is as long and straight as possible. This requires some maneuvers to gain length and correct dorsal chordee. After the initial reconstruction, some children will return after puberty for cosmetic "touch up" procedures to correct minor residual defects of the urethra, glans, or corpora.

## Continence

Regardless of the type of initial anatomic reconstruction, most children with exstrophy will ultimately require some type of procedure to address urinary incontinence secondary to the lack of a normal sphincter mechanism. The ability of the bladder to grow and achieve a reasonable (approximately 100 mL) capacity appears to portend a good prognosis. Children who reach this size are candidates for bladder neck reconstruction which carries the hope of dryness with volitional voiding. Patients with small bladders that do not grow and those who have suboptimal outcomes following a bladder neck reconstruction may still achieve continence through bladder augmentation. Bladder augmentation incorporates a bowel segment into the native bladder in order to increase capacity and the potential to store urine. Depending on the degree of incontinence, procedures designed to tighten the bladder outlet may be done in conjunction. These range from bladder neck narrowing procedures to complete transaction and closure. Once the bladder is augmented and the bladder neck altered, effective emptying usually requires the use of intermittent catheterization. Because exstrophy children have sensate genitalia and anatomically abnormal urethras, self-catheterization via the urethra may be difficult. The creation of a catheterizable stoma using either appendix or a small piece of bowel alleviates these troubles. A very small minority of children, mostly girls, will achieve continence without any of these procedures.

## Ongoing Role of Primary Care Physician

### Growth

Children with exstrophy are prone to growth retardation and decreased bone mineralization [5]. Short stature may be even more pronounced in children who have undergone bladder augmentation with intestinal segments and suffer from chronic metabolic acidosis, but the evidence on this is conflicting. Routine monitoring of growth with standard charting is recommended with the addition of electrolytes in patients who have undergone bladder augmentation. Patients with poor growth should be further evaluated with bone mineral density testing and consideration for endocrinology referral in abnormal cases.

## Renal Development

Children with bladder exstrophy require routine annual surveillance of their kidneys starting at the time of a baseline ultrasound done at birth. Prior to reimplantation, nearly all children with exstrophy have vesicoureteral reflux (VUR) and are maintained on a daily dose of antibiotic prophylaxis. Pyelonephritis following reconstructive surgeries is a cause for further evaluation to exclude obstruction. Renal/bladder sonogram is the preferred screening exam as this provides excellent initial information regarding the status of the kidneys with no radiation exposure. Subsequent work-up can be tailored by the pediatric urologist based on the results of the ultrasound.

## Recognition of Potential Surgical Complications

Children with exstrophy typically require several surgeries before achieving an acceptable functional and cosmetic result. In the short-term, most patients are seen at regular intervals by the pediatric urologist following a major reconstructive surgery. Pediatricians should have a low threshold for contacting the surgeon with concerns during this time. In the long-term, however, pediatricians play a critical role in the recognition and triage of postsurgical complications that might develop between routine visits.

In the newborn, after primary or delayed closure, frequent urinary infections may indicate obstruction to the free flow of urine from outlet stenosis. Prolapse of the bladder mucosa or frank bladder dehiscence may also occur when the initial closure fails.

The incidence of long-term complications and need for surgical revision following reconstruction of the lower urinary tract are very high (30–40 %). Bladder stones are quite common, particularly when the bladder has been augmented with bowel. Patients typically complain of symptoms of cystitis (frequency, urgency, dysuria) and may report blood or particulate material on catheterization. Children with augmented bladders should perform a mechanical saline irrigation on a scheduled basis following surgery. Routine urine cultures are difficult to interpret in patients who have undergone bladder augmentation and perform intermittent catheterization, as these specimens are nearly universally colonized with bacteria. Cultures should be obtained for symptomatic cystitis and clinical evidence of pyelonephritis. Upper tract imaging is always warranted in patients with the latter, especially following a ureteral reimplantation. Stomal stenosis is a common long-term complication in children with exstrophy who require a catheterizable channel. Other stomal problems include prolapse, bleeding, parastomal hernia, and polyp formation. Pediatricians should make a point of examining these stomal sites and always inquire about catheterization schedules and habits.

## Psychological Aspects

Children with bladder exstrophy face a significant chronic health condition that imparts many unique demands [6]. Exstrophy patients face challenges in practical life and relationships. They must confront anxiety regarding their physical differences and the potential for multiple surgical procedures. Ultimately the quality of life of children with exstrophy is determined not only by the outcome of their medical and surgical care but by their ability to develop essential coping mechanisms. While the strong resilience of many of these patients is reassuring and gratifying, recent reports of increased post-traumatic stress disorders (PTSD) and suicidal ideations are a cause for significant concern. Active surveillance of mental health is recommended with specialist referral for those in need.

## Fertility/Sexual Issues

Concerned parents will often have questions regarding the potential for future fertility and sexual relationships. Males with bladder exstrophy are likely infertile but are candidates for advanced reproductive techniques such as intracytoplasmic sperm injection. Females with exstrophy have successfully carried and delivered children. Females are particularly prone to uterine prolapse, and for this reason, delivery by cesarean section is recommended. Although a number of familial cases of bladder exstrophy have been reported, the genetics is not well understood. A 1:70 transmission rate to progeny from an affected parent has been cited [7]. The long-term sexual health of men and women with exstrophy is the focus of ongoing study. From an anatomical standpoint, the reconstructed male phallus can be expected to be shorter and wider with some level of upward deflection but suitable for vaginal intercourse. The exstrophic female vaginal canal and internal genitalia is usually normal. The configuration of the external genitalia is a reflection of the surgical reconstruction. Stenosis of the vaginal introitus is possible with obvious implications on intercourse. As stated above, exstrophy patients also face significant issues of self-esteem and anxiety that must be overcome in developing sexual relationships.

## Conclusions

The birth of a child with exstrophy marks the start of a lifelong journey and the promise of a formidable surgical undertaking that usually starts within days and lasts through adolescence. Bladder exstrophy tends to be an isolated defect, and thus, a quality surgical repair and diligent surveillance for potential complications portend the hope for an excellent quality of life. In this challenging group of patients, the importance of cooperation between specialists and primary care providers could not be greater.

## References

1. Kiddoo DA, Carr MC, Dulczak S, Canning DA. Initial management of complex urological disorders: bladder exstrophy. Urol Clin North Am. 2004;31(3):417–26, vii-viii.
2. Gearhart JP, Ben-Chaim J, Jeffs RD, Sanders RC. Criteria for the prenatal diagnosis of classic bladder exstrophy. Obstet Gynecol. 1995;85(6):961–4.
3. Gearhart JP, Mathews RI. Exstrophy-Epispadias. In: Wein AJ, editor. Campbell-Walsh urology. 9th ed. Philadelphia: Saunders; 2007. p. 3497–553.
4. Gearhart JP, Jeffs RD. The use of parenteral testosterone therapy in genital reconstructive surgery. J Urol. 1987;138(4 Pt 2):1077–8.
5. Canturk F, Tander B, Tander B, et al. Bladder exstrophy: effects on bone age, bone mineral density, growth, and metabolism. Bone. 2005;36(1):69–73.
6. Wilson CJ, Pistrang N, Woodhouse CR, Christie D. The psychosocial impact of bladder exstrophy in adolescence. J Adolesc Health. 2007;41(5):504–8.
7. Shapiro E, Lepor H, Jeffs RD. The inheritance of the exstrophy-epispadias complex. J Urol. 1984;132(2): 308–10.

# 16 Daytime Wetting

Julian Wan

## Introduction

Nocturnal enuresis is often considered one of the most embarrassing problems a child can face in childhood. Because it occurs at night and at home, however, it is possible often to limit the social effect, albeit at times by making social sacrifices. Families can keep their children out of overnight school field trips or sleepovers. They may turn down camp-out invitations. They work out discreet solutions with chaperones and camp counselors. Daytime incontinence on the other hand can be quite vexing to both the child and family. If it seems to occur particularly in a sporadic fashion or with little warning, it can be very frustrating. The child and family may feel "caught" by the wetting and have a sense of being powerless to prevent future occurrences. This chapter is a survey of the primary causes of daytime incontinence in children. It will review the general concepts underlying the basic approach to evaluating and treating a child who has daytime wetting. Specific conditions that cause daytime incontinence will be discussed and guidance offered on targeted therapies.

J. Wan, M.D. (✉)
Department of Urology, Division of Pediatric Urology, CS Mott Children's Hospital, 1500 East Medical Center Drive, 3875 Taubman Center, Ann Arbor, MI 48109, USA
e-mail: juliwan@umich.edu

## Natural History of Continence Control

Normal bladder control in a child requires several basic parts of the anatomy to be complete and normal. There must be an intact neural system. The coordination of voiding is mediated in the pontine micturition center of the brain stem. External sphincter relaxation is synchronized to occur just prior to detrusor contraction. There must be a normal and intact urinary system. These two components are sufficient to have a physiologically safe system. Healthy babies and pre-toilet-trained children, for example, store and void using just these two components without any consequences [1]. In addition to these two components, continence requires that there is a conscious perception of what are occurring during storage and voiding and an understanding of the social norms associated with continence. In a sense, every normal child already has the mechanism of continence but has to learn when and where it is appropriate to void.

Babies and pre-toilet-trained children store urine under low pressure until the volume reaches the bladder functional capacity at which point the external sphincter relaxes, the bladder neck opens, and the detrusor contracts. These actions occur in a synchronized sequence that is essentially reflexic. It is involuntary, and there is little social awareness as anyone who has ever been

R. Rabinowitz et al. (eds.), *Pediatric Urology for the Primary Care Physician*, Current Clinical Urology, DOI 10.1007/978-1-60327-243-8_16, © Springer Science+Business Media New York 2015

voided upon while changing a baby's diaper can attest. Adults in contrast perceive when their bladders are becoming full and have awareness typically *long before* the functional capacity is reached. They can then choose to voluntarily initiate the voiding process. Likewise they can inhibit or delay the voiding reflex for often extended periods of time until it is socially convenient to void.

The transition from the pattern of babies and incontinent children to the adult pattern passes through several phases. First, the child must be able to sense bladder fullness and link the sensation to a mental perception of fullness. This usually occurs around age 1–2 years. Next, the child must have awareness and perception of the external sphincter. The earliest means of continence control is squeezing the external sphincter in response to a detrusor contraction. This may be an extension of voluntary control over the guarding reflex [2]. It may be also at this period of time, around age 2–4 years, that avoidance maneuvers such as the Vincent's curtsy can occur [3]. This is the maneuver wherein a child tucks the heel under the perineum and sits on it. This action presses up against the perineum thereby tightening the pelvic muscles. By age 3–5 years, most children have developed an adult pattern of voiding. They are aware of bladder fullness and perceive what that sensation means. They can inhibit the micturition reflex temporarily until it is socially appropriate and can initiate voiding even when bladder volume is less than the functional capacity. By age 6 years, the vast majority of children (>75 %) have achieved daytime continence, and the majority are dry at night [4].

Children before they can be expected to void like adults, therefore, must be able to do the following. They must have awareness of bladder fullness and understand what that sensation means. They must be able to void before they are compelled to void at their functional capacity. They must understand or want to understand the social norms of continence. Many of the problems we encounter in children struggling to achieve daytime relate to a failure to fully achieve these capabilities.

## Structure of this Chapter

This chapter focuses on daytime continence issues. Often daytime continence problems occur simultaneously with nighttime wetting or other issues. Separate chapters elsewhere cover topics that are often associated with daytime wetting, including classic or monosymptomatic nocturnal enuresis; neurogenic bladder; incontinence in patients with renal failure; wetting after failed prior continence procedures; wetting associated with bowel problems; wetting after chemotherapy, radiation therapy, and trauma; adult and recalcitrant nocturnal enuretics; and wetting due to congenital or anatomical anomalies.

General concepts related to the evaluation of any child with daytime wetting problems will first be discussed. Specific causes of daytime wetting will then be covered. Finally treatment techniques will be discussed, particularly those which related to changing toilet habits and voiding patterns.

## A Practical Approach Toward Evaluation

### General Concepts

Most children achieve some degree of daytime continence by age 5 years old. If they do not achieve any significant period of continence (6 months or more), they are defined as having primary daytime incontinence. Children who have achieved at least 6 months or more of continence before becoming incontinent are defined as having secondary incontinence. About 70 % of affected children have primary incontinence [5]. This differentiation is important. Secondary incontinence is usually the result of a change in a previously normal function and supports the assumption that the internal anatomy and function is inherently normal in the past. It implies that something new has occurred that has altered the normal state. When searching for a cause, it should logically therefore be aimed at discerning what has changed recently in the child's life. Has there been some social upheaval such as a death, birth, divorce, job loss, or other major events? Did they move? Has the child been enrolled into a new school? Is there a new member in the household?

Children who have never been continent for a sustained period of time may have a variety of causes. Some may have congenital anomalies which were previously unrecognized until the child failed when attempting to achieve continence [6]. Occasionally there are children who have only just gained control of their bladders and may have done very well for 6–12 months before relapsing and having wetting episodes. Up to 10 % of children fall into this category [6]. The vast majority of these children later do regain control and typically do not have any underlying conditions. It is not known why this relapse occurs. It has been speculated that it may simply represent that the achievement of control is not a fixed event but can have a spectrum wherein some children gain stable persistent control a bit earlier, and others don't achieve this until 6–12 months later. Another point to remember is our adult perceptions are unlike that of a child. We view the achievement of toilet control as a developmental building block leading to other accomplishments. Some inexperienced parents mistakenly expect that each child will automatically hit their developmental landmarks and proceed as if on an agenda. Their child may be very interested in the toilet, the whole toileting process, or the kiddie potty, but in much the same way as they can be very interested in a particular toy. They can be fascinated for a short intense period of time, but that does not necessarily mean they are achieving continence; 6 months later they are no longer as interested much as they can lose interest in a toy.

Other studies suggest that intermittent periods of urgency, frequency, and incontinence may be normal in otherwise healthy children up to age 7 [5, 7, 8]. Some experts therefore advocate taking a less aggressive and more patient approach until the child is in primary school. Girls are more commonly affected than boys in general across age groups [9]. Several risk factors have been associated with daytime wetting although definite causative links have not been established. They include a strong family history in parents and siblings, social upheaval or disturbance (social trauma such as a death of parent, sibling, loss of home, divorce, and refugee status), neuropsychiatric pathology, mild and minor neuropsychiatric dysfunction (attention-deficit disorder, hyperactivity disorder), general developmental delay, and physical and sexual abuse.

Families with children now live more complex and busier lives than they did in the past. There are more social pressures to have better and earlier toilet control. Many day care centers, for example, will not accept a child until daytime continence is achieved. As physicians we must try to be sure the expectations of the families are reasonable and that our evaluation is appropriate and measured. A general strategy when addressing wetting is to divide the patients into three categories depending on when the wetting occurs. This separates the patients into these groups: wetting only at night, wetting in the day and night, and daytime-only wetting. Though there are always exceptions, one can use these observations to help organize an evaluation and treatment process. For patients who are wet only at night, it suggests that when the children are awake and conscious, they are able to understand what is occurring in their bladders and act accordingly. It is when they are unconscious that there are problems, and so one could argue teleologically that the underlying anatomy is probably intact and functional. For patients who are wet day and night, one has to consider nearly all of the possible causes of wetting. The occurrence of wetting regardless of the state of consciousness suggests that whatever is probably occurring does so below the level of the child's mind or volition. Finally in cases of daytime-only wetting, one is left with the interesting situation that wetting occurs only when the children are conscious. When they are asleep, they are dry, and so one must conclude that their unconscious selves do a better job at maintaining continence than when they are awake. The old saying reminds us that, "one should never say never." These basic observations are not foolproof but help to provide a framework for the subsequent approach.

The initial evaluation of any child with daytime incontinence is no different than those with any sort of voiding disorder. It should begin with a detailed voiding and bowel history, a physical exam, and a urinalysis. In some cases other non-invasive testings such as uroflow, postvoid residual (PVR) using ultrasound, or pad or diaper weighing have value. In a few specific diagnoses, more invasive testing with x-ray imaging, urodynamics, and cystoscopy may be warranted. In the vast majority of cases, however, daytime wetting can be effectively evaluated and treated without resorting to testing beyond the history, physical, and urinalysis.

## Directed History

Whenever possible the history must be obtained from both the child and the parents or guardians. The history should start from the beginning and include birth history, noting prematurity, time, if any, spent in the neonatal care unit, and if the child was sent home with auxiliary care such as home oxygen. If positive these findings suggest that there may be a risk of developmental delay. One should also inquire if the prenatal ultrasound noted any abnormalities in the urinary system. Occasionally a duplicated system or even a posterior urethral valve can be overlooked particularly if the child had some other concomitant illnesses which preoccupied the family and treating physicians [10]. The rest of the general history should inquire as to any known neurological and congenital abnormalities. Is the child achieving the expected development milestones? Is the child otherwise voiding and defecating in a normal manner? Young and inexperienced parents may not always be sure what is normal and have only their own habits and behavior to use. Be sure when conducting the history that the interviewer's understanding of what is "normal" is similar to what the parents report as "normal." For parents who do not have much experience and who do not have grandparents or more experienced parents to consult with, their understanding can be naïve and primitive. Any urine coming out may be misconstrued as being "normal" voiding. Be sure to inquire specifically about wetting outside of daytime wetting. Patients with both day- and nighttime wetting encompass a wider possibility of causes than those who only have daytime wetting. Families and patients (particularly older children and adolescents) sometimes focus more on what is most socially annoying to them and so downplay or ignore wetting at other times, inadvertently making the evaluation less clear.

The past medical and surgical history should include any surgical procedures especially those involving the back, central nervous system (CNS), bowel, genitalia, bladder, kidney, or urethra. Significant illnesses such as meningitis should be noted along with any documented urinary tract infections. For older children and adolescents, sexual development and menarche should be noted. The family history should note any familial disorders and history of familial voiding issues. The current family structure and living situation should be recorded in the social history, noting any recent sudden changes. A general review of systems should be done looking for any other issues. Children who have other major health issues early in life can be delayed developmentally simply because they have spent a large amount of their life sick, in the hospital, or recuperating from treatment.

There should be a detailed voiding and bowel history. The age of toilet training (if achieved) should be noted and the course of the daytime wetting described. A toileting diary can be helpful in gathering accurate data. Elaborate surveys are not needed, and a simple grid noting the date and time of toilet use is more than sufficient. Specific data should include the frequency and pattern of voiding and defecation and when wetting occurs. These tools are needed because the recall of toilet habits is not always reliable despite well-meaning patients and guardians. When asked about basic information such as how often the child voids, these parents often do not know because they are unaware of the actual pattern of toilet use once the child has some semblance of control and independence. Be especially wary when the parents give the nondescript answer of "normal." What is normal of an adult is not normal for a child. The normal adult frequency of voiding is only 3 or 4 times from the time they arise in the morning to the time they turn in to bed at night. For primary school-age children, such a frequency is very low. In a survey of normal children in the primary school-age range, only 10 % voided as infrequently as 4 times per day [11]. Seek out details about the nature of voiding. Does the child use avoidance maneuvers (also called holding maneuvers)? These are repetitive actions which are often observed by the family such as squatting down on a toy or heel of the foot (Vincent's curtsy), crossing the legs, or dancing about (doing the "potty dance"). Does the child have to run to the bathroom at the last moment? When does the wetting occur? Is it the same time of day each time? Are there activities which are associated with wetting? Is the wetting associated with giggling and laughing? Finally when the child does void, is the stream strong and straight? Does it deflect or angle off? Is there hesitation or straining?

In addition to voiding frequency and pattern, one needs to know about bowel habits. Is the child constipated? Does he/she strain at stool? How often does the child have a bowel movement? Has the child needed help in the past with bowel movements? The typical child has a bowel movement every day or every other day. If the time between bowel movements is greater than that be suspicious of constipation. Ask about the size and consistency of the stool. Very large bowel movements (e.g., the parents report that the child can clog the toilet or have to break up the bowel movement prior to flushing) are also suspicious of constipation. Is the child also suffering from fecal soiling? If so, how often is this happening and for how long?

## Pertinent Physical Examination

The physical examination should begin with a global sense of development. If the child is in primary school, is the child at an age-appropriate grade? Does the child strike you as being appropriate in terms of affect and behavior? Can the child perform basic tasks and follow and understand the questions directed toward him/her during the exam? The physical examination should include testing of perineal sensation and reflexes (can the child plantar and dorsiflex?). Is the anal sphincter tone normal? Particular attention should be paid to the back, genitals, and urethra. Funny tufts of hair along the back and irregular clefts or grooves especially those who run deep and whose base cannot be visually inspected are noteworthy and suggest an occult spinal dysraphism. Asymmetry of the buttock, anal verge, legs, and feet is an additional sign. When examining the abdomen, note if the bladder or colon is palpable. Note the underwear; sometimes the history is grossly underestimated, and the underwear bearing signs of past episodes of wetting and soiling is a far more accurate record.

## Urinalysis

A basic urinalysis is needed during the initial evaluation of every child for daytime wetting. The usual parameters should be examined (specific gravity, pH, dipstick testing for glucose, protein, nitrites, leukocytes, and hemoglobin). If the urine is suspicious, microscopy is recommended along with culture and antibiotic sensitivities. An inconclusive or ambiguous dipstick does not rule out a UTI—only a true culture can do that.

## Ancillary Diagnostic Tools

### Toilet Diary

The toilet diary is probably the most useful ancillary tool. Once the child has a modicum of control and independence, the parents often have only a very rudimentary sense of the actual daily habit and routine. It is typically a social disruption (i.e., extra laundry, difficulty enrolling in day care or after-school care) which triggers the initial consultation. The toilet diary is a useful tool in two ways. First, it is a diagnostic tool in helping to determine the actual pattern and frequency of voids. Second, once a treatment plan has been created, the toilet diary can serve as a way of tracking progress and ensuring that there is good compliance with the treatment regimen. For younger children up to early primary school age, the parents should help the children to fill in the data. Remember to be considerate of the child; don't make the child take the diary to school where inadvertent discovery by classmates could be devastating. Have the child track the habits on a separate slip of paper or notebook. Once at home the data could be transferred onto the main diary.

### Pad Testing

Some authors advocate the use of pad weighing to help to quantify wetting [12]. Pad weighing is clearly less subjective, but in most cases, their use is not necessary. Unlike in adult urology where chronically wet women and men have used pads historically as a primary means of management, the use among children with daytime-only wetting is limited. Other researchers have not found much utility with pad weighing with children; frankly the long-term goal of the patients and parents is usually no wetting, so quantification is usually not an issue [13].

### Uroflow and Postvoid Residual

Uroflow is a noninvasive means of measuring how rapidly the child is voiding. The child is asked to void with a full bladder into a special toilet or container which is equipped with a sensor so that the rate of urine flow can be tracked. The typical normal child will have a bell-shaped curve. The test is an excellent screening test but lacks specificity. In patients who have reports of hesitancy or slow stream, it may help identify anatomical issues such as a stricture or posterior urethral valves. Unfortunately it is not very specific, and so patients with poor flow due to poor bladder activity may not be differentiated. When ordering this test, be sure the child's bladder is full and there is an adequate volume. Ideally the voided volume should be at least 50 % of the estimated capacity by age [14]. For example, if the patient is 8 years old, one would like at least a voided volume of 150 mL (8+2=volume estimate by age +2 in ounces ≈ 300 mL). Uroflow may be of practical value in patients being treated with biofeedback. It is an effective noninvasive way of judging relaxation of the sphincter and pelvic muscles. The availability of inexpensive ultrasound devices dedicated to measuring bladder volume makes it possible to measure PVR noninvasively. The usual PVR is close to zero; although some normal children will have small PVRs of 5–7 mL. If the PVR is elevated it must be interpreted in terms of the estimated bladder capacity. Volumes which are over 30 mL and which are more than 10–15 % of the estimated bladder capacity may be significant [15–17].

These tests are simple to perform and noninvasive and do not use ionizing radiation. These advantages, however, should not lead to widespread indiscriminate use. They are most useful when applied to a patient with report of a poor or hesitant stream. The finding of a poor uroflow with a concomitant elevated PVR with daytime wetting would justify further more invasive testing. Likewise if the diagnostic picture assembled from the history, physical exam, and toilet diary is unclear or contradictory, it may be helpful to do these tests. For example, if the toilet diary suggests that the child is voiding regularly and frequently and, yet, there is still wetting between voids, one has to wonder about the efficacy and completeness of each void.

## Invasive Testing

Invasive testing is usually not required to evaluate and treat the vast majority of patients. Their use is most effective when the noninvasive methods have not been able to clarify the situation or if there is a specific question which cannot be resolved by any other less invasive method. Symptoms which indicate a need for further invasive evaluation include recurrent or febrile UTI, continuous incontinence, prior urological surgery, or known GU anomaly. Findings of occult spinal dysraphism at physical exam and abnormal uroflow and marked elevated PVR (suggesting some bladder dysfunction or significant obstruction) all need further evaluation. These tests include voiding cystourethrogram (VCUG), urodynamics, and more complex imaging such as magnetic resonance imaging (MRI).

## Voiding Cystourethrogram and Nuclear Medicine Renal Scans

The VCUG is usually indicated in children who have recurrent culture-proven UTI and can detect vesicoureteral reflux, abnormal bladder necks, and outlet obstructions (valves and strictures). It may also show nonneurogenic detrusor-sphincter dyssynergia, a situation where in the bladder and sphincter muscle act out of synch and work against each other. There is currently much discussion in the pediatric urology world as to the best approach to evaluating a child with recurrent UTI. Some advocate working up the bladder (so-called "bottom-up" approach) first with a VCUG. Others recommend working up only those who are susceptible to renal scarring (so-called "top-down" approach) by ordering a nuclear medicine renal scan [18, 19]. In this particular situation because wetting is the primary issue, at this time, it would be the author's opinion that until further evidence becomes available, the "bottom-up" approach starting with a VCUG should be considered when faced with both wetting and UTIs. The advantage is that not only would VUR be detected, but other issues of interest such as strictures, posterior valves, and completeness of emptying could be assessed.

## Urodynamics

Formal urodynamic studies (UDS) like other invasive studies are usually not necessary in the vast majority of children [20]. For neurologically normal children and those who have not had prior urological reconstructive surgery, urodynamics are rarely necessary. These studies attempt to recreate or simulate what happens to the child during urine storage, emptying, and ideally at time of wetting. The behavior of the bladder and urethra is tracked during this recreation. This monitoring is achieved by placing special catheters which have pressure sensors into the urethra and bladder or rarely suprapubically. These tests include the cystometrogram, urethral pressure profile, pelvic floor electromyography, and bladder and Valsalva leak point pressures. They can be done individually or in concert; fluoroscopy can also be added to visualize the behavior of the bladder and urethra. These tests can be done individually but usually are combined in concert to obtain the most information. The nuances of these tests and how they are carried out are beyond the scope of this chapter, but typically they can be carried out as an outpatient and do not last more than an hour or two. For children who are sensate and who may be anxious about being catheterized, it is sometimes necessary to put the child under general anesthesia very briefly and place and secure the urodynamic catheters before waking up the child for testing. The child must be fully awake for the test to be of value.

There are four main indications for urodynamics in children with daytime wetting. The first indication is to help diagnose neurogenic bladder disorders. If there are symptoms and signs (known prior history, back abnormalities, neurologic deficits) which raise the suspicion of neurogenic dysfunction, then urodynamics should be carried out. The primary study is the cystometrogram; additional tests are added depending on the nature of the voiding dysfunction. For children with daytime-only wetting, the principal concerns are with the parameters of bladder compliance, bladder activity, and bladder sphincter coordination. Bladder compliance refers to the ability of the bladder to accommodate increases in urine storage with minimal or no increase in pressure. The normal bladder will fill and expand over time with only a small increase in storage pressure. Patients with neuropathic bladders can have poor bladder compliance resulting in sporadic wetting when the bladder pressure is sufficiently high. Patients with neurogenic bladders can be overactive with contractions which occur at volumes less than the functional capacity and outside of volitional control. The other extreme, underactivity or hypoactivity, can also occur; these patients will fill well beyond their expected capacity but cannot generate a normal voiding contraction. Finally, normal emptying and storage occurs in synchronization with the urinary sphincter mechanism. During normal filling, the sphincter mechanism is active to help preserve continence. When normal capacity is reached, the normal sequence is to have the sphincter mechanism relax and open prior to the contraction of the bladder. In some cases of neuropathic bladder and all cases of nonneurogenic neurogenic bladder, this coordination is lost, and the bladder and sphincter mechanism contracts and relaxes out of sequence. At times they contract simultaneously and end up working against each other. This lack of coordination is termed detrusor-sphincter dyssynergia and is commonly seen when there is some neuropathology between the sacral spine and pontine micturition center.

The second use of urodynamics is when there is some specific anatomical condition suspected to be associated with wetting. For example, if daytime wetting is only associated with straining, coughing, or heavy lifting, urodynamics can help both not only to quantify the degree of exertion needed to cause wetting but also to offer insight into a possible cause. True stress incontinences are very rare among children, but if the history and findings suggest this possibility, then urodynamics would be worthwhile.

The third application of urodynamics is in the diagnosis of patients with nonneurogenic neurogenic bladder (see later discussion) [21, 22]. This is a condition which by definition is a diagnosis of exclusion. Afflicted children present with physical findings on imaging studies consistent with severe obstruction or neuropathology, yet all workup fails to find any such issues. The etiology is believed to be a severe bladder sphincter dyssynergia.

Finally urodynamics are needed to help puzzle out patients with daytime wetting who have failed all prior conventional treatments. They may serve to help confirm the absence of more severe concerns thereby giving resolve and reassurance to carry on with other therapies. When all conventional treatments have been unsuccessful and more invasive and irreversible therapies are being contemplated, urodynamics should definitely be carried out.

### Other Studies

When history, physical findings, symptoms, and signs justify, a MRI scan of the lumbosacral spine should be carried out looking for a tethered cord or other occult neuropathology. Kidney and bladder ultrasound (USN) is commonly done to rule out any occult anatomical issue such as a duplex system with an ectopic insertion. Unless there is compelling evidence on imaging studies, history, or physical exam of urethral pathology or bladder obstruction, cystoscopy has no role in the evaluation of daytime wetting.

## Differential Diagnosis

The International Children's Continence Society Standardization Committee document recognizes eight conditions as possible causes of nonneurogenic daytime wetting [23]. They can usually be diagnosed, and treatment can be begun with only a good history, physical exam, and some basic noninvasive methods. If there is no clinical improvement, more invasive methods can then be carried out (See Table 16.1).

### Pseudo-Daytime-Only Wetting

Before discussing the differential diagnosis in detail, one should be aware of conditions which can mimic daytime-only wetting. These conditions can be grouped under the heading of pseudo-daytime-only wetting. They should be distinguishable by a thorough history and physical exam. Occasionally they may present mislabeled as a case of daytime-only wetting.

**Table 16.1** Differential diagnosis of daytime-only wetting

| |
|---|
| Pseudo-daytime-only wetting |
| Duplicate ureter with ectopic insertion |
| Obstruction of urethra or bladder neck |
| Extraordinary urinary frequency syndrome |
| Urinary retention |
| Physical and sexual abuse |
| Urethral prolapse |
| Hypospadias and epispadias in girls |
| Overactive bladder |
| Infrequent voiding |
| Dysfunctional voiding |
| Underactive (hypoactive) bladder |
| Nonneurogenic neurogenic bladder |
| Dysfunctional elimination syndrome |
| Giggle incontinence |
| Vaginal voiding |

### Duplicate Ureter with Ectopic Insertion

During fetal development complete ureteral duplication can occur. Rather than a single ureter, there are two distinct ureters from the kidney carrying urine down toward the pelvis. The upper pole ureter can insert outside of the bladder. It can end up draining into the urethra, bladder neck, uterus, or vagina. These upper pole moieties can be quite small and poorly developed yet be sufficient enough to create wetting. The result of this ectopic insertion is a continuous slow drip by drip leakage. The patient paradoxically will report normal voiding and emptying yet will have continuous wetting. This condition can only occur in girls. Embryologically, the ureter cannot insert below the bladder neck and pelvic diaphragm in boys. The diagnosis can be suspected on ultrasound (USN) which can show an elongated kidney with two distinct renal pelves. Confirmatory testing includes intravenous urography (IVP), computed tomography (CT), or MRI. Nuclear medicine renal scans (dimercaptosuccinic acid [DMSA] or mercaptoacetyltriglycerine [MAG3]) can also be used. The definite treatment is surgical. The upper pool moiety can be removed (heminephrectomy), or the upper pole ureter can be connected the lower pole pelvis (ureteropyelostomy). Occasionally, it may be preferable to reimplant the ectopic ureter into the bladder.

### Obstruction of the Urethra or Bladder Neck

Patients with true obstruction of the urethra or bladder neck (stricture, posterior urethral valve, or rhabdomyosarcoma of the bladder neck or prostatic urethra) can present with dribbling incontinence after voiding in the daytime. Typically there will be a weak force of stream or in severe cases near-complete retention. The diagnosis is confirmed by VCUG. Treatment is dependent on the diagnosis; posterior valves and strictures are usually initially treated by endoscopic incision, and masses are typically staged by biopsy. Final therapy with the tumors is usually dependent on the clinical stage and pathological grade.

### Extraordinary Urinary Frequency Syndrome

Occasionally children up to about age 10 years will present with only markedly increased urinary frequency but with no pathological cause. This condition is termed extraordinary urinary frequency syndrome. The number of voids can be as high as 10–12 times when awake, sometimes several times in an hour, and often the children will even wake up and void at night. There is no history of UTI, and the force of stream is otherwise normal. There are no other associated issues. Usually the condition is self-limiting and resolves within 6 months. There is no known etiology, but some type of social change (new school, new sibling, etc.) has been found in many cases [24, 25].

### Urinary Retention

Complete retention with overflow wetting can occur in children and is often due to a combination of constipation, infrequent voiding, and urinary infection. Extrinsic or intrinsic masses while rare should be remembered as possible diagnoses. For young preschool-age children, bladder neck or prostatic rhabdomyosarcoma can obstruct normal urinary flow. For girls, external compression due to hydrometrocolpos can present with retention. Finally very large ovarian cyst can cause a marked sense of urgency and be confused with a distended bladder; USN will usually help to differentiate these conditions.

### Physical and Sexual Abuse

Physical and sexual abuse can manifest as urinary problems; occasionally only as daytime wetting. Some studies have suggested that up to one in five children prior to puberty experience some form of abuse [26]. Remember that many cases of abuse will not always have obvious physical signs. A lack of physical signs does not rule out abuse. Usually there is dramatic change in behavior. There may be regression of milestones and fearful behavior. In older school-age children, phobias, acting out, sleep disturbances, and overtly sexual behavior have all been reported. In addition to voiding issues, the most common symptoms are generalized vague complaints, such as headaches or stomachaches. A good history and keeping an open mind to this possibility are critical. When evaluating patients with voiding disorders, one must always consider the possibility of sexual abuse as an underlying cause of secondary voiding dysfunction, particularly in older children. Inquiring about the possibility of abuse should be included in the history. Many jurisdictions in the United States mandate reporting of suspicion by all physicians. Typically parents are aware of why you have to ask about this possibility. If the history leads to a suspicion of abuse, many facilities will have an established protocol. Often there are specific teams of physicians, nurses, and social workers who will carry forward the investigation.

## Urethral Prolapse, Hypospadias, and Epispadias in Girls

Young girls, particularly African-American girls, can prolapse their urethras [27]. No specific cause has been identified. There is laxity in the lining of the urethra and it rolls out. Ischemia and edema develop, and the girl may present with dysuria, poor emptying, and a dribbling incontinence. It is hard to miss this diagnosis because there is a characteristic edematous "doughnut"-shaped urethral opening on visual inspection. The treatment can be conservative with sitz baths to help reduce the swelling, hoping for natural reduction. When that fails, surgical resection is necessary.

Finally, epispadias and hypospadias are rare malformation anomalies of the female urethra and bladder neck. Usually this results in an incompetent continence mechanism and nearly continuous leakage of urine. A good physical exam should be sufficient with confirmatory testing on VCUG and MRI. Treatment usually requires surgery to reconstruct the bladder neck or to close it off and building a catheterizable channel.

## Overactive Bladder

The constellation of symptoms comprising urgency and frequency with or without incontinence is defined as being overactive bladder (OAB). The frequency must be greater than seven times per day. Overactive detrusor contraction during filling is the causative factor. In the history, avoidance maneuvers such as squatting, heel sitting, pressing on the perineum or genitalia, or walking on tiptoes are commonly reported. They occur as the child tries to suppress the urgency and thereby prevent wetting. For some children with recurrent wetting, the problem can worsen through the day owing to loss of concentration and fatigue. It may occur during the night leading to nocturia but not always nocturnal enuresis. Children with this problem often diminish their fluid intake to minimize wetting. Another form termed "dry OAB" manifests as a strong urge but is associated with little or no actual voided urine. There is only a tremendous sense of urgency. It can be equally disruptive causing the child to hurry to the bathroom but with no relief from voiding. This form usually occurs more commonly in older patients and the elderly. No specific single cause is known. The current theories suggest that overactivity maybe a manifestation of more generalized issues in the body which can affect also the bowel, mood, and behavior [28, 29].

A thorough history and a toilet diary will quantify the urinary frequency, small voided volumes, and urgency incontinence. Fluid intake in older children will often be low, and the urine specific gravity will be high. With normal voiding and emptying of the bladder, no further investigations are necessary before empiric therapy has begun. The only critical exception is if the child has had recurrent UTIs together with bladder problems. In these cases, assessment with renal and bladder ultrasound should be performed and, depending on the age of the child, a VCUG to look for VUR.

It is imperative to obtain a good bowel history. Constipation can both be a contributing factor and a side effect. Forceful contractions of the pelvic floor during avoidance maneuvers may lead to postponement of defecation. A constipated child will often be also an infrequent voider. Constipation and fecal soiling are often found in children with OAB, and this condition has to be treated simultaneously.

Treatment in children should always start with the standard approach addressing each of these concerns. From the toilet diary look to see if there is a pattern which could be accommodated by adjusting the child's daily activity. If a scheduled voiding pattern and normalizing habits do not correct the symptoms after 3–4 weeks or if there are tremendous social pressures on the child, anticholinergic drugs should also be started. Establishing a normal voiding pattern by promoting good habits and eliminating avoidance maneuvers along with judicious use of anticholinergic drugs are the foundations of any treatment of OAB. If the initial treatment is unsuccessful particularly if the results seem to call into question the original diagnosis, further UDS are indicated. The main concern is to exclude any other pathology, particularly occult neuropathy.

Should the condition prove to be recalcitrant to conventional therapy, other options such as neuromodulation and biofeedback can be offered. Sacral nerve neuromodulation has been used effectively in adults and older children [30, 31]. Biofeedback can also be used to help retrain the pelvic muscles; the aim being to teach the child how to fully relax the sphincter and pelvis. Many of these methods are invasive (with rectal or vaginal sensors) and require a lot of cooperation from the child and family. In some cases a less invasive approach using electromyography patches can be used. The child is taught to relax the pelvic muscles and to learn what contraction and relaxation feels like. Recently there have been successes reported with adapting computer video games to this use. The child's ability to control the pelvic muscles is tracked and used to manipulate game play [32]. For the most difficult cases, those who are unresponsive to any treatment, endoscopic suburothelial botulinum toxin type A injections to the detrusor muscle have been used, but this approach is not yet a standard therapy and is an off-label use (see below for further discussion).

The treatment of children with OAB is nearly always done as an outpatient. There have been reports of inpatient treatment or group treatments, but usually these methods have been only done in Europe and are not translatable at this time to a North American practice environment [33]. There are few studies of any rigor on the efficacy of any therapy only in OAB. Of the results available, signs and symptoms seems to disappear in about 50 % of the children. If pharmacotherapy is added, the cure rate seems to increase to 70 %, but the long-term stability without recidivism remains in question [33].

## Infrequent Voiding

Some children will wait until there is an overwhelming sense of urgency before attempting to void. They are not reacting to the earlier sense of mere fullness. This infrequent voiding pattern causes them to rush to the bathroom. Usually they are too late, and urge incontinence occurs. It has been theorized that the strong sphincter activity in infrequent voiding is a behavioral maladjustment of the guarding reflex and not a primary bladder/sphincter dysfunction [2, 34]. Usually this syndrome is considered an acquired disorder due to a combination of detrusor overactivity and voluntary overcompensation with the sphincter mechanism. The history will include urgency and incontinence with avoidance maneuvers, delay of voiding, and few voids per day. In the most cases, flow is often normal, and emptying is complete; testing with uroflow and bladder scan is usually not needed. In some extreme cases where there has been long-term distention, the PVR may be elevated. No invasive investigations are recommended in the initial phase. Treatment should start with standard the institution of a scheduled voiding program with 6–7 voiding efforts during the time the child is awake. The parents or guardians are asked to pick events which naturally punctuate the day into small chunks. These chunks do not have to be perfectly equidistant in time, but should be regular events. By choosing to schedule voiding attempts at these moments, there is no excuse that the child was too busy; it is easier to enforce and remember, and there are built-in reminders due to the regularity of these events. Mealtimes, coming and going to school, favorite morning or afternoon activity, bath time, and bedtime are all excellent choices to pick from. Children are encouraged to go to the toilet even if they do not feel any need; parents and guardians are instructed in front of the child not to negotiate, bargain, or otherwise alter this schedule. They are told never to ask the child if he or she "feels like going to the bathroom." If the patient had an accurate sense of this feeling, they would not be in the office seeking consultation. This treatment is usually the only one needed for improvement.

### Dysfunctional Voiding

Dysfunctional voiding refers to overactivity in the external sphincter or the pelvic floor during voiding, often with incomplete emptying as a result. The overactivity can be seen as a *staccato* flow pattern caused by intermittent contractions of pelvic floor activity during the voiding. This action results in dips in flow rate and coincides with high bladder pressure. It can also be seen as fractionated voiding with complete interruption of the stream. This pattern occurs if the detrusor contraction is weak, and so the urine flow comes to a complete halt when the pelvic floor contracts. To speed up micturition, these children often start to strain.

Because of incomplete emptying, UTIs are common. In addition to incontinence and straining at voiding, constipation is a common symptom. The number of daily voids can be normal or infrequent. There can also be urgency owing to the fact that most of the affected children also show signs of overactivity. Dysfunctional voiding can be suspected from the history and bladder diary alone. The uroflow is an easy noninvasive method to confirm the diagnosis. The PVR is often increased. In patients with dysfunctional voiding and a history of UTI, ultrasound of the kidneys and bladder is needed, and a VCUG to determine if VUR and renal damage are present. Urodynamic investigation is often indicated, especially if there is poor emptying. It is important to determine if the bladder problems are secondary to some form of neuropathology or if the bladder is hypocontractile.

Like other functional concerns, treatment should start with the standard advice on normalizing toilet habits, treatment of constipation, and antibiotic prophylaxis if there are recurrent UTIs. In children with decreased daytime voiding frequency (four or fewer), the number of micturitions should be increased to by a scheduled voiding program. Basic relaxed voiding training is often not enough to help these children keep their pelvic floor relaxed during voiding. Treatment is aimed at inducing full relaxation of the sphincter during voiding, with no residual urine. Strategies to achieve these goals include pelvic floor muscle awareness and timing training, repeated sessions of biofeedback visualization of pelvic floor activity, and relaxation. When large PVRs are present, especially in combination with recurrent UTIs, VUR, or renal scarring, clean intermittent self-catheterization (ISC) may be indicated. In these cases, α-blockers can also be an appropriate alternative before clean ISC is introduced.

Treatment efficacy can be measured by tracking improvement of bladder emptying and resolution of associated symptoms. Although some studies have evaluated the effects of the above-discussed treatment options in patients with dysfunctional voiding, only one was randomized [35]. From the studies available, it seems that standard therapy alone has a cure rate of approximately 50 % of patients with dysfunctional voiding. With addition of biofeedback, the cure rate would probably increase to 60–70 %.

### Underactive (Hypoactive) Bladder

The term underactive bladder (also known as a hypoactive or lazy bladder) is the counterpart to the OAB. This diagnosis is given only after confirmatory urodynamics show that detrusor activity is absent or diminished during voiding. The child empties the bladder in an abnormal fashion by abdominal straining. The bladder capacity is typically higher than normal, and the PVR can be markedly elevated; values of 50 % or more are not uncommon. The symptoms are usually infrequent voiding, straining and intermittent flow, recurrent UTI, incontinence, and often constipation. Treatment is aimed at improving bladder emptying. Clean ISC is the procedure of choice. Intravesical electrostimulation has been described, but it is not yet recommended as a routine procedure for children [36]. Intermittent catheterization achieves two goals: effective emptying and prevention of further detrusor muscle distention.

## Nonneurogenic Neurogenic Bladder

The nonneurogenic neurogenic bladder was first discussed by Hinman and colleagues in 1973. These patients present with the symptoms, signs, and findings on imaging studies consistent with a neuropathic bladder or a severely obstructed one. Paradoxically, there is no detectable neuropathology or obstruction. It is currently believed to be an extreme form of dysfunctional voiding; the patient is literally fighting against himself or herself. The history usually includes daytime and nighttime wetting, recurrent UTIs, and encopresis or constipation. Imaging of the upper and lower urinary tracts typically shows hydroureteronephrosis. In most cases, a thorough evaluation with renal scintigraphy, VCUG, and urodynamics is recommended. The VCUG typically shows a grossly trabeculated bladder (so-called Christmas tree bladder), and VUR is seen in half of patients [21, 22, 37]. Half of the patients have renal damage. A long futile past medical history with multiple failed surgeries aimed at correcting VUR can occur before the correct diagnosis is finally made. Urodynamics will show findings consistent with a neurogenic bladder; hyperreflexia with detrusor-sphincter dyssynergia is the classic finding. Due to the nature and rarity of the condition, it is a diagnosis of exclusion. A careful neurological exam and an MRI of the spinal cord must be done to rule out a neurogenic cause.

The management of nonneurogenic neurogenic bladder depends on the severity of the findings. It is similar to the approach used to treat neurogenic bladder dysfunction. Clean ISC and anticholinergic drugs are the mainstays of treatment. If the patient is noncompliant with clean ISC because of urethral discomfort, a catheterizable stoma (Mitrofanoff continent stoma) can be created. Temporary urinary diversion or augmentation cystoplasty may be necessary, if bladder compliance is poor. These can be quite challenging cases, and often the key is early recognition before unnecessary and ineffectual surgeries have been performed.

## Dysfunctional Elimination Syndrome

When bowel dysfunction is found simultaneously with nonneurogenic voiding problems, it is termed dysfunctional elimination syndrome. The common neural pathways to the brainstem that control and relax the pelvic floor musculature may provide a theoretical basis for both systems being affected. Typically constipation and infrequent voiding are present. It is more often seen in girls and is associated with recurrent UTI and VUR [38]. The workup follows the same pattern as for other types of bladder dysfunction, with the additional attention paid to bowel habits. Treatment of voiding habits is conducted simultaneously with treatment of the bowel problems. Correcting the constipation will often improve the bladder symptoms, and biofeedback therapy often is an important part of treatment.

## Giggle Incontinence

In some children, giggling can trigger partial or complete bladder emptying [39]. This can occur in childhood, adolescence, and adulthood. Termed *enuresis risoria*, it is well known enough to generate the saying, "I laughed so hard, I peed my pants." Usually the patient does not have any other lower urinary tract symptoms. The cause is unknown, but it has been suggested that laughter via central mechanisms allows the micturition reflex to "escape" central inhibition.

There is no simple treatment. Most children as they grow older simply outgrow it. The standard approach is to have the child empty the bladder prior to situations where laughter or giggling is expected, but this is simpler said than done. Biofeedback and pelvic floor muscle exercises to strengthen awareness of the muscles have been also advocated [40]. CNS stimulatory drugs, such as methylphenidate (Ritalin™), have been reported be effective [41].

## Vaginal Voiding

Some girls who otherwise are continent will experience mild wetting soon after normal voiding, due to trapping of urine in the vagina. Termed vaginal reflux, usually there is no other issue except vaginal entrapment of urine. The condition is not associated with other lower urinary tract symptoms. It may be due to labial adhesions or an inappropriate position on the toilet. The classic presentation is that of a girl who does not spread her legs enough during voiding and who is sitting on the front edge of the toilet seat. Small girls who may be afraid of falling backward into the toilet seem particularly prone. The treatment is usually simple: change how the girl sits on the toilet. If there are labial adhesions, these need to be treated. Initial therapy can be with topical estrogen ointment; recalcitrant cases should be divided surgically.

## General Treatment Recommendations

### Constipation Therapy

Constipation needs to be treated whenever it occurs in conjunction with daytime wetting. The parents and child should plan on a regular time each day to try to defecate. Sometimes a cycle exists that must be undone before regularity can be restored. Hard stools can lead to painful defecation; the pain in turn makes the child reluctant to defecate which only worsens the constipation. Treatment is aimed at both an acute solution and a long-term solution. In the long term, a diet rich in fiber is recommended. We suggest a plan of commonly available fiber-rich foods which can be rotated in order to provide variety. Increased fluid intake with water is also recommended. Laxatives are usually necessary until the situation can be managed by diet alone. In some cases they have to be used indefinitely. Usually we prefer to use osmotic laxatives such as polyethylene glycol (MiraLAX™) because they can both be used acutely to empty out the colon and at smaller doses for long-term management. We usually recommend 1.5 g/kg/day up to 34 g. Other options include mineral oil (15–30 mL/kg/day up to 200 mL in 12 h) or hypertonic enemas.

### Normalize Bladder Habits

Any plan of treatment for daytime wetting in general requires good bladder habits. These plans must necessarily take into account the particular nuances of each patient's situation. As noted above any such plans must correct any bowel issues. In addition there are several other general requirements. First, the patient and parents or guardians must fully understand the plan and be able and willing to cooperate. It does little good to work up a plan if the child and adults involved are not interested in participating. In cases where the child is not developmentally able to play a part (that is, it is not a psychological or psychiatric issue which can be treated simultaneously), treatment might have to be deferred or delayed until the point the child is able to participate. Any treatment plan will not work instantly nor will it yield results in just a few days. Both the patients and the adults must have a realistic understanding of how long it might take and how much effort it will require. Second, the patient should be asked to cease any and all avoidance maneuvers. Dancing about, doing the "potty dance," Vincent's curtsy, and crossing one's legs habitually should be stopped, and they should be regarded as a reminder that the child should go to the bathroom and try to void [3]. Third, the child should have good toilet mechanics. For girls, this means sitting in a comfortable situation which allows them to spread their legs and to fully relax their pelvic muscles. Many girls especially those who are small often "perch" on the edge of the toilet and sit in a manner which presses their legs together because of a lack of stability. Potty chairs can be useful in small children but for older girls, having them sit facing the tank may be a solution. The tank will give the girls something to hold onto for stability, and the wider sitting stance will open the legs apart and help facilitate relaxation of the pelvic muscles. For boys, be sure that they actually take the time to unzip their pants and take their time voiding. Fashion comes in and out of favor, and so one has to be aware of habits which can affect voiding. Some boys rather than opening the fly will instead push their pants downward and guide the penis up and over the edge of the pants to void. Fourth, voiding should become regular in frequency. The patient should try to void regularly throughout the day and not wait until there is a strong urgency. A regular pattern should be established. The majority of children and most adults do not easily follow a schedule based on the clock. Children's lives are typically dictated by adults, and their day is more similar to cultures based on event time. Their day is punctuated by events such as waking, breakfast, start of school, gym or recess, lunch, end of school, and favorite afternoon activity such as sports/music practice, dinner, and bedtime. These events usually occur regularly throughout the day even if they are not perfectly spaced. The gap time between the end of one event and the start of the next event is the ideal time for the child to go to the bathroom. There is no excuse of interrupting a favorite event, and it is an unobtrusive opportunity to void. Fifth, the child and adults are asked to help track the habits and behavior by maintaining a voiding diary. This serves to not only track progress or the lack thereof in a reliable fashion but also as a gentle reminder to stick to the plan. Collectively, these general recommendations are termed urotherapy (see Table 16.2) [36].

## Additional Therapies

### Biofeedback

Biofeedback is often used in conjunction with a comprehensive rehabilitation program. It is a broad general term applied to techniques by which physiologic activity is conveyed to the patient as visual or acoustic signals, providing the patient with information about physiologic processes. In brief, a series of repetitive exercise or activities are done by the child with the goal of improving better control of the pelvic floor muscles and sphincter. The aims are to improve both the resting tone of the pelvic muscles and the ability to fully relax. Biofeedback may be used for the management of filling (detrusor overactivity) and voiding (dysfunctional voiding owing to pelvic floor muscle overactivity) phase abnormalities. In relation to the filling phase, it can help the child to recognize involuntary detrusor contractions, and in relation to the voiding phase, it can help the child to identify how to relax the pelvic floor muscles.

**Table 16.2** Urotherapy options

| General treatment recommendations |
|---|
| Correct constipation |
| Normalize bladder habits |
| Stop avoidance maneuvers |
| Additional options |
| Biofeedback |
| Neuromodulation |
| Clean intermittent catheterization |
| Anticholinergic drugs |
| Alpha-adrenergic blocking drugs |
| Botulinum toxin type A |

Typically this training is done by having the child repetitively contract and relax the pelvic floor and sphincter muscles. This activity can be tracked invasively using an anorectal or vaginal probe or less invasively by surface patch electromyography electrodes. Biofeedback may be performed using a cystometrogram for children with involuntary detrusor contractions. In this situation, the child is taught how to recognize early and inhibit involuntary detrusor contractions, by watching the pressure curve during cystometry. When an involuntary contraction occurs, the child is encouraged to try consciously to suppress the contraction. This form of biofeedback is very invasive and time consuming and has limited use as routine treatment. If there is an indication for a cystometric investigation (e.g., in a patient with therapy-resistant urge syndrome), it can be used to teach the patient at the same time.

Biofeedback in the treatment of dysfunctional voiding is widely used and has been reported to be effective [42]. It is performed either by using uroflow only or in combination with pelvic floor electromyography. The technique teaches the child how to relax the pelvic floor muscles during micturition: the child sits on a toilet with a flow transducer, watching the flow curve and the electromyogram online on a computer monitor, trying to empty completely in one relaxed continuous portion. As noted earlier, efforts to make the process more interesting and tolerable to the child have included linking the training to a video game. Other such approaches of linking an interactive interface with the biofeedback training may help improve patient compliance and cooperation [32]. Estimation of PVR should always be checked after each voiding to see whether or not progress with the emptying ability is made.

### Neuromodulation

Neuromodulation has been used in adults for various lower urinary tract symptoms. The invasive nature of the procedure (anal, genital, or urethral probe) makes it less applicable for children. In OAB, stimulation of inhibitory pathways via an anal probe has been used, and in the underactive bladder, the detrusor has been activated through intravesical stimulation [43, 44]. Another technique is transcutaneous electrical nerve stimulation with surface electrodes. The inhibitory nerves to the bladder are stimulated via cutaneous receptors to the sacral root (S3). Some benefits have been shown, but no controlled studies are available. These techniques are applicable only to children in whom other treatment modalities have failed [30, 31].

### Clean Intermittent Self-Catheterization

In children with an underactive detrusor, bladder emptying can often be achieved with timed and double voiding. If this does not provide adequate results, clean ISC, which long has been used to manage neurogenic bladders, may be tried [45]. Fortunately outside of situations with retention or when the bladder has to be blocked down using anticholinergics to prevent high storage pressures, ISC does not play a major role in most children with daytime wetting. The key limitation with clean ISC is the invasiveness of the procedure. The problem in the long run is not just the discomfort but coping with the situation. The acceptance and training period is often worse than for children with neuropathic bladder dysfunction. Long-term compliance in these otherwise healthy children is also often lower.

## Pharmacotherapy

### Anticholinergic Drugs

Anticholinergic drugs aimed at the muscarinic receptors remain one of the mainstays of therapy for OAB. The blockade of parasympathetic muscarinic receptors inhibits activity of the bladder detrusor and limits or completely blocks overactivity. Treatment has been shown to increase bladder capacity, increase bladder compliance, and decrease detrusor contractions in neurogenic detrusor overactivity.

In functional overactivity, pharmacotherapy is instituted when modification of habits and behavior does not work. The use of medications as the primary treatment in children with daytime incontinence with bladder overactivity can be carried out empirically. Medication alone is rarely successful and almost always has to be part of a coordinated effort along with behavioral modification. We do not support pharmacotherapy alone, but emphasize the importance of standard urotherapy together with the use of drugs.

When anticholinergic drugs are used, there is always a risk of increase in PVR. The development of a UTI or poor urinary stream should cause the PVR to be rechecked. Other common side effects include sun sensitivity, dry mouth, blurring of vision, constipation, and flushing. Occasionally, overheating (hyperpyrexia) may occur, particularly when the child is exposed to hot weather. CNS side effects (hallucination, irritation) have also been described. They are usually rare and warn of overdosage.

Currently the most widely used anticholinergic drug is oxybutynin hydrochloride. In addition to the anticholinergic effects, the agent has musculotropic relaxant effects and local anesthetic properties [46]. In the treatment of OAB, oxybutynin can be used in oral doses of 0.1–0.15 mg/kg twice daily. Efficacy of oxybutynin in OAB has been described in only a few open studies. While there have been comparative studies with other medications, there are no large-scale placebo-controlled studies that are available in children [47].

Tolterodine is another anticholinergic drug used mainly for the treatment of OAB in adults. Several studies have been performed in children and showed a satisfactory safety profile [48]. Its chemical structure reduces penetration of the blood–brain barrier, thereby limiting some side effects. Trospium chloride and propiverine are other commercially available anticholinergics, but there are no large studies in children about their efficacy and tolerability.

### α-Adrenergic Blocking Agents

Alpha-adrenergic blockers (e.g., doxazosin, prazosin) have been prescribed to treat dysfunctional voiding and incomplete bladder emptying. It is hoped that they would help relax the overactive pelvic floor and sphincter. Theoretically it should work much as it has been applied to treat benign prostatic hypertrophy in adult men. No large-scale controlled prospective study using these drugs in children has been conducted, but the evidence of their efficacy from case series is promising and optimistic [49].

### Botulinum Toxin

Botulinum toxin type A is currently used in children mainly with neurogenic detrusor overactivity but has also been used for nonneurogenic OAB [50]. The initial results are interesting. One study of 20 patients who underwent injection of botulinum toxin A resulted in 12 months of suppression of overactivity. Injection into the external sphincter is also possible in cases with pelvic floor overactivity. Results from a study with botulinum toxin type A in nonneurogenic conditions in children have been published more recently, with some positive results [51]. The use of botulinum toxin in the nonneurogenic bladder regarding OAB and dysfunctional voiding shows promise but remains an off-label use which needs further study before being incorporated into the usual treatment options. In particular further understanding of its mechanism of action and its durability are needed.

### Antibiotics

All children with symptomatic UTI should be treated with appropriate antibiotic therapy. If a child has an underlying voiding disorder associated with recurrent UTIs, prophylactic antibiotic therapy is recommended during the treatment period. Trimethoprim-sulfamethoxazole, nitrofurantoin, and trimethoprim alone have proven to be successful in this role. If the patient is prone to infection, it can confuse matters; one is not sure if the symptoms are due to the infection or the ongoing voiding issues. We usually suggest that the patient be kept on a course of prophylactic antibiotics until the treatment plan is well in place, then it could be tapered off.

## References

1. de Groat WC, Araki I, Vizzard MA, Yoshiyama M, Yoshimura N, Sugaya K, Tai C, Roppolo JR. Developmental and injury induced plasticity in the micturition reflex pathway. Behav Brain Res. 1998; 92:127–40.
2. Park JM, Bloom DA, McGuire EJ. The guarding reflex revisited. Br J Urol. 1997;80:940–5.
3. Vincent SA. Postural control of urinary incontinence. The curtsy sign. Lancet. 1966;2:631–2.
4. Jansson UB, Hanson M, Sillen U, Hellstrom AL. Voiding pattern and acquisition of bladder control from birth to age 6 years—a longitudinal study. J Urol. 2005;174:293–8.
5. Jarvelin MR, Vikevainen-Tervonen L, Moilanen I, Huttunen NP. Enuresis in seven-year-old children. Acta Paediatr Scand. 1988;77:148–53.
6. Oppel WC, Harper PA, Rider RV. The age of attaining bladder control. Pediatrics. 1968;42:614–26.
7. Hellström AL, Hanson E, Hansson S, Hjälmås K, Jodal U. Micturition habits and incontinence in 7-year-old Swedish school entrants. Eur J Pediatr. 1990;149:434–7.
8. Sureshkumar P, Jones M, Cumming R, Craig J. A population based study of 2,856 school-age children with urinary incontinence. J Urol. 2009;181:808–16.
9. Swithinbank LV, Carr JC, Abrams PH. Longitudinal study of urinary symptoms in children. Scand J Urol Nephrol Suppl. 1994;163:67–73.
10. Bomalaski MD, Anema JG, Coplen DE, Koo HP, Rozanski T, Bloom DA. Delayed presentation of posterior urethral valves: a not so benign condition. J Urol. 1999;162:2130–2.
11. Bloom DA, Seeley WW, Ritchey ML, McGuire EJ. Toilet habits and continence in children: an opportunity sampling in search of normal parameters. J Urol. 1993;149:1087–90.
12. Hellstrom AL, Andersson K, Hjalmas K, Jodal U. Pad tests in children with incontinence. Scand J Urol Nephrol. 1986;20:47–50.
13. Bael AM, Lax H, Hirche H, Gabel E, Winkler P, Hellstrom AL, van Zon R, Janhsen E, Guntek S, Renson C, van Gool JD, the European Bladder Dysfunction Study. Self-reported urinary incontinence, voiding frequency, voided volume and pad-test results: variables in a prospective study in children. BJU Int. 2007;100:651–6.
14. Koff SA. Estimating bladder capacity in children. J Urol. 1983;21:248.
15. Pederson JF, Bartrum RJ, Grytter C. Residual urine determination by ultrasonic scanning. Am J Roentgenol Radium Ther Nucl Med. 1975;125: 474–8.
16. Jansson UB, Hanson M, Hanson E, Hellstrom AL, Sillen U. Voiding pattern in healthy children 0 to 3 years old: a longitudinal study. J Urol. 2000;164: 2050–4.
17. Williot P, McLorie GA, Gilmour RF, Churchill BM. Accuracy of bladder volume determinations in

children using a suprapubic ultrasonic bi-planar technique. J Urol. 1989;141:900–2.
18. Ross JH, Kay R. Pediatric urinary tract infection and reflux. Am Fam Physician. 1999;59:1485–6.
19. Preda I, Jodal U, Sixt R, Stokland E, Hansson S. Normal dimercaptosuccinic acid scintigraphy makes voiding cystourethrography unnecessary after urinary tract infection. J Pediatr. 2008;151:581–4.
20. Bael A, Lax H, de Jong TPVM, Hoebeke P, Nijman RJM, Sixt R, Verhulst J, Hirche H, van Gool JD, European Bladder Dysfunction Society. The relevance of urodynamic studies for urge syndrome and dysfunctional voiding: a multicenter controlled trial in children. J Urol. 2008;180:1486–93.
21. Allen TD. The non-neurogenic neurogenic bladder. J Urol. 1977;117:232–8.
22. Hinman F, Baumann FW. Vesical and ureteral damage from voiding dysfunction in boys without neurologic or obstructive disease. J Urol. 1973;109:727–32.
23. Nevéus T, von Gontard A, Hoebeke P, Hjalmas K, Bauer S, Bower W, Jorgensen TM, Rittig S, Walle JV, Yeung CK, Djurhuus JC. The standardization of terminology of lower urinary tract function in children and adolescents: report from the Standardisation Committee of the International Children's Continence Society. J Urol. 2006;176:314–24.
24. Zoubek J, Bloom DA. Extraordinary urinary frequency. Pediatrics. 1990;85:1112–4.
25. Coriglinao T, Renella R, Robbiani A, Riavis M, Bianchetti MG. Isolated extraordinary daytime urinary frequency of childhood: a case series of 26 children in Switzerland. Acta Paediatr. 2007;96:1347–9.
26. Ellsworth PI, Merguerian PA, Copening ME. Sexual abuse: another causative factor in dysfunctional voiding. J Urol. 1995;153:773–6.
27. Hillyer S, Mooppan U, Kim H, Gulmi F. Diagnosis and treatment of urethral prolapse in children: experience with 34 cases. J Urol. 2009;73:1008–11.
28. Franco I. Overactive bladder in children. Part 1: pathophysiology. J Urol. 2007;178:761–8.
29. Franco I. Overactive bladder in children. Part 2: management. J Urol. 2007;178:769–74.
30. Oerlemans DJAJ, van Kerrebroeck PEV. Sacral nerve stimulation for neuromodulation of the lower urinary tract. Neurourol Urodyn. 2008;27:28–33.
31. Bosch JLHR, Broen J. Sacral nerve neuromodulation in the treatment of patients with refractory motor urge incontinence: long-term results of a prospective longitudinal study. J Urol. 2000;163:1219–22.
32. Herndon CDA, Decambre M, McKenna PH. Interactive computer games for treatment of pelvic floor dysfunction. J Urol. 2001;166:1893–8.
33. Vijverberg MA, Elzinga-Plomp A, Messer AP, van Gool JD, de Jong TP. Bladder rehabilitation, the effect of a cognitive training programme on urge incontinence. Eur Urol. 1997;31:68–72.
34. Lettgen B, von Gontard A, Olbing H, Heiken-Lowenau C, Gaebel E, Schmitz I. Urge incontinence and voiding postponement in children: somatic and psychosocial factors. Acta Paediatr. 2002;91:978–84.
35. Klijn AJ, Uiterwaal CS, Vijverberg MA, Winkler PL, Dik P, de Jong TP. Home uroflowmetry biofeedback in behavioral training for dysfunctional voiding in school-age children: a randomized controlled study. J Urol. 2006;175:2263–8.
36. Hellstrom AL, Hjalmas K, Jodal U. Rehabilitation of the dysfunctional bladder in children: method and 3-year followup. J Urol. 1987;138:847–9.
37. Hinman F. Urinary tract damage in children who wet. Pediatrics. 1974;54:142–50.
38. Chen JJ, Mao W, Homayoon K, Steinhardt GF. A multivariate analysis of dysfunctional elimination syndrome, and its relationships with gender, urinary tract infection and vesicoureteral reflux in children. J Urol. 2004;171:1907–10.
39. Glahn BE. Giggle incontinence (enuresis risoria). A study and an aetiological hypothesis. Br J Urol. 1979; 51:363–6.
40. Richardson I, Palmer LS. Successful treatment for giggle incontinence with biofeedback. J Urol. 2009; 182:2062–6.
41. Berry AK, Zderic S, Carr M. Methylphenidate for giggle incontinence. J Urol. 2009;182:2028–32.
42. Porena M, Costantini E, Rociola W, Mearini E. Biofeedback successfully cures detrusor-sphincter dyssynergia in pediatric patients. J Urol. 2000;163: 1927–31.
43. Gladh G, Mattsson S, Lindstrom S. Anogenital electrical stimulation as treatment of urge incontinence in children. BJU Int. 2001;87:366–71.
44. Gladh G, Mattsson S, Lindstrom S. Intravesical electrical stimulation in the treatment of micturition dysfunction in children. Neurourol Urodyn. 2003;22: 233–42.
45. Lapides J, Diokno AC, Silber SJ, Lowe BS. Clean, intermittent self-catheterization in the treatment of urinary tract disease. J Urol. 1972;107:458–61.
46. Diokno AC, Lapides J. Oxybutynin: a new drug with analgesic and anticholinergic properties. J Urol. 1972;108:307–9.
47. Curran MJ, Kaefer M, Peters C, Logigian E, Bauer SB. The overactive bladder in childhood: long-term results with conservative management. J Urol. 2000;163: 574–7.
48. Hjalmas K, Hellstrom AL, Mogren K, Lackgren G, Sternberg A. The overactive bladder in children: a potential future indication for tolterodine. BJU Int. 2001;87:569–74.
49. Cain MP, Wu SD, Austin PF, Herndon CDA, Rink RC. Alpha blocker therapy for children with dysfunctional voiding and urinary retention. J Urol. 2003;170: 1514–7.
50. Hoebeke P, De Caestecker K, Vande Walle J, Dehoorne J, Raes A, Verleyen P, Van Laecke E. The effect of botulinum-A toxin in incontinent children with therapy resistant overactive detrusor. J Urol. 2006;176: 328–30.
51. Radojicic ZI, Perovic SV, Milic NM. Is it reasonable to treat refractory voiding dysfunction in children with botulinum-A toxin? J Urol. 2006;176:332–6.

# 17 Tumors of the Lower Genitourinary Tract in Children and Adolescents

Armando J. Lorenzo, Joao Luiz Pippi Salle, and Martin A. Koyle

## Introduction

Tumors of the lower genitourinary tract are fortunately relatively rare in children. This is particularly true when compared to the incidence of such neoplasms in adult populations exposed to different risk factors, presenting with a different profile in terms of malignant potential and underlying histology. Similarly, when considering pediatric tumors, the lower urinary tract is an uncommon primary site. Thus, in most primary care settings, the provider will encounter few patients who are ultimately found to have such problem. Nevertheless, many children with benign conditions present with similar symptomatology or physical exam findings. This poses a difficult situation whereby the healthcare provider needs to rule out a rare disorder without exposing children to unnecessary, invasive, or expensive tests, while accurately selecting those that need further specialized management.

Besides rare, the differential diagnosis of tumors affecting the lower genitourinary tract can be somewhat extensive and includes benign conditions with little clinical significance along with malignancies that can be life threatening and require early intensive therapy. Accurate assessment, proper evaluation, and prompt referral can favorably impact prognosis by avoiding unnecessary delays in the initiation of pathology and stage-specific management.

In this chapter we aim to describe the most important considerations in the differential diagnosis for patients with these conditions, summarizing the diagnostic algorithm and appropriate management in preparation for referral when indicated.

## Clinical Presentation

Children with lower urinary tract tumors usually present with signs and symptoms triggered by mass effect (i.e., obstructive symptoms) or local invasion and disruption of the urothelium (such as hematuria). Occasionally, the diagnosis is suspected due to unexpected findings on imaging studies obtained for a seemingly unrelated complaint (most commonly, evaluation of a urinary tract infection). Similarly though, abnormalities detected during the evaluation of common genitourinary complaints—most commonly symptoms secondary to a urinary tract infection—may be concerning for a neoplasm yet

A.J. Lorenzo, M.D., M.Sc., F.R.C.S.C., F.A.A.P., F.A.C.S.
Hospital for Sick Children, University of Toronto, Toronto, ON, Canada

J.L.P. Salle, M.D., Ph.D., F.A.A.P., F.R.C.S.C. (✉)
Division of Urology, Department of Surgery, Sidra Medical and Research Center Doha, State of Qatar
e-mail: psalle@sidra.org

M.A. Koyle, F.A.A.P., F.A.C.S.
Division of Urology, Hospital for Sick Children, Toronto, ON, Canada

R. Rabinowitz et al. (eds.), *Pediatric Urology for the Primary Care Physician*, Current Clinical Urology,
DOI 10.1007/978-1-60327-243-8_17, 

end up representing inflammatory reaction that subsides with treatment.

On history it is important to define the symptomatology and ascertain the duration of the problem. Understandably, this is occasionally limited to the developmental stage of the child and his/her ability to provide reliable information. For most cases, the complaints are either the development of hematuria (sometimes described as a change or darkening of the urine), suprapubic pain, or lower urinary tract symptoms—obstructive (such as urinary hesitancy, decreased or intermittent stream, sensation of incomplete emptying) or irritative (dysuria, urinary frequency, urgency). Less frequently patients present acutely with urinary retention, have constitutional symptoms (related to an underlying malignancy, anemia due to bleeding, or renal insufficiency), or have complaints secondary to the presence of metastatic disease. It is important to keep in mind that the presence of hematuria in a child should lead the healthcare provider to consider other important medical problems not necessarily related to urinary tract neoplasms (such as nephrological conditions).

As discussed in the following paragraphs, some entities are seen in association with specific medical conditions or prior surgical interventions. In particular, prior exposure to chemotherapy or radiation should heighten the suspicion for a recurrence or secondary malignancy: thus, a more aggressive evaluation of these patients should be conducted even in the setting of seemingly mild symptoms. Similarly, exposure to immunosuppressants, commonly used in children following transplantation, increases the risk of specific inflammatory conditions that may mimic a tumor (such as BK virus cystitis) or increase the long-term risk of tumors that may involve the genitourinary tract. Lastly, a history of prior reconstructive surgery with bowel (i.e., augmentation cystoplasty) has been associated with the latter development of malignancies. These patients may be at increased risk due to multiple factors, most notably chronic inflammation from catheterization, recurrent infections, and irritation from mucus and stones. Lastly, a known history

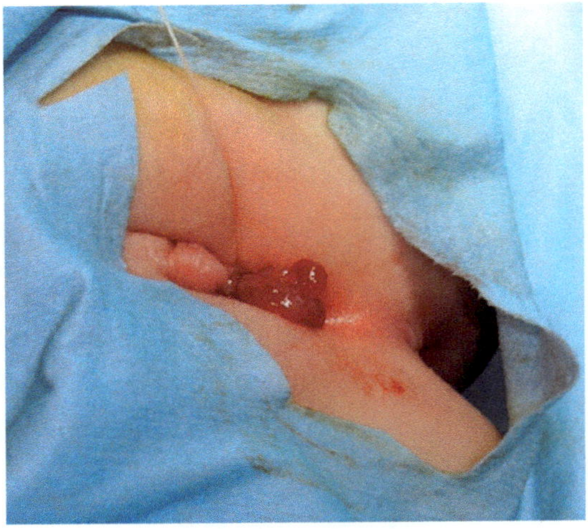

**Fig. 17.1** Transurethral extension of bladder mass, with tumor clearly visible on physical exam (exam under anesthesia prior to cystoscopy). This child was found to have a large bladder rhabdomyosarcoma

of any syndrome should be considered, as some tumors are specifically seen in association with some of them.

Physical examination is frequently unremarkable, especially on gross inspection. The presence of scars may point toward previous urinary tract surgeries, information that may be relevant in some cases. In addition, as with all patients with suspected neoplasms, it is important to palpate areas of lymph node involvement. A focused exam may detect a palpable mass in the suprapubic region (either reflecting mass effect by the tumor and/or bladder distention from involvement of the outlet). Similarly, extension through the urethra may allow for direct visualization of the mass (Fig. 17.1). It is imperative to perform a full genital exam and a rectal exam. In some younger children or even in older, anxious children, this may require sedation or even an anesthetic.

Although the differential diagnosis is extensive for both types of complains, common features deserve to be highlighted in order to improve the diagnostic threshold and avoid delayed diagnosis: If a child presents with symptoms that cannot be otherwise explained (e.g., negative workup for a urinary infection) and if the problems persists or worsens despite a proposed intervention (such as the empiric administration of antibiotics) or in the setting of inconclusive previous workups for similar complaints, the child should be considered for more extensive evaluation, including a "screening" ultrasound of the abdomen and pelvis.

Laboratory evaluations may aid in the differential diagnosis and management. One of the most important ones is a properly collected urine specimen for microscopic evaluation and culture. Despite having lower urinary tract symptoms, the classic finding is "sterile" hematuria. Thus, the implications of such report should include the presence of an inflammatory condition caused by a microorganism difficult to culture (such as *Mycobacteria*) or that requires specific culture conditions (such as *Adenovirus* and other viruses) or that the presence of blood is related to vascular friability and disruption by the tumor.

The initial imaging modality is an abdominopelvic ultrasound (also limited in some institutions to a kidney and bladder ultrasound), which often is considered more of a screening exam rather than the definitive study. Advantages include its widespread availability, acceptable cost, noninvasiveness, and lack of ionizing radiation exposure. These advantages usually outweigh the limitations of the study, which include that it is operator dependent, is affected by patient movement or body habitus, and has limited ability to detect small lesions or reliably report on important features (such as contrast uptake). With the addition of Doppler interrogation, the radiologist is able to report on the presence of blood flow in some circumstances. Subsequent imaging modalities are obtained to better define the site of origin, involvement of contiguous structures, and evidence of local and distant spread. Commonly, these include CT scan and magnetic resonance imaging. Increasingly, many favor the use of the latter in pediatric patients due to its better anatomical definition and the lack of radiation. Indeed, exposure to radiation has been increasingly questioned, and CT scans are an important source in everyday medical practice. It should be remembered that radiation exposure confers a cumulative effect, and children with malignancies are bound to be exposed to many imaging studies following their diagnosis. Thus, studies that expose the patient to radiation (in particular CT scans) should be requested only after careful consideration of other modalities.

Once radiologically defined, the next step involves obtaining a tissue sample, which is commonly done in conjunction with an exam under anesthesia and cystourethroscopy and, in females, vaginoscopy and speculum exam. During this evaluation, a rectal or bimanual exam can be conducted (given that this evaluation is often limited in children during a clinic visit for the obvious reasons noted earlier). It is recommended to obtain biopsies through the easiest access route (favoring in some occasions percutaneous over endoscopic) and avoid excessive use of cautery to limit the resulting distortion of the tissue. Nevertheless, there are some circumstances in which a biopsy may not be warranted and may be potentially associated with significant risks. These include patients with a suspected pheochromocytoma, in whom manipulation of the mass may lead to acute surge in catecholamine release and potentially life-threatening hypertensive crisis or arrhythmias. Also, if the mass has the visual appearance of a hemangioma (friable, red, and grossly composed of large blood vessels), tissue sampling may lead to significant bleeding which may be difficult to control.

## Epidemiology

The importance of lower urinary tract tumors is certainly not related to its incidence but the potential for malignancy. Although it is unclear if the problem is underreported (particularly for benign tumors or nonneoplastic conditions), the rarity of these problems is highlighted on all reports on the subject. Furthermore, by comprising a wide range of histological types, each particular diagnosis generates few patients even in large healthcare databases. For example, in the National Cancer Institute-maintained Surveillance, Epidemiology, and End Results (SEER) database, only a total of 140 cases were extracted on an analysis that explored 30 years worth of data collection. This report—included in the Reference section and limited to malignant tumors in patients younger than 18 years of age—indicates the predominance of rhabdomyosarcoma and urothelial neoplasms. While rhabdomyosarcoma is predominant in younger children (prepubertal), papillary urothelial neoplasms increase in incidence in the older age groups. Importantly, these databases as well as collective reports from multi-institutional study groups continue to show promissory improvements in morbidity and mortality as years go by and experience increases.

## Differential Diagnosis

Admittedly the differential diagnosis is extensive, yet entails a few relatively common pathologies. In general, the first step to consider is differentiation between benign and malignant processes along with remembering the possibility of non-neoplastic etiologies (i.e., inflammatory or "pseudotumors"). The different conditions are rarely specifically suspected at presentation (and thus diagnosis relies heavily on pathology evaluation). In the following paragraphs we will discuss specific pertinent diagnoses, with particular considerations for each entity along with its management:

## Rhabdomyosarcoma

This tumor leads the list of malignant lower urinary tract tumors in the pediatric population, representing one of the most common and best-studied solid genitourinary neoplasms in children. Commonly diagnosed before 5 years of age, these neoplasms have a 3:1 male predominance. Due to the relative rarity of the diagnosis, absence of screening protocols, and unspecific symptoms, most patients present with rather large masses with impressive involvement on imaging studies (Fig. 17.2). In addition, not uncommonly these children have a history of prior evaluations and potential delays in diagnosis. The possibility of missing this neoplasm is one of the main reasons for ultrasound evaluation of young patients with lower urinary tract symptoms that lack a clear etiology.

The etiology of this neoplasm is far from elucidated. There are some conditions that appear to confer an increased risk; these include neurofibromatosis and Costello, Beckwith–Wiedemann, and Li–Fraumeni syndromes. Considering the infrequent occurrence of these syndromes, affected children are monitored in specialized clinics with

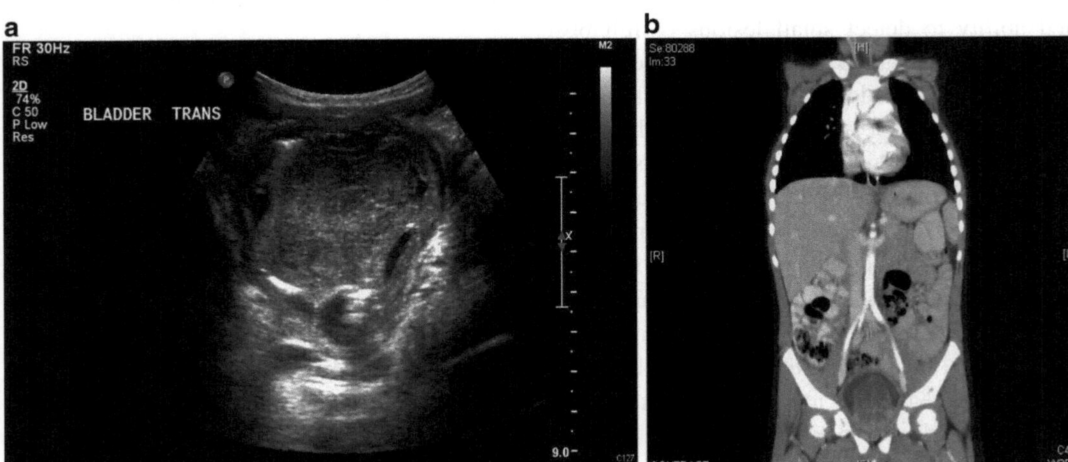


**Fig. 17.2** Bladder/prostate rhabdomyosarcoma diagnosed in a 4-year-old boy who presented with progressive difficulty to void and subsequent urinary retention. Initial ultrasound showed a large bladder mass occupying most of its lumen (**a**). The patient subsequently underwent evaluation with CT scan (**b**), which failed to disclose any evidence of metastatic disease. Biopsy obtained during diagnostic cystoscopy showed large friable mass. Pathology confirmed the diagnosis of embryonal rhabdomyosarcoma

protocols aimed at early identification of malignancies (e.g., patients with Beckwith–Wiedemann are also screened regularly for the development of Wilms' tumors and hepatoblastomas).

There are no specific findings on history or physical exam that may particularly increase the suspicion for a lower urinary tract rhabdomyosarcoma. Perhaps the only exceptions are the extrusion of tumor material through a natural orifice (classically described for embryonal botryoid genitourinary rhabdomyosarcoma, as shown in Fig. 17.1) and the detection of cutaneous involvement by metastatic disease, which in young children is generally due to either neuroblastoma or rhabdomyosarcoma. Commonly, the child presents with symptoms suggestive of urinary tract obstruction, hematuria, or a palpable abdominal mass. By virtue of their young age, patients are unable to reliably relate the duration or character of their symptoms, although commonly families describe a rather fast progression over time. By the time an imaging study is obtained (initially ultrasound in most cases), the detection of a mass is straightforward, as the neoplasm is usually greater than 5 cm in size and locally invasive. The exact location and involvement is harder to define and relies on axial imaging with CT scan or, preferably, magnetic resonance imaging. Even then, the primary organ of origin may be hard to define, as seen with male patients with a neoplasm that may be arising from the bladder neck/trigone or prostate. Even during cystoscopy the anatomical distortion may preclude this differentiation, yet allows confirming the growth originating in the urinary tract and, more importantly, allows for generous sampling for histological analysis. This information is then used to properly diagnose and stage the patient, who should be subsequently enrolled in one of the large multi-institutional trials (Children's Oncology Group in North America, formerly the Intergroup Rhabdomyosarcoma Studies). Risk stratification is the basis of multimodal therapy and is protocol based considering the tumor type (according to the International Classification of Rhabdomyosarcoma, including embryonal, alveolar, anaplastic, and undifferentiated), primary tumor site, tumor size, and presence of nodal involvement or metastatic disease. Importantly, these parameters are predictors of survival. In children who appear to have disease amenable to resection allowing preservation of function, exploration and attempt at surgical removal are offered. Otherwise, neoadjuvant chemotherapy and sometimes radiation therapy are given. These protocols change over time, and upon diagnosis it is wise to review management guidelines available from the different study groups. Important concepts to keep in mind are the benefit of a multidisciplinary approach (i.e., multimodal therapy) and the goal of avoiding radical surgical resection while preserving survival standards.

An important management consideration for children that present with urinary retention is the use of indwelling transurethral catheterization over suprapubic access. Any attempt at percutaneous catheterization of the bladder can lead to upstaging or spillage and should be considered in very rare circumstances as a "last resort" measure. Indeed, many patients may have persistent problems with bladder emptying even after the initiation of chemotherapy, and urethral catheterization is frequently required to avoid urinary retention and cystitis due to incomplete evacuation of urine with chemotherapy by-products (such as acrolein in children treated with cyclophosphamide).

## Urothelial Neoplasms (Including Urothelial or Transitional Cell Carcinoma and Papillary Urothelial Neoplasm of Low Malignant Potential)

While a very important diagnostic consideration (and the reason for aggressive evaluation of hematuria) in older patients, in children these tumors are fortunately infrequent. This age-related difference may highlight yet to be defined discrepancies in genetic predisposition and/or environmental exposures. Interestingly, there has been a "diagnostic shift" in recent years with the better recognition and improved classification of these neoplasms; thus, the apparent increase in

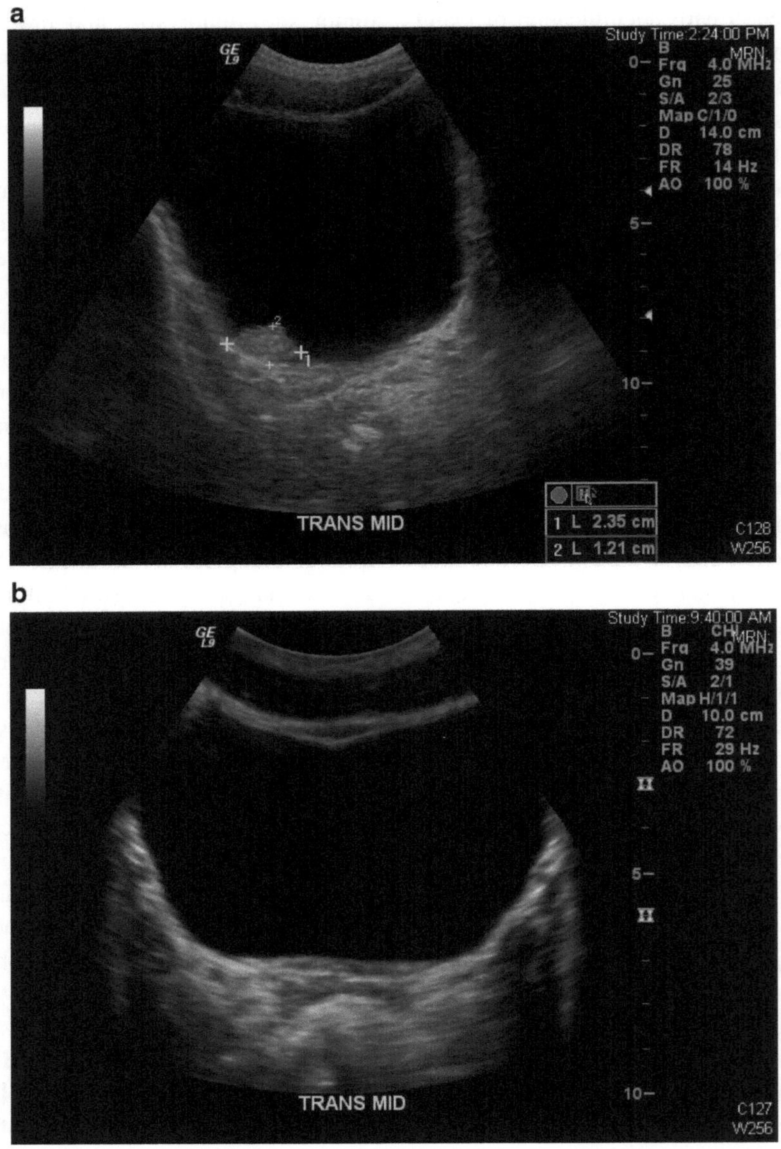


**Fig. 17.3** Urothelial neoplasm (later confirmed as a papillary urothelial neoplasm of low malignant potential on pathology) diagnosed in a 15-year-old teenager who presented with asymptomatic microhematuria detected during a routine physical exam and "well-child" visit. Ultrasound demonstrated a mass in the bladder wall growing toward the lumen (**a**, arrow). The patient subsequently underwent cystoscopy and transurethral resection. Follow-up ultrasounds have not shown any evidence of recurrence (**b**)

reports may be a reflection of better diagnostic capabilities and improvements in histological discrimination.

Upon evaluating the histological pattern and propensity for invasion and metastasis, children appear to have a more "benign" course and higher likelihood of cure with resection than the adult counterparts. Pediatric cases tend to be detected during the workup of hematuria, whereby an ultrasound demonstrates a mass within the bladder (Fig. 17.3). In contrast to patients with rhabdomyosarcoma, the age of presentation tends to be older (adolescents) and favors male gender, and the associated symptomatology is less striking.

Most reported cases represent papillary urothelial neoplasms of low malignant potential, term coined from the rich experience with urothelial carcinoma in adults, and—as the name implies—are likely associated with a very favorable prognosis. In general, the likelihood of recurrence is low and the need for intravesical chemo or immunotherapy appears unwarranted for most. The exception to this favorable course is the development of urothelial carcinoma following exposure to chemotherapeutic agents, in particular cyclophosphamide. Patient with history of such exposure are at risk for high-grade and/or invasive urothelial carcinoma; the development may lapse years following exposure, and occurrence of hemorrhagic cystitis during therapy may be a risk factor for subsequent tumor formation.

The diagnosis is usually suspected following ultrasound evaluation of a child with gross or microscopic hematuria. Rarely, it is an unexpected finding in patients with irritative voiding symptoms or recurrent urinary tract infections. Due to the small size of most lesions, the value of axial imaging (such as CT scan or magnetic resonance imaging), is limited. Nevertheless, for large tumors or when there is concern for invasion (i.e., high-grade neoplasm), axial imaging is warranted. Initial management includes diagnostic cystoscopy and resection for histological evaluation and subtyping, achieved in most cases through the same endoscopic transurethral approach. Whenever possible the goal should be complete eradication of all visible tumor. In the same setting it is customary to obtain a urine sample by barbotage to send for cytological evaluation. Although traditionally these samples are sent for cytology, the diagnostic yield of this test for diagnosis and subsequent monitoring is limited considering the low-grade nature of most lesions. If the resulting diagnosis is papillary urothelial neoplasm of low malignant potential or "low-grade" urothelial carcinoma, no further adjuvant therapies are offered, yet the child is customarily followed regularly for recurrence. The long-term outcome of these patients remains relatively unknown but somewhat worrisome considering the known increase in risk with age and likelihood of recurrence with other urothelial neoplasms. Surveillance with cystoscopy is difficult to implement considering that most pediatric cases would require anesthesia. In the absence of strict guidelines, evaluation should include at the very least monitoring for recurrent hematuria and ultrasonography. Exceptional cases with invasive or "high-grade" malignancies are difficult to manage, most commonly treated in consultation with healthcare providers with experience in adult patients (following "age-tailored" or empiric protocols).

## Adenocarcinoma

Even though a very rare bladder neoplasm, it is relevant in pediatrics due to its interesting association with conditions encountered in children, namely, bladder exstrophy, augmentation techniques employing segments of bowel, and the presence of urachal abnormalities. These conditions have been associated with the later development of bladder malignancies, including adenocarcinoma. Importantly, although the association is herein described for adenocarcinoma, reports have included other malignancies including urothelial carcinoma. Carcinogenesis in these patients is likely multifactorial and includes the effect of chronic inflammation and recurrent infections among many potential triggers. Unfortunately, in general, the prognosis is not favorable. Due to the rarity and relative recent knowledge of the association, current practice has not included effective screening protocols. Moreover, as the population with these problems ages, the expectation is that the problem may become more frequent. Healthcare providers who interact with these patients as they grow into adulthood should counsel them about the importance of avoiding additional risk factors (i.e., smoking), regular monitoring which may include cystoscopy, and early evaluation of any worrisome signs or symptoms (such as unexplained hematuria).

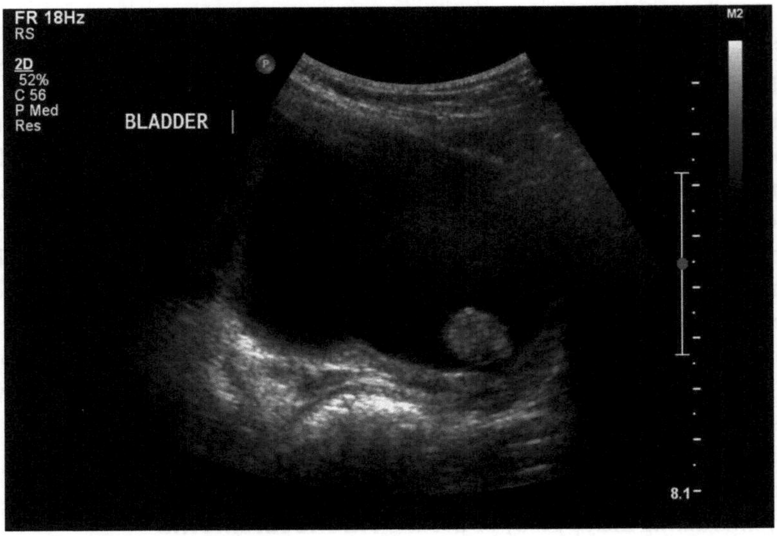


**Fig. 17.4** Bladder mass (*arrow*) found on routine follow-up of a patient that had prior bladder surgery (ureteral reimplantation). The child was asymptomatic. Following cystoscopic evaluation and transurethral resection, pathology was consistent with a nephrogenic adenoma without evidence of malignancy

## Nephrogenic Adenoma (or Nephrogenic Metaplasia)

This rare bladder lesion is considered a benign response of the urothelium, resulting in urothelial metaplasia and the development of papillary lesions. Within the urinary tract, it is most commonly found in the bladder and associated with a prior insult such as infections, chronic inflammation, trauma, or surgery (Fig. 17.4). On occasion the tumors are also encountered in other parts of the urinary tract, such as the urethra. Patients present clinically with hematuria and dysuria and an otherwise unremarkable examination. Bladder lesions can attain a large size prior to establishing the diagnosis, as prior normal genitourinary imaging studies may be relied upon (particularly in patients with recent surgical intervention). The presence of a mass is confirmed with ultrasonography. Cystourethroscopy usually reveals a tumor similar in gross appearance to urothelial carcinomas. As the distinction cannot be done by visual inspection alone, histology is essential to confirm the diagnosis.

Complete resection can be achieved endoscopically in many cases, although some reports indicate the need for open removal. Although malignant transformation has not been reported, recurrence is not uncommon. Thus, surveillance with ultrasonography is advised.

## Inflammatory Tumors

These benign reactive proliferative conditions have the radiological and endoscopic features of a submucosal neoplasm, thus are difficult to differentiate from a malignant process without adequate histological evaluation. Even then, differentiating these tumors from malignant lesions (rhabdomyosarcoma, leiomyosarcoma, and lymphoma) can be difficult, yet has critical implications for management. No known etiological factors explain their occurrence or define an increased risk. Two different histological patterns are included under this category: inflammatory myofibroblastic tumor (also known as inflammatory "pseudotumor" or inflammatory pseudosarcoma) and inflammatory eosinophilic tumor (sometimes referred to as eosinophilic cystitis in cases with diffuse bladder infiltration).

Inflammatory myofibroblastic tumors (Fig. 17.5) are fortunately rare in children, present in different anatomical sites, and potentially difficult to

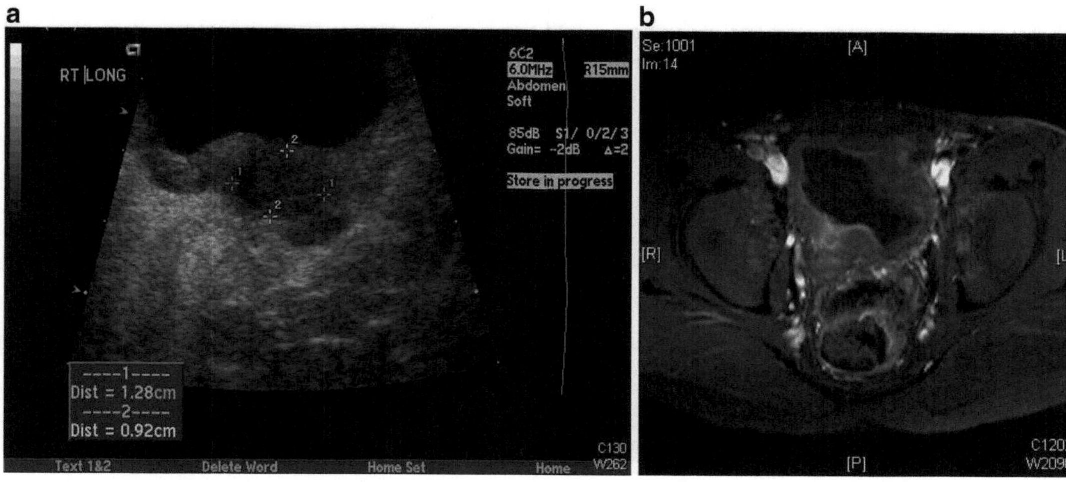


**Fig. 17.5** Bladder tumor encountered in a teenage boy who underwent evaluation for unspecific lower abdominal pain. Ultrasound showed focal thickening of the posterior wall (**a**, *arrow*), worrisome for a malignant process. This finding was corroborated by magnetic resonance imaging (**b**). Resection with extensive sampling showed the presence of a myofibroblastic tumor without any changes indicative of a malignant neoplasm. The child remains asymptomatic with no evidence of recurrence 2 years after the initial evaluation and extensive endoscopic resection

manage. Despite their perceived "benign" nature, surgical intervention—including open resection or endoscopic debulking with bladder preservation—is recommended in most cases due to concern for malignancy and local invasion with functional embarrassment. In addition, removal may be the only option for controlling persistent or recurrent hematuria. Rare reports have raised the possibility of observation prior to radical resection, recommendation that should be considered in children with tumors in difficult anatomical locations (such as the bladder trigone), in whom removal and subsequent reconstruction may be particularly challenging.

Eosinophilic tumors (Fig. 17.6) are occasionally associated with peripheral eosinophilia or allergic tendencies. Besides surgical resection, based on the specific histopathological finding of tissue infiltration by eosinophils, medical management with antihistaminics, leukotriene receptor antagonists, or corticosteroids may be implemented. Due to the presence of histological changes consistent with a granulomatous reaction in some children, it is important to rule out other conditions (principally tuberculous cystitis and histiocytosis).

## "Pseudotumors"

Some conditions can have some of the symptoms and diagnostic features of a tumor without representing a true neoplasm. Inflammatory processes of the bladder are the most frequent ones and can be particularly worrisome on imaging studies, some ultimately requiring tissue sampling for microscopic evaluation. These occur most frequently following surgery or have an infectious etiology (including viral, see Fig. 17.7). The challenge remains as the process of differentiating from true neoplasms and avoiding invasive procedures.

In some circumstances, intraluminal collections—such as blood clots, mucus, or fungal balls—can be occasionally mistaken for a tumor (Fig. 17.8). Clear demarcation from the mucosa and movement of the "mass" with change in position of the child are suggestive of such pathologies. Similarly, lack of blood flow on Doppler interrogation may aid in the diagnosis. Moreover, patients with a large clot may have a history of passing fragments in the urine (along with gross hematuria). Not uncommonly, these children have important comorbidities,

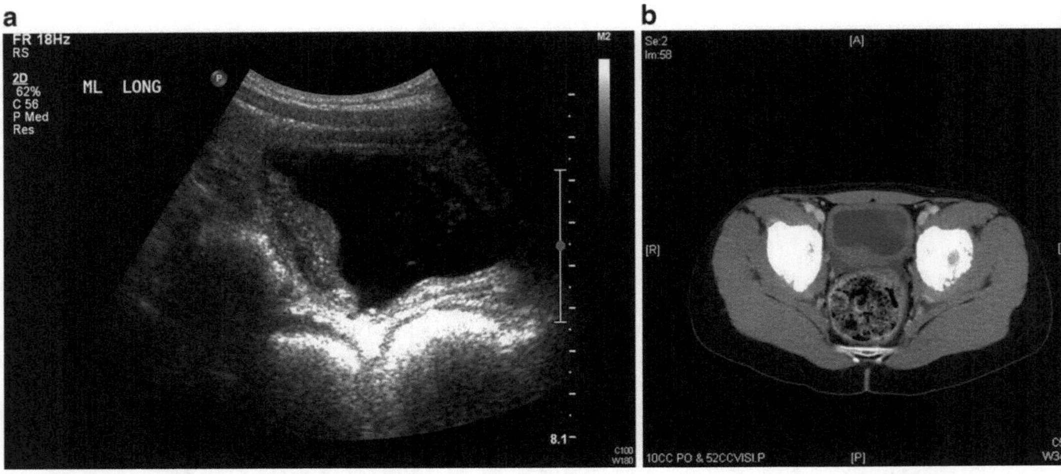


**Fig. 17.6** Focal bladder wall thickening detected on ultrasound evaluation of a child with persistent hematuria and negative urine culture. Ultrasound showed persistent focal thickening on serial exams (**a**). The findings were corroborated on a CT scan (**b**). Cystoscopy and biopsy were diagnostic for an eosinophilic bladder tumor

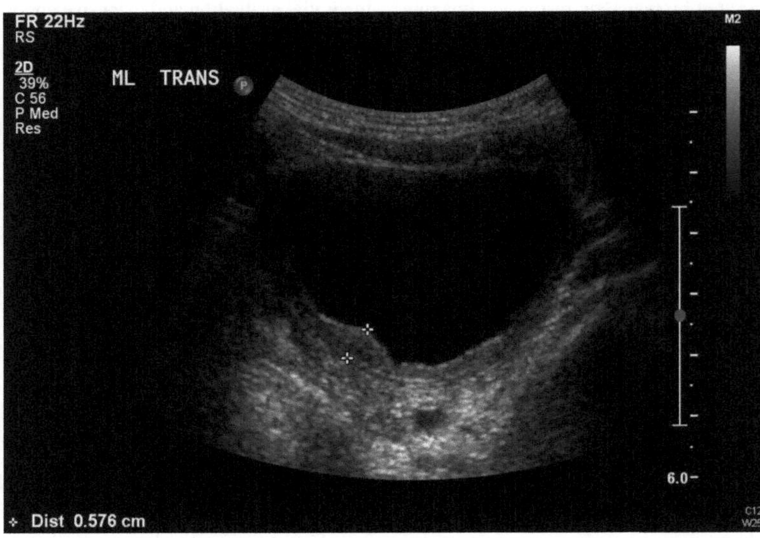


**Fig. 17.7** Bladder wall thickening detected on ultrasound evaluation of a child who presented with acute onset of gross hematuria and lower urinary tract symptoms. Ultrasound showed focal thickening most prominent in the posterior wall (*arrow*). Urine cultures returned negative. The patient experienced resolution of his symptoms and a follow-up ultrasound was normal. The findings were subsequently confirmed to be due to adenoviral cystitis

such as exposure to chemotherapeutic agents or immunosuppression (following solid organ or bone marrow transplantation). Initial management entails supportive measures, drainage (if associated with obstruction), and antibiotic coverage. If urine microscopy or previous cultures suggest the presence of a fungal infection, coverage (empiric or specific) has to be appropriately tailored. Patients who fail to respond to these interventions need to be considered for endoscopic or open exploration for evacuation.

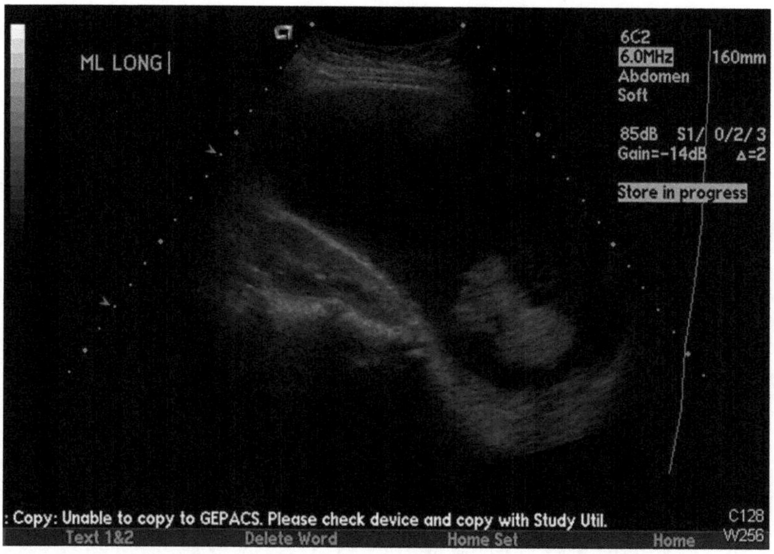


**Fig. 17.8** Free-floating "mass" in a child with hematuria following bone marrow transplantation. Intraluminal clot was evacuated during cystoscopy

## Hemangioma

This benign tumor accounts for a minority of lesions encountered in the bladder and may occur sporadically or part of a syndrome, such as Klippel–Trenaunay or Proteus. Three histological subtypes have been characterized: cavernous (the most common), capillary, and arteriovenous. These vascular tumors range in size from less than 1 cm to more than 10 cm, but are usually detected when ~1 cm. Most pediatric patients with bladder hemangiomas present with gross hematuria. On ultrasound clots may be difficult to differentiate from the mass; thus, Doppler evaluation may be of value in suspicious cases (Fig. 17.9). Cystoscopy often reveals the lesion located on the posterior and lateral bladder walls. In many cases endoscopic treatments are the procedures of choice, with surgical resection reserved for more extensive clinical scenarios. Due to the potential extension into the bladder wall, some advocate magnetic resonance imaging for patients with large lesions or evidence of detrusor involvement on ultrasound.

## Polyps

Congenital fibroepithelial polyps are rare lesions detected in children during the evaluation of obstructive lower urinary tract symptoms or incidentally discovered on imaging studies (Fig. 17.10). Location at the level of the bladder neck and/or posterior urethra creates an impediment to the flow of urine, thus the explanation of the symptoms. Being often pedunculated, the polyp may be intermittently detected in the bladder as it may migrate toward the urethra following micturition. Endoscopic removal is curative and recurrences following complete resection are uncommon.

## Neurofibroma

This diagnosis should be considered in patients with a genetic predisposition, almost exclusively seen in children with generalized neurofibromatosis type 1. Although genitourinary involvement in this condition is rare, the most common

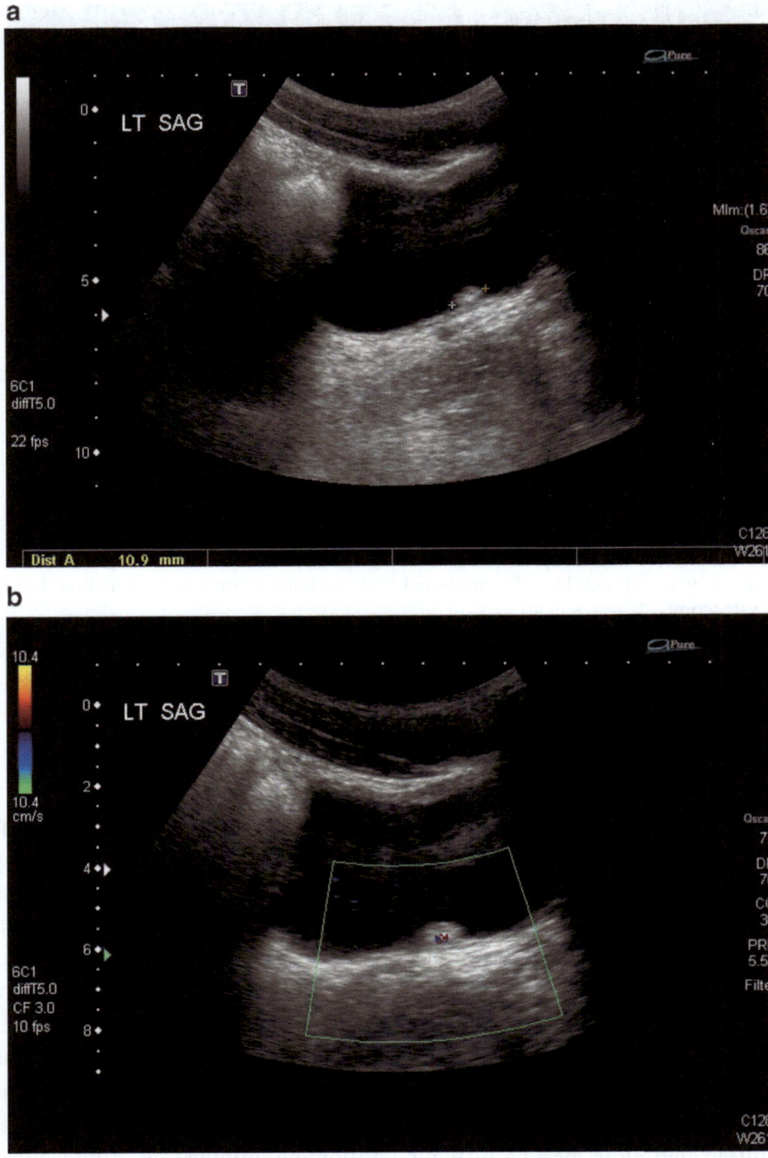


**Fig. 17.9** Small bladder mass detected during workup of recurrent gross hematuria in an otherwise asymptomatic child. A well-defined mass was detected on ultrasound (**a**, *arrow*), which appeared to have rich blood supply on Doppler evaluation (**b**). Cystoscopy showed small, well-defined friable mass consistent with a hemangioma. It was completely ablated with laser through a cystoscope

presentation is related to neurofibromas of the bladder. These tumors are thought to originate from the nerve sheaths of the bladder's autonomic nerve plexus. Due to the rarity of the problem and lack of guidelines, management is tailored based on the symptoms and presence of functional compromise. Involvement can be quite extensive (Fig. 17.11), and individualized strategies for surgical resection have been reported (including transurethral resection, partial cystectomy, and total cystectomy with diversion). Although malignant transformation is a concern,

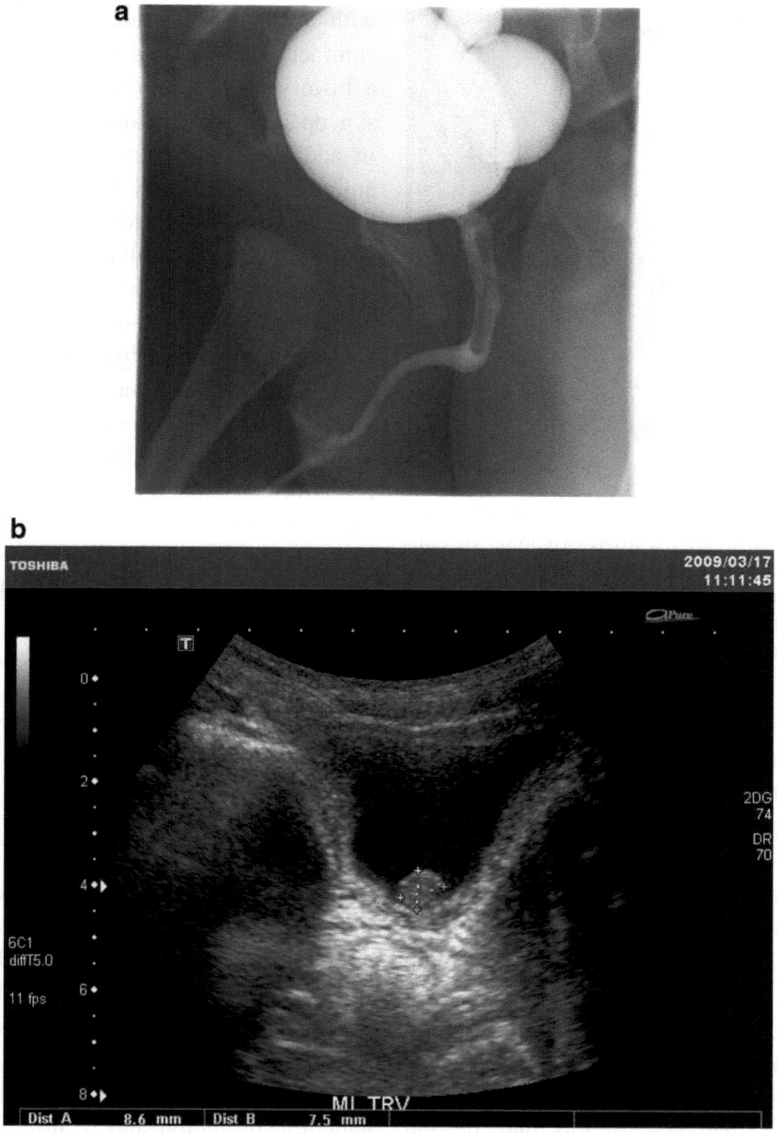


**Fig. 17.10** Prostatic urethral polyp detected during the evaluation of hematuria and obstructive lower urinary tract symptoms. Note filling defect in the urethra during voiding (panel **a**, *arrow*). Ultrasound evaluation (**b**) with a full bladder can be interpreted as a bladder mass. The diagnosis was confirmed with cystoscopic evaluation and transurethral resection

it appears to be almost exclusively detected in adulthood. Importantly, patients with neurofibromatosis may be at increased risk for rhabdomyosarcoma and have a more aggressive pattern of disease; thus, a high index of suspicion should be exercised, and the diagnosis of a neurofibroma should be considered keeping in mind the possibility of a bladder malignancy.

## Leiomyoma and Leiomyosarcoma

These tumors represent two ends of the bladder smooth muscle neoplastic spectrum and are overall rare. Both are far less common than rhabdomyosarcoma, which is the main diagnostic consideration in the pediatric patient population. The benign lesion, leiomyoma, appears well

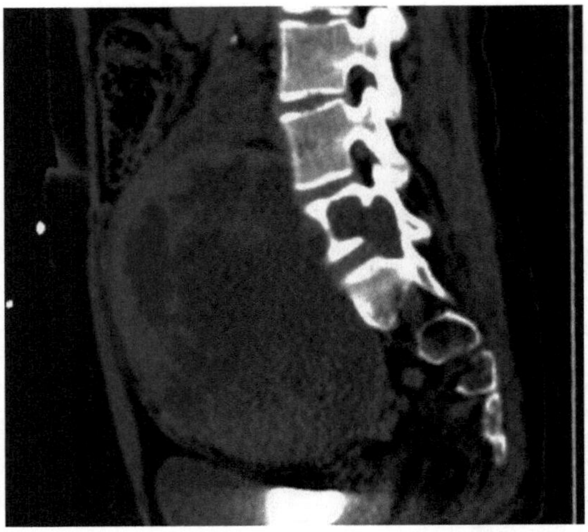

**Fig. 17.11** Large pelvic neurofibroma in an adolescent with neurofibromatosis type 1, progressive lower abdominal distention, and urinary frequency. Mass involvement of most of the pelvis is better appreciated on sagittal CT scan reconstruction. Note the involvement of the foramina and vertebral body (*arrow*)

defined on imaging studies and may be associated with mild or absent symptoms. Management centers on resection to eradicate the mass and histological evaluation (Fig. 17.12). Experience in adult patients suggests that transurethral resection may be considered in some cases and, if the lesion is considered benign, offered as the main modality for removal. Adjuvant therapy protocols for the leiomyosarcoma are limited due to the rarity of the disease, although reports suggest a favorable response to multimodal therapy. Case reports suggest that these tumors may present with intraperitoneal rupture (including one originating in the urachus); thus, the diagnosis should be suspected in the rare setting of hemoperitoneum, urinary ascites, and a bladder mass on imaging studies.

## Pheochromocytoma

Bladder involvement is an uncommon extra-adrenal site for this unusual tumor. The curious symptomatology that can be elicited in these patients relates to pressure elicited on the mass with changes in bladder volume and detrusor contraction. Thus, an astute clinician may detect a history of headaches, sweating, palpitations, syncope, or visual disturbances with micturition. In addition, manifestations related to catecholamine production may be encountered (such as hypertension, tachycardia). Although commonly sporadic, certain familial syndromes portent an increased risk of developing pheochromocytomas, namely, multiple endocrine neoplasia, neurofibromatosis, von Hippel–Lindau disease, and Sturge–Weber syndrome. The definitive preoperative diagnosis of a pheochromocytoma relies on imaging studies and demonstration of elevated levels of catecholamines or their metabolites in blood or urine (Fig. 17.13). Due to the risk of triggering a hypertensive crisis or life-threatening arrhythmia, if suspected these lesions should not undergo preoperative biopsy unless absolutely necessary. Surgical resection after adequate hydration and systemic adrenergic blockade is the preferred treatment option.

## Inverted Papilloma

This urothelial papillary neoplasm with distinctive histopathological characteristics is more commonly diagnosed in adults, with only a handful of case reports in the pediatric literature. The majority of patients present with hematuria and/or irritative bladder symptoms. Even though the lesion is considered benign, rare cases of malignant transformation and recurrences have been reported. Thus, long-term monitoring is warranted until more data is accrued on the natural history of the disease.

## Malakoplakia

This is a rare granulomatous inflammatory disease that can affect the genitourinary tract and is often misdiagnosed as a malignant process. Presentation during childhood is uncommon. The disease is thought to result from inadequate killing of bacteria by macrophages or monocytes that

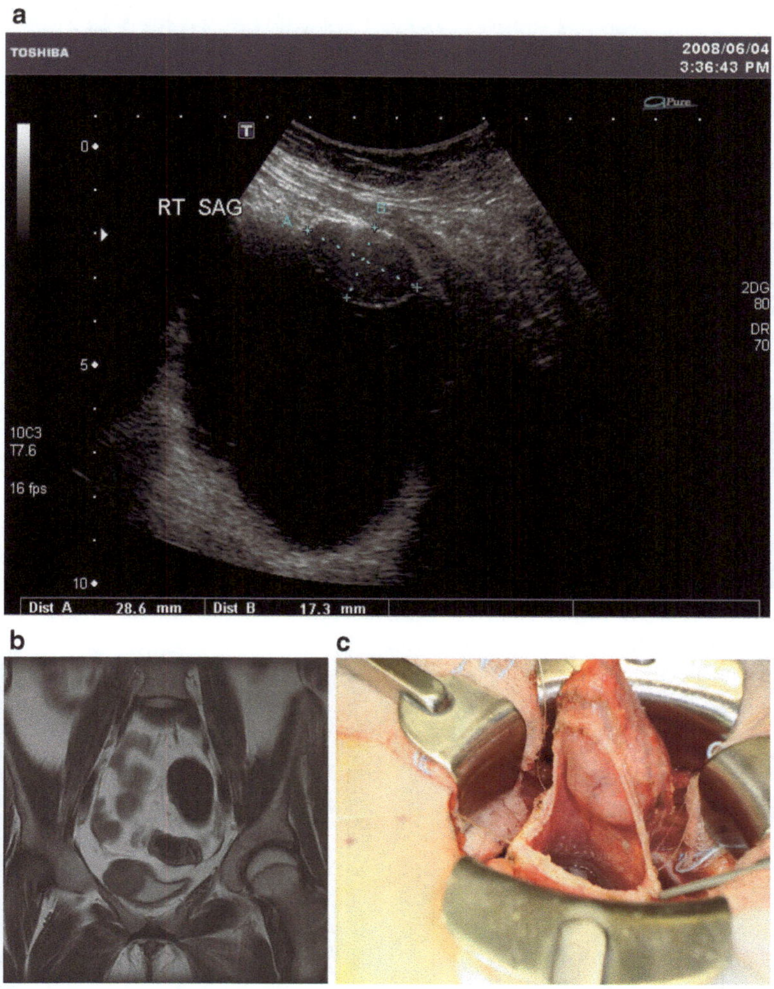


**Fig. 17.12** Bladder mass detected incidentally during workup of lower abdominal pain. A well-defined mass was detected on ultrasound (**a**) and subsequent magnetic resonance imaging (**b**). Cystoscopy showed an intact urothelium and biopsy was inconclusive. Partial cystectomy was conducted (**c**). Pathology was reported as a leiomyoma

exhibit defective phagolysosomal activity. Thus, patients tend to have a history of recurrent urinary tract infections. The condition is detected as a thickened bladder wall, irregularity of the mucosa, or polypoid masses on ultrasound evaluation obtained during the workup of these infections. On cystoscopy the lesions of malakoplakia characteristically appear as soft yellow-brown plaques with central ulceration and peripheral hyperemia. Biopsy is essential for establishing the diagnosis, relying on the detection of foamy histiocytes and Michaelis–Gutmann bodies (which are considered pathognomonic for malakoplakia). Medical management consists of cholinergic agonists and prolonged antimicrobial coverage. In patients who fail medical management, surgical resection should be considered.

## Lower Urinary Tract Involvement by Other Neoplasms

The lower urinary tract is close to other anatomical structures, which may be the site of benign or malignant tumors that invade or displace the bladder, ureter, or urethra. Example of one such tumor

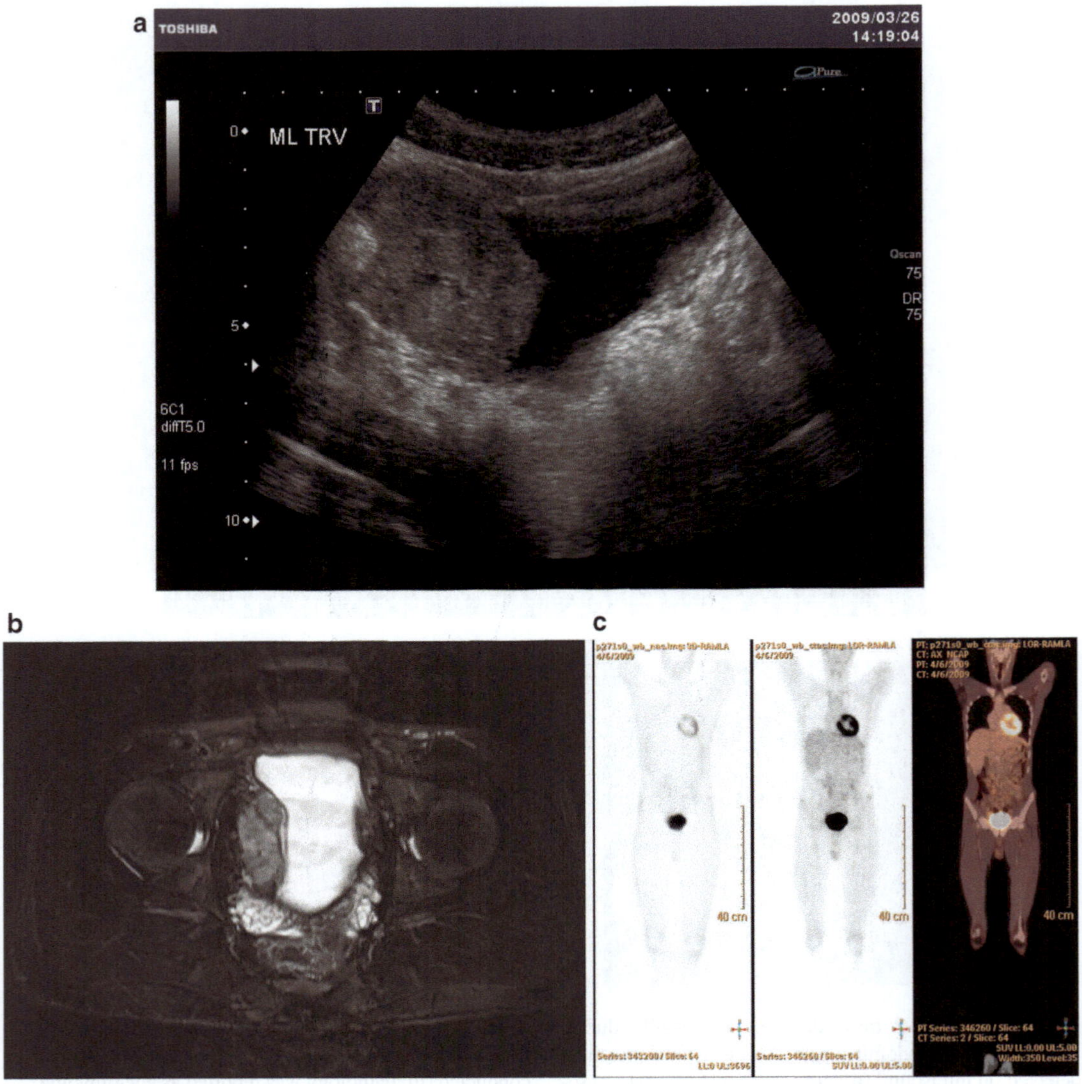


**Fig. 17.13** Bladder pheochromocytoma diagnosed in a teenager who presented with palpitations and episodes of syncope during micturition. Initial ultrasound evaluation showed a large mass in the lateral aspect of the bladder (**a**). The patient underwent further evaluation with magnetic resonance imaging (**b**) and PET scan (**c**). Laboratory examination confirmed the active production of catecholamines; thus, biopsy was not conducted and he underwent partial cystectomy. Pathology confirmed the diagnosis. Following surgery he experienced complete resolution of his initial symptomatology

is sacrococcygeal teratomas, which can attain a large size and push aside many pelvic structures. In addition, hematological malignancies can rarely present with direct bladder involvement, with associated symptoms such a hematuria. Although the differential diagnosis for this situation can be extensive (including many uncommon tumors), one stands out as particularly interesting: Patients with a Wilms' tumor may present with symptoms related to direct invasion and extension down the collecting system (i.e., an uncommon manifestation of a relatively common pediatric tumor, see Fig. 17.14). The child may develop hematuria, obstructive symptoms, and even pass small tumor fragments in the urine. Evaluation of the lower urinary tract is of importance, as the striking renal mass may be thought to be explanation enough for the symptoms.

a b

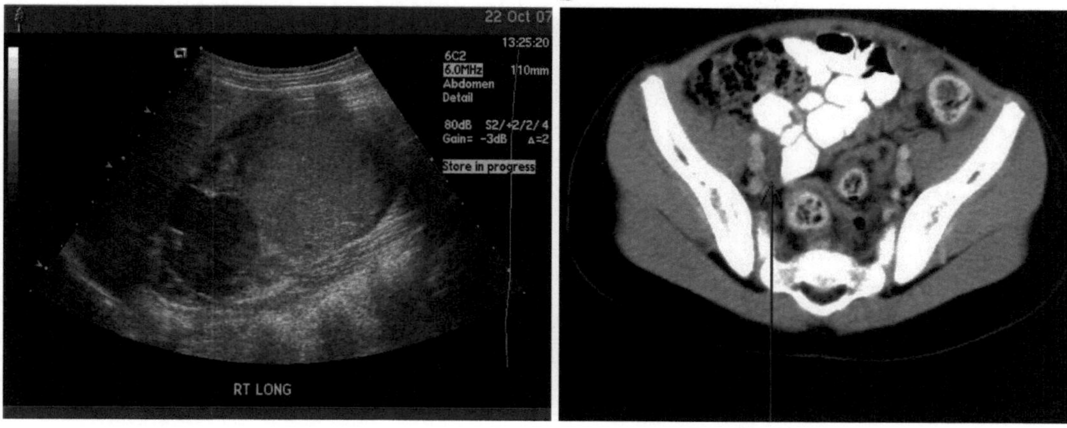


**Fig. 17.14** Patient with history of hematuria and abdominal distention was found to have a renal mass on renal ultrasound (**a**). On a subsequently obtained CT scan, the mass was noted to extend down to the renal pelvis and lower urinary tract (note ureteral involvement, panel **b**, *long arrow*). Pathology confirmed the presence of a Wilms' tumor with urothelial (botryoid) extension

This particular situation—called urothelial or botryoid extension—should alert the clinician to adequately pay attention to images of the distal ureter and bladder. Furthermore, the surgical intervention may have to be appropriately tailored in order to avoid transection of the ureter with tumor inside of it.

## Management and Referral

Most children present in stable condition. Consequently, for these patients initial management is safely conducted in a primary care setting. As previously discussed, the first issue is differentiating common benign conditions from the rare yet potentially more morbid or life-threatening ones. For those found to have any evidence of a lower urinary tract tumor, the decision on how to proceed is based on the most likely diagnoses, the child's comorbidities, and the result of the initial workup (including laboratory evaluations and imaging studies). The decision to refer should then be fairly straightforward; aside from those who have findings that can be clearly explained by a condition treatable in a primary care setting (such as a urinary tract infection in an immunocompetent patient), it is reasonable to contact and refer to a specialist, such as a pediatric surgeon or urologist. In the unusual circumstances where the underlying medical condition is complex (as patients who have previously undergone a transplant or children on chemotherapy), it is prudent to arrange for a visit with the patient's healthcare provider responsible for the management of the main comorbidity (oncologist, rheumatologist). Clearly, in situations where there is evidence of obstruction, severe hematuria, post-renal dysfunction, or systemic compromise, the patient should be acutely transferred to a facility able to provide the adequate level of care.

## Suggested Reading

Alanee S, Shukla AR. Bladder malignancies in children aged <18 years: results from the Surveillance, Epidemiology and End Results database. BJU Int. 2010;106(4):557–60.

Quigley R. Evaluation of hematuria and proteinuria: how should a pediatrician proceed? Curr Opin Pediatr. 2008;20:140–4.

Husmann DA, Rathbun SR. Long-term follow up of enteric bladder augmentations: the risk for malignancy. J Pediatr Urol. 2008;4(5):381–5.

Wu HY, Snyder 3rd HM, Womer RB. Genitourinary rhabdomyosarcoma: which treatment, how much, and when? J Pediatr Urol. 2009;5(6):501–6.

# Pediatric Hernias and Hydroceles

# 18

Steve S. Kim and Howard M. Snyder III

## Introduction

Pediatric inguinal hernias and hydroceles represent the clinical manifestations of a patent processus vaginalis (Fig. 18.1), whereby incomplete fusion and obliteration permit access of intraperitoneal contents to the groin and/or scrotum. Hernias represent the protrusion of bowel, omentum, and other intraperitoneal contents (fallopian tube, ovaries, etc.) down the patent processus vaginalis which present as intermittently palpable groin and/or scrotal masses. The term *incarcerated* hernia is used to describe a situation where the hernia sac contents fail to spontaneously reduce from the groin and scrotum requiring prompt medical attention. A *strangulated* hernia represents a situation where entrapped viscera undergo ischemic necrosis representing a true surgical emergency. Hydroceles reflect the presence of intraperitoneal fluid, rather than visceral organs within the processus vaginalis. *Non-communicating* hydroceles represent retained fluid within the groin or scrotum which does not freely communicate with the intraperitoneal cavity thus posing little risk for the sequelae of incarceration or strangulation. *Communicating* hydroceles, however, reflect a persisting connection with the intraperitoneal cavity which poses a distinct risk for future incarceration and strangulation.

S.S. Kim, M.D.
Assistant Professor of Clinical Urology Keck School of Medicine, University of Southern California Children's Hospital Los Angeles, Division of Urology, 4650 Sunset Blvd Mailstop #114, Los Angeles, CA 90027, USA
e-mail: stkim@chla.usc.edu

H.M. Snyder III, M.D. (✉)
Division of Urology, Department of Pediatric Urology, The Children's Hospital of Philadelphia, 34th Street and Civic Center Boulevard, 3rd Floor, Wood Center, Philadelphia, PA 19104, USA
e-mail: snyderh@email.chop.edu

## Incidence

Pediatric inguinal hernias and hydroceles are commonly encountered within the scope of a pediatric primary care practice, and therefore it is essential that pediatric providers are familiar with their diagnosis and management. Inguinal hernias occur in approximately 1–2 % of all live births and are more commonly found in males than females (4:1) [1, 2]. Hernias are also associated with prematurity with as many as 30 % of premature infants with a birth weight of less than 1,000 g identified as having a clinical hernia [2]. With regard to laterality, there is a higher incidence of inguinal hernias on the right side (60 %) versus the left side (30 %), with 10 % presenting bilaterally [3]. The peak incidence of hernias is within the first month of life with a third of all hernias presenting within the first 6 months of life [4]. Accordingly, the risk of incarceration is highest early on in infancy with a steep decline after the first year of life.

R. Rabinowitz et al. (eds.), *Pediatric Urology for the Primary Care Physician*, Current Clinical Urology, DOI 10.1007/978-1-60327-243-8_18, 

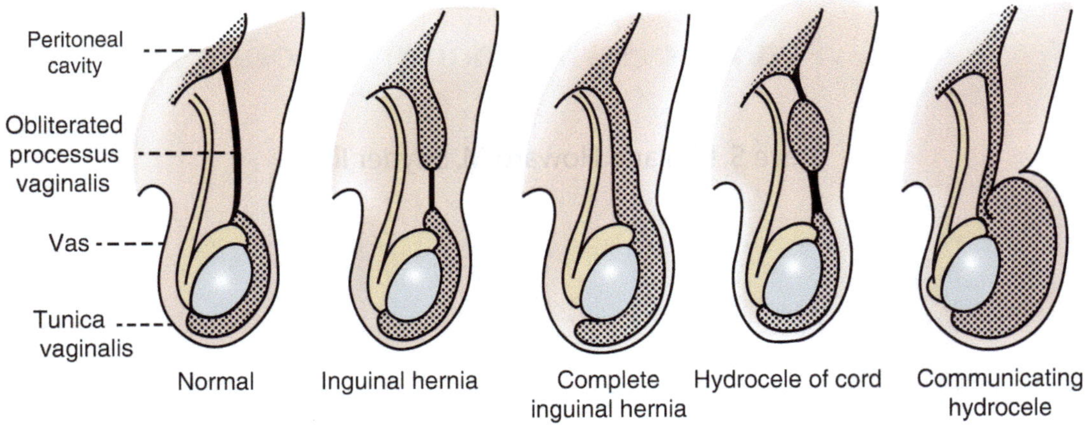


**Fig. 18.1** Anomalies of the inguinal canal and scrotum that may result from anomalous closure of the processus vaginalis (Adapted from [5])

## History

A careful history is critical in documenting pediatric hernias and hydroceles due to their intermittent nature. Frequently, a diagnosis is made primarily by history rather than on physical exam. Hernias and hydroceles are typically seen as a bulge or swelling of the groin and/or scrotum which are associated with increased intra-abdominal pressure (crying, Valsalva, etc.). As the swelling may be intermittent in nature, it is not uncommon that the hernia or hydrocele may not be clinically appreciable on physical exam, and therefore it becomes imperative to obtain a good history. Both clinical hernias and communicating hydroceles are frequently seen while a child is in the upright position or increases intra-abdominal pressure by coughing or straining. Hernias and hydroceles may not be associated with any significant discomfort or pain. However, when pain or discomfort is associated with a frank hernia, one must consider the possibility of visceral compromise with either an incarcerated or strangulated hernia. Symptoms worrisome for a bowel obstruction or ischemic compromise may include excessive crying, inconsolability, vomiting, or obstipation. Other useful information includes conditions that may be associated with increased intra-abdominal pressure such as the presence of ventriculoperitoneal shunts or peritoneal dialysis catheters which may contribute to a hernia.

## Physical Examination

A careful physical examination of the child suspected to have a hernia or a hydrocele should be performed in the supine position. In older children, it may also be possible to perform an examination in the erect position. In boys, the testes should be inspected to ensure that the diagnosis is not other causes for a groin or scrotal mass such as an undescended testis, a varicocele, or a testicular or paratesticular tumor. Maneuvers can be used to elicit increases in intra-abdominal pressure which may facilitate a diagnosis of a clinical hernia or hydrocele. In cooperative children, asking the child to strain, cough, or to sit up may increase intra-abdominal pressure sufficient enough to reveal a clinical hernia. Additionally, a thickened spermatic cord or "silk glove sign" may be identified when palpating the cord against the pubic tubercle indicating the likely presence of a patent processus vaginalis. Hydroceles can be palpated as fluid within either the scrotal sac or, in the case of hydroceles of the spermatic cord, loculated within the inguinal canal. In distinguishing a non-communicating from communicating hydrocele, in the latter, one is often able to squeeze fluid back and forth into the intraperitoneal cavity confirming the suspicion of a patency. Additionally, a comparison of bilateral spermatic cord structures may reveal evidence of thickened cord structures suggestive of a communicating hydrocele.

## Evaluation and Management

The evaluation of a child suspected to have a hernia or communicating hydrocele is largely based on history and physical examination. Laboratory studies are unnecessary in making a diagnosis of a hernia. Radiographic imaging studies are typically not required in making a diagnosis, but ultrasonography can be useful in both confirming a diagnosis of a hernia and ruling out other potential inguinal or scrotal pathology which may mimic a hernia.

In the management of hernias and hydroceles, it is paramount to be able to distinguish those situations which require immediate attention and surgical intervention. Suspected cases of strangulated hernias which present with inguinal masses which are painful to touch and accompanied by signs of systemic toxicity (leukocytosis, fever, hemodynamic instability, etc.) require emergent surgical intervention without delay. In the absence of systemic toxicity worrisome for a strangulated hernia, incarcerated hernias should undergo a trial of manual reduction. Oftentimes this requires the use of sedation to achieve sufficient relaxation of a child, in combination with Trendelenburg positioning, to achieve a manual reduction of an incarcerated hernia. In cases of a strangulated hernia, these efforts are unsuccessful and warrant immediate surgical repair. In those children where manual reduction is accomplished, it is recommended that the surgical repair be undertaken in an expedient fashion. In the absence of incarceration, reducible clinical hernias and communicating hydroceles should be surgically corrected in a prompt manner to avoid the possibility of incarceration.

Non-communicating hydroceles are frequently encountered early on in infancy and should be followed expectantly. A majority will spontaneously resolve during the first year of life. Persisting non-communicating hydroceles beyond 1 year of age may be considered for elective surgical repair given the decreasing likelihood of spontaneous resolution. A secondary onset of a hydrocele not present at birth typically occurs between 2 and 6 months of life. Non-communicating hydroceles which do not wax and wane in size may be followed and then referred after 1 year of age for surgical evaluation.

The surgical approach to the pediatric hernia or hydroceles differs from that of adults. Because of the etiology based on a congenitally patent processus vaginalis, pediatric hernia and hydrocele repairs are typically carried out through an inguinal incision which affords the ability to dissect and to perform a high ligation of the hernia sac. In the absence of an emergent situation, these procedures can be typically carried out on an outpatient basis in a majority of cases and are associated with minimal pain and morbidity.

## Conclusions

Pediatric inguinal hernias and hydroceles are a common clinical entity encountered in pediatric practice. Hernias and hydroceles in children are a result of a congenitally patent processus vaginalis. A thorough history and physical examination are key to making the diagnoses. Incarcerated and strangulated hernias require immediate or emergent intervention.

## References

1. Tam P. Inguinal hernia. In: Listen J, Irving JM, editors. Neonatal surgery. 3rd ed. London: Butterworths; 1990. p. 367.
2. Scherer L, Grosfeld J. Inguinal hernia and umbilical anomalies. Pediatr Clin North Am. 1993;40:1121.
3. Borkowski S. Common pediatric surgery problems. Nurs Clin North Am. 1994;29:551–62.
4. Holder T, Ashcraft K. Groin hernias and hydroceles. In: Holder T, Ashcraft K, editors. Pediatric surgery. Philadelphia: WB Saunders; 1980. p. 594–608.
5. Welch KA, Randolph JG, Ravitch MM, et al., editors. Pediatric surgery, vol. 2. 4th ed. St Louis: Year Book; 1986. p. 780.

# Retractile Testes

# 19

Robert A. Mevorach, William C. Hulbert Jr., and Ronald Rabinowitz

## Introduction

From birth to adulthood, testicles should be easily palpated within the scrotum on routine office evaluation. Testes palpated above the scrotal sac raise questions of descent and concerns for future fertility and predisposition to testicular cancer. The retractile testis, which is a normal testis that has an active cremasteric reflex, is clinically unrelated to a truly undescended testis but may be difficult to distinguish by initial examination.

This chapter will provide practical guidance to help assure that retractile testes are defined early in development and segregated clinically from those that are truly undescended testes (UDTs). This clarity assures that each boy receives appropriate management, and each parent is spared the stress that may accompany misdiagnosis.

R.A. Mevorach, M.D., F.A.A.P., F.A.C.S.
Chesapeake Urology, Owings Mills, Maryland, MD, USA
e-mail: rmevorach@cua.md

W.C. Hulbert Jr. , M.D., F.A.A.P., F.A.C.S. • R. Rabinowitz, M.D., F.A.A.P., F.A.C.S. (✉)
Division of Pediatric Urology, Department of Urology, University of Rochester Medical Center, Rochester, NY, USA
e-mail: william_hulbert@urmc.rochester.edu; ron_rabinowitz@urmc.rochester.edu

## Definition

The "retractile testis" is defined as a testicle that is located along the normal route of testicular descent (abdominal, inguinal, suprascrotal) that can be manipulated into a dependent position in the scrotum and dwells there, after traction is removed, for a finite period of time after the reflex abates and before the reflex returns. Structural problems often associated with UDTs—abnormalities of epididymal appearance and attachment, as well as a patent processus vaginalis, are found at the low rates as are seen in the general population in children with retractile testes. The commonly accepted etiology of unilateral or bilateral retraction appears to be an overactive cremasteric reflex arc (Fig. 19.1). This etiology is empirically borne out by the increased incidence of retractile testes among boys with cerebral palsy, who commonly display generalized hyperreflexia. Certain authors have suggested that the cremasteric muscle itself may be abnormal, as muscle reflex latencies would not allow for prolonged retraction in normal skeletal muscle fibers.

The retractile testicle will eventually occupy the scrotum without significant manipulation at or before pubertal development in boys, but some residual cremasteric hyperreflexia may occasionally persist into adulthood. While clinical issues may arise, retractile testes should be viewed as requiring ongoing observation, not routine intervention. In contrast, UDTs require intervention

R. Rabinowitz et al. (eds.), *Pediatric Urology for the Primary Care Physician*, Current Clinical Urology, DOI 10.1007/978-1-60327-243-8_19, © Springer Science+Business Media New York 2015

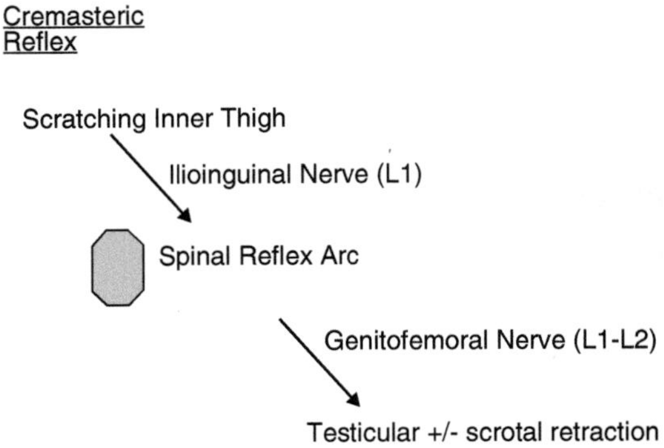


**Fig. 19.1** Cremasteric reflex arc

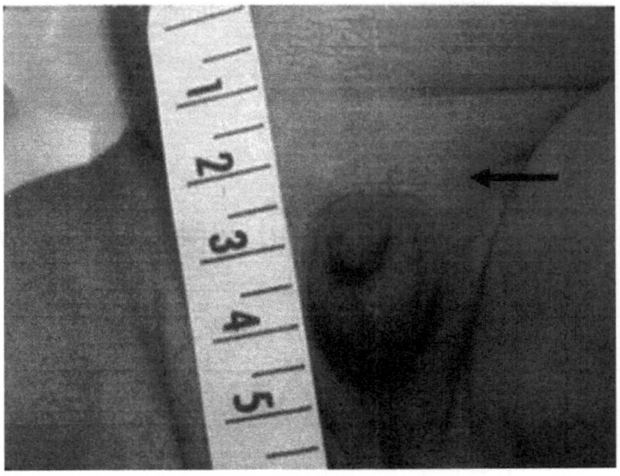

**Fig. 19.2** View of a 3-month-old external genitalia. The right descended testis is associated with a left undescended testis (*arrow*) and a hydrocele that simulates a scrotal testis

and should not be managed by observation, once diagnosed.

There remains some controversy in the literature regarding the clarity of the line that separates retractile from UDTs. A key to this ongoing debate may be the concept of an "acquired" UDT (aUDT). By definition, an aUDT is simply a testis that was once clearly palpable within the scrotum but, with overall growth and development, has later proven to be undescended. By these criteria, a diagnosed retractile testis that *ascends* could prove the case for a pathologic continuum between retractile and UDT, instead of two distinct entities. Arguing against this idea is a recent report on 172 patients from the Division of Pediatric Urology at Vanderbilt University. The authors showed that only 3.2 % of retractile testes underwent secondary ascent over 6 months to 8.5 years of observation. Of these, 13/19 (68 %) had a patent processus vaginalis repaired at the time of surgery, a finding typically associated with a true UDT. Although authors still disagree on whether retractile testes are merely less typical UDTs waiting to ascend, all would agree with the need for a careful genital examination of every boy, and specialty referral if questions arise.

## History

Birth history may guide expectations, as premature infants are more likely to have UDTs. Additionally, an accurate account of a scrotal examination from birth records or prior examiners in the older boy may steady one's resolve through a difficult exam.

Retractile testicles may begin their "hit or miss" positional observations at birth, with parents often reporting visualization of the testes within the scrotum during sleep or in warm baths. Hydroceles that give an appearance of scrotal fullness, with or without UDTs, may confound this evidence for a true scrotal position for the testis after birth (Fig. 19.2). Many times, the question of proper scrotal position is not even brought up until 4–6 months of age, after Leydig cell testosterone stimulation, mediated by the perinatal pHCG (placental human chorionic gonadotropin) and the 3-month LHRH (luteinizing hormone-releasing hormone) surge, is completed. This physiologic "mini-puberty" interferes with normal reflex-mediated testicular retraction, following which serum testosterone levels assume their prepubertal nadir. Reported "ascent" of the testis that often occurs at this time of lower hormone level is indistinguishable by history alone from certain ectopic or otherwise UDTs because their possible resting positions may have significant overlap (Fig. 19.3).

However, simply asking the older child "how many testes do you have in the scrotum" often answers the question of retractile versus UDTs.

In the older child and adolescent, there may be reports of discomfort as the testis draws backward through the external inguinal ring.

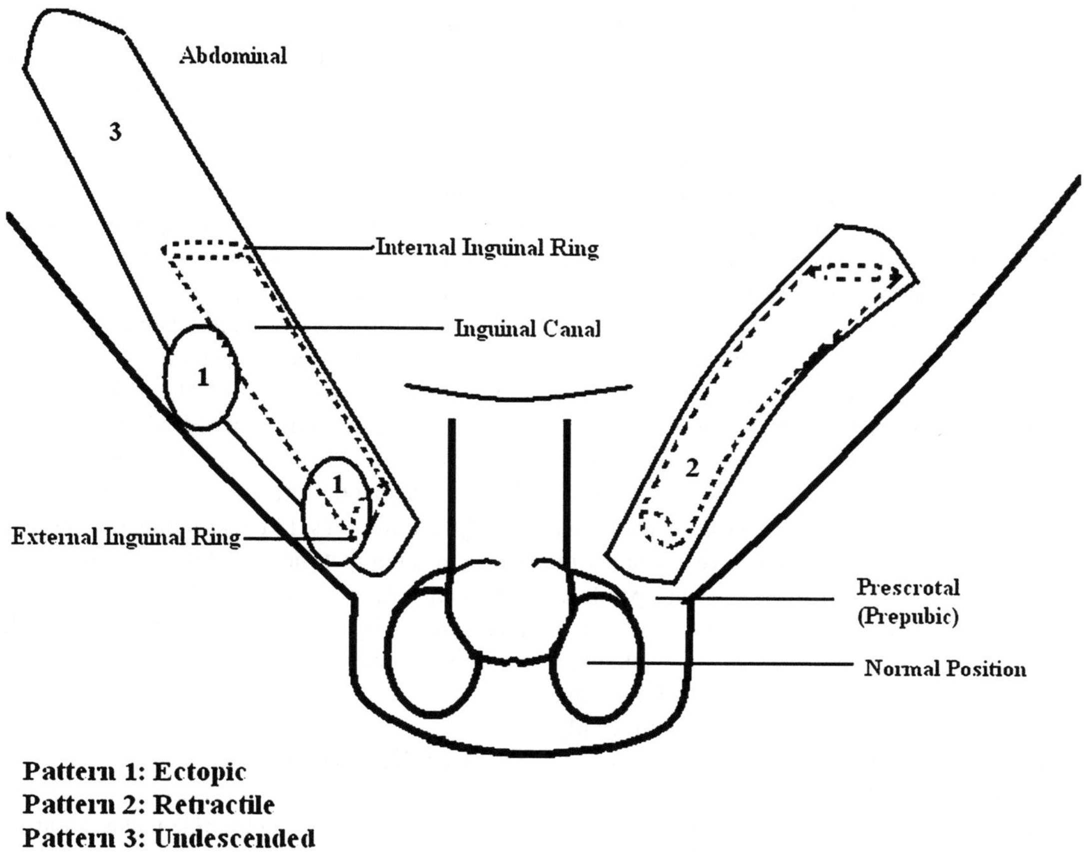


**Fig. 19.3** Patterns of retractile testes

Boys can often demonstrate their individualized and learned technique for returning the testis to its normal location, but presentation for acute scrotal pain is not uncommon. Some of these patients benefit from formal orchidopexy in that setting. Even though retractile testes may demonstrate considerable vertical mobility, there is neither literature nor experience that indicates a propensity for torsion of such a spermatic cord.

Conditions associated with retractile testes are few and include:

- Cerebral palsy
- Hypopituitarism
- Hyperthyroidism
- Attention-deficit/hyperactivity disorder (ADHD)
- Klinefelter syndrome
- Down syndrome
- Chiari II malformations

## Physical Examination

The physical examination should begin with a general assessment of the appropriateness of secondary sexual characteristics for the boy's chronological age.

A warm room, a relaxed child, and a gentle examiner are the basis for accurate testicular examination. While these elements seem to align themselves less often than the "stars" do, repeated reassurance and persistence will normally win the day. Positioning choices—recumbent, seated with legs crossed, reclining on a parent's lap, standing, squatting—all have their advocates, but speak more to examining style and personal preference than any particular merit.

Every examination of a boy should begin with the elements that are likely routine in their perception and therefore least threatening. Begin with a clothed child, reveal new areas to be examined as needed, and re-cover as you move onward. Abdominal examination should precede inguinal and genital exams. Asking permission from children who understand "please" can create tremendous trust, but a reliable examination may be difficult in spite of experience and effort. With a child in a supine frog-legged position, move to the internal ring of the uninvolved side in unilateral cases, or the visibly lesser affected testis in bilateral instances. Gently pushing down caudad beginning at the midpoint between the anterior-superior iliac spine and the pubic tubercle prevents retraction of the testis into the inguinal canal, and assures palpation of the descended, and most undescended, testes. Observe for signs of hernia or hydrocele (enlarged scrotum, patulous external ring, thickened spermatic cord) even if none is easily palpable, as this may influence counseling or planned intervention and follow-up. Once the testis is milked into the scrotum, gently cradle it in place between thumb, index, and middle finger after confirming a normal gonad. Once the reflex abates, release the testis without moving either the abdominal or scrotal hand and observe for a 2–3 s count. A retractile testis will not ascend until the abdominal muscles contract, or the inner thigh is touched, stimulating a cremasteric reflex. Repeat attempts may be needed, and engaging the child in "mental mathematics" can assist in relaxing abdominal musculature and attaining a reliable exam. Some authors have attempted to be more quantitative in their approach to retractile testes by measuring the distance from the pubic tubercle to the mid-testes. When the distance at rest is greater than 4 cm (most are 5–8 cm), this system, described by Scorer, would confirm a descended testis, but universal application and prospectively controlled studies are lacking.

## Gonadotropin-Releasing Hormone (GnRH) or HCG Stimulation in Diagnosis

As greater than 95 % of retractile testes maintain their scrotal position at puberty, it followed that stimulation of the normal boy with either gonadotropin-releasing hormone (GnRH) agonists or HCG for a few weeks could serve as a diagnostic tool. A positive result would reassure physician and parents of the likely pubertal expectations, and no ill effects were expected with such a limited use. Accordingly, up until the past few years, occasional specialists used varied but similar regimens to induce descent, and aside from a brief period of aggressive behavior, prolonged erections, genital discomfort, penile growth, and injection pain, no concerns were apparent. Unfortunately, recent reports implicate GnRH and HCG in increased apoptosis of testicular germ cells and potential negative impact on future fertility, when used as an adjunct in UDTs. Even with debate ongoing, it would seem that the use of these medications for diagnostic purposes would best be avoided and replaced by serial observation until the risk potential is defined.

## Diagnostic Imaging

Although ultrasonography (US) can identify 97 % of inguinal and scrotal testes, there are currently no defining criteria for differentiating between retractile and UDTs by any imaging modality. Further, recent literature would support a referral to a pediatric urologist as the next step in evaluation of any boy with concern of testicular maldescent, prior to any diagnostic imaging, since imaging is rarely needed in the evaluation.

## When to Refer

At any point in the ongoing care of a boy, a scrotal position for the testis must be achieved on examination. If exam conditions were suboptimal for achievement of this, then a repeat attempt in the near term should be arranged. When there remains any doubt regarding testicular location, specialty referral is appropriate. As guidance, many pediatric urologists have chosen to begin operative intervention on UDTs as early as 3–4 months of age on a routine basis and most are addressed well before 2 years of age.

Early diagnosis forms the basis for ongoing observation and the accurate diagnosis of the retractile testis is essential to this management.

Boys, particularly those postpubertal, having pain associated with cephalad displacement of the testis and the need for manual replacement of the testis into the scrotum for relief of that discomfort, warrant non-emergent surgical counseling and intervention. While there have been attempts at disruption of the continuity of the cremasteric fibers as attempts to abate retraction, only a formal orchidopexy with medial relocation of the internal ring has been successful in the authors' experience to resolve this complaint. The surgery is extensive and often has a prolonged recovery time for the older male.

## Conclusion

Retractile testes are defined by an uncompromised physical examination and periodic reevaluation for confirmation from infancy to adolescence. Changes in the position of any testis should be assessed and referred until proper scrotal location is achieved.

## Suggested Reading

Agarwal PK, Diaz M, Elder JS. Retractile testis—is it really a normal variant? J Urol. 2006;175(4):1496–9.

La Scala GC, Ein SH. Retractile testes: an outcome analysis on 150 patients. J Pediatr Surg. 2004;39(7): 1014–7.

Lewis K, Lee PA. Endocrinology of male puberty [Review] [20 refs]. Curr Opin Endocrinol Diabetes Obes. 2009;16(1):5–9.

Miller OF, Stock JA, Cilento BG, McAleer IM, Kaplan GW. Prospective evaluation of human chorionic gonadotropin in the differentiation of undescended testes from retractile testes. J Urol. 2003;169(6): 2328–31.

Rabinowitz R, Hulbert WC. Late presentation of cryptorchidism—the etiology of "testicular reascent". J Urol. 1997;157(5):1892–4.

Stec AA, Thomas JC, DeMarco RT, Pope 4th JC, Brock 3rd JW, Adams MC. Incidence of testicular ascent in boys with retractile testes. J Urol. 2007;178(4 Pt 2): 1722–4; discussion 1724–5.

# 20 Undescended Testes

Jack S. Elder

## Introduction

The most common congenital abnormality of the male genitalia is an undescended testis (UDT), also known as cryptorchidism (Fig. 20.1). At birth, approximately 4.5 % of boys have a UDT. Because testicular descent occurs late in gestation, 30 % of premature males have a UDT, whereas the incidence is 3.4 % at term. Many undescended testes descend spontaneously during the first 3 months of life, and by 3 months the incidence decreases to 1 %. Cryptorchidism is bilateral in 10 % of cases. There is some evidence that the incidence of cryptorchidism is increasing. Although cryptorchidism usually is considered to be a congenital condition, an increasing number of older boys with a previous normal exam are being diagnosed with a UDT. Typically, these boys have a scrotal testis that "ascends" to a low inguinal position, and therefore require an orchiopexy. Some boys have secondary cryptorchidism after repair of an inguinal hernia. This complication is most common in neonates and young infants and affects as many as 1–2 % of patients undergoing hernia repair.

J.S. Elder, M.D. (✉)
Division of Pediatric Urology, Massachusetts General Hospital, 55 Fruit Street, Boston, MA 02114, USA
e-mail: jack.s.elder@gmail.com

The process of testicular descent is regulated by an interaction between hormonal and mechanical factors, including testosterone, dihydrotestosterone, Müllerian-inhibiting factor, insulin-like factor 3, the gubernaculum, intra-abdominal pressure, and the genitofemoral nerve. The testis develops at 7–8 weeks gestation. At 10–11 weeks, the Leydig cells produce testosterone, which stimulates differentiation of the Wolffian (mesonephric) duct into the epididymis, vas deferens, seminal vesicle, and ejaculatory duct. At 32–36 weeks, the testis, which is anchored at the internal inguinal ring by the gubernaculum, begins its process of descent. The gubernaculum distends the inguinal canal and guides the testis into the scrotum. Following testicular descent, the patent processus vaginalis (hernia sac) normally involutes.

In newborns with a UDT, spontaneous testicular descent may occur because of hormonal events. At birth, the serum testosterone is low, approximately 60 ng/dl, because of suppression of the fetal hypothalamic-pituitary-testicular axis by circulating maternal estrogens in utero. Following delivery, with absence of the inhibitory estrogens, there is a rebound surge of luteinizing hormone (LH) and follicular-stimulating hormone (FSH), resulting in a temporary burst of testosterone, which causes some undescended testes to descend to the scrotum. By 3–4 months, the serum testosterone returns to baseline. Consequently, if the testis has not descended by 4 months, it will remain undescended.

R. Rabinowitz et al. (eds.), *Pediatric Urology for the Primary Care Physician*, Current Clinical Urology,
DOI 10.1007/978-1-60327-243-8_20, © Springer Science+Business Media New York 2015

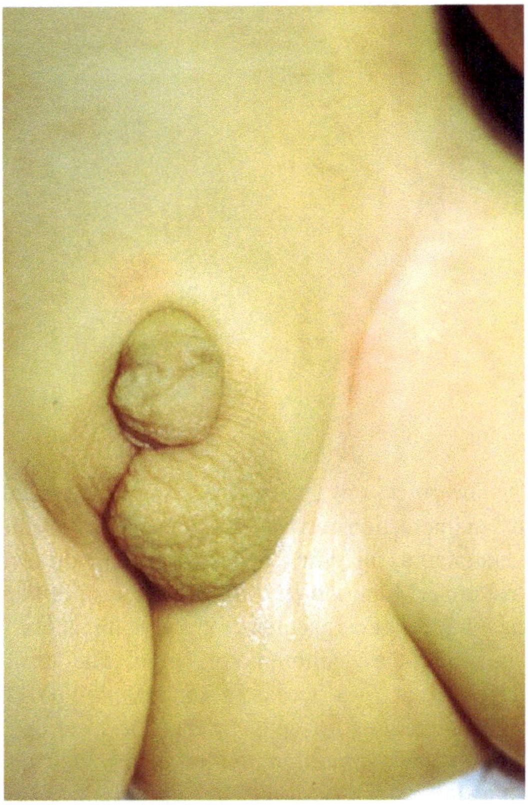

**Fig. 20.1** Infant with a right undescended testis. Note underdevelopment of right hemiscrotum

## Classification

The position of a UDT is described as abdominal (nonpalpable), peeping (abdominal but can be pushed into the upper part of the inguinal canal; usually nonpalpable), inguinal, gliding (can be pushed into the scrotum but retracts immediately to the pubic tubercle), and ectopic (superficial inguinal pouch or, rarely, perineal). Most undescended testes are palpable just distal to the inguinal canal over the pubic tubercle.

A retractile testis may be misdiagnosed as a UDT. In these boys, the testis may be in the inguinal canal or even nonpalpable, and difficult to manipulate into the scrotum. However, with relaxation, the testis resides in the scrotum. Boys older than 1 year of age frequently have a brisk cremasteric reflex; and if the child is anxious or ticklish during a scrotal examination, the testis may be difficult to manipulate into the scrotum. Retractile testes are not considered to be true undescended testes, and generally do not need treatment. However, many need ongoing monitoring, because as many as 1/3 eventually "ascend" to an undescended position, necessitating surgical treatment.

## Nonpalpable Testis

Approximately 10 % of undescended testes are nonpalpable. Of these, 50 % are viable testes in the abdomen or high in the inguinal canal, and 50 % are atrophic or absent, almost always in the scrotum, secondary to spermatic cord torsion in utero (vanishing testis). If the nonpalpable testis is abdominal, it will not descend after 3 months of age.

## Consequences of a UDT

The risks of having a UDT include infertility, testicular cancer, incarcerated inguinal hernia, testicular torsion, testicular trauma, psychological consequences of having an empty scrotum, and sexual dysfunction (if the child has anorchia).

## Infertility

The primary reason for performing an orchiopexy is to maximize potential for fertility. At birth, the testes contain germ cells, which are precursors to mature sperm. Normal spermatogenesis involves gradual maturation of primordial germ cells into gonocytes. At 3–5 months of age, the gonocytes become Ad spermatogonia. These cells eventually become type B spermatogonia and primary spermatocytes, and at puberty spermatogenesis occurs. In a UDT, exposure to the core body temperature interferes with the gradual maturation of gonocytes into mature sperm. Although the number of gonocytes in a UDT in a 2-month-old boy is normal, at 6 months, the gonocyte-to-Ad spermatogonia ratio is lower than normal. Over time, the number of germ cells gradually decreases in a UDT, reducing its potential for fertility. A recent prospective randomized clinical trial demonstrated that ultimate testicular size of undescended testes subjected to orchiopexy at 6 months was significantly larger than testes undergoing orchiopexy at 3 years of age. Undescended testes also have a reduced number of Leydig cells, which produce testosterone, although the serum testosterone in boys with a UDT is normal. Finally, fibrosis of the testicular interstitium also occurs over time. In the postpubertal testis, no spermatogenesis is observed, and the histologic appearance is Sertoli cell only.

In unselected men, 93 % are fertile. In men who underwent a unilateral orchiopexy as a child, approximately 90 % are fertile, similar, though slightly lower than the control population, presumably because the contralateral testis usually functions normally. In men who underwent bilateral orchiopexy, however, only 65 % are fertile. Factors which are associated with infertility include older age at orchiopexy and testicular position, with abdominal testes exhibiting more severe histologic changes than ectopic testes. In addition, as many as 1/3 of boys have a structural abnormality of the epididymis where sperm maturation and storage occur (Fig. 20.2). Furthermore, experimental studies have demonstrated that extensive mobilization of the vas deferens, which is common during surgical correction of high undescended testes, can lead to denervation of the vas and infertility.

## Testicular Cancer

Testicular cancer is the most common malignancy in young adult men, and it occurs most often in men age 15–40 years, with a lifetime risk of 0.3–0.7 %. An association between germ cell cancer of the testis and UDT has been recognized for more than a century.

The secondary reasons for performing an orchiopexy in boys with a UDT are to move the testis to a position where it can be palpated easily and to diminish the risk of developing a germ cell tumor. Recent meta-analyses have clarified the ultimate risk of malignancy in boys with a UDT. The relative risk of testicular cancer is 2.75–8 times higher

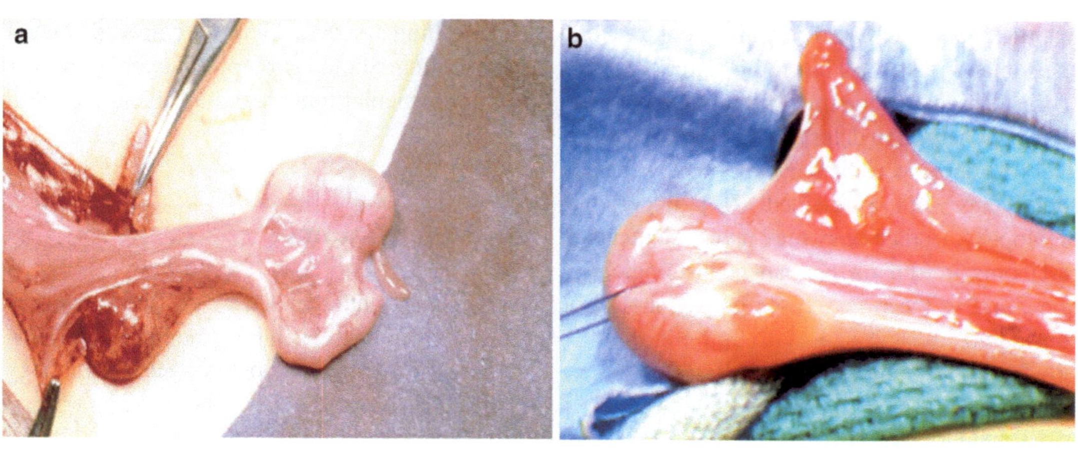

**Fig. 20.2** Structural abnormalities of the epididymis in boys with an undescended testis. (**a**) Long-looping epididymis. (**b**) Disjunction of the epididymis from the testis, preventing sperm from the affected testis to enter the reproductive tract

than in the general population. If surgical correction by orchiopexy is performed by age 10–12 years, the risk is only 2–3 times higher, whereas if the orchiopexy is performed beyond age 12 years, the risk is 6–8 times higher. It is uncertain whether undescended testes that were abdominal are at higher risk for malignant change compared with testes that were inguinal at the time of orchiopexy. Screening for testicular cancer in boys with a history of a UDT should begin around age 15 years, and adolescents and young men should be taught to perform monthly testicular self-examination. Ultrasound screening of the formerly cryptorchid testis is unnecessary, unless induration is detected, or if the young man has known microlithiasis (calcium deposits) of the testis.

The type of germ cell testicular tumor that occurs varies with the previous surgical history. In men with a UDT that becomes malignant, the most common testis tumor is a seminoma, which generally is treated by radical orchiectomy and radiation therapy. On the other hand, if the man has undergone an orchiopexy and the testis is in the scrotum, the most common tumor type is a non-seminomatous tumor, which is treated by radical orchiectomy and systemic chemotherapy in most cases.

In men who have undergone a unilateral orchiopexy, many have thought that the contralateral normal descended testis also is at increased risk for malignancy. However, recent studies suggest that there is no increased risk in the contralateral testis unless it also has been or is undescended.

Testis biopsy at the time of orchiopexy generally is not helpful in determining whether a boy is likely to develop testicular cancer. However, in adolescents with a retained UDT undergoing orchiopexy, testis biopsy may reveal elements of carcinoma in situ on permanent histologic sections, and in these rare cases biopsy should be considered.

## Inguinal Hernia

Before descent of the testis from an abdominal to a scrotal position occurs, an elongated pocket of peritoneum extends down the inguinal canal, and the testis normally slides along this pathway, called the processus vaginalis. When the testis reaches the scrotum, the processus vaginalis regresses. If the processus vaginalis persists and remains patent, an inguinal hernia or communicating hydrocele is common.

In boys with a UDT, the processus vaginalis usually remains patent, causing an increased risk of having an inguinal hernia. Approximately 85 % of boys with a congenital UDT undergoing an orchiopexy have a patent processus vaginalis, and excision with closure of the processus vaginalis (i.e., hernia repair) usually is necessary at the time orchiopexy. In addition, up to 6 % of inguinal hernias are associated with a UDT; consequently, the position of the testis in boys with an inguinal hernia should be determined.

Since boys with a UDT have a patent processus, they are at risk for developing a symptomatic hernia, and because the channel tends to be narrow, they can present with an incarcerated hernia.

## Testicular Torsion

Under normal circumstances, the testis is fixed in the scrotum and cannot rotate more than 90–180°. With a UDT, however, the testis is essentially floating freely along the inguinal canal, and spontaneous rotation of the spermatic cord can occur, resulting in testicular torsion. Although this condition is rare, sudden onset of inguinal pain and swelling associated with an empty ipsilateral hemiscrotum should prompt emergency evaluation for testicular torsion and incarcerated inguinal hernia.

## Testicular Trauma

An inguinal undescended or retractile testis is subject to rupture by blunt traumatic injury by compression against the pubic bone. Orchiopexy avoids this risk.

## Psychological Consequences

Most boys with a UDT have underdevelopment of the scrotum on the affected side. Preoccupation with an empty scrotum or embarrassment with peers can occur in boys with a UDT. If there is a solitary testis, it usually undergoes hypertrophy, and adolescent boys can have a distinctly asymmetric appearance. In this situation, insertion of a testicular prosthesis should be considered.

## Sexual Dysfunction

Adolescent and adult males with a history of cryptorchidism generally have a normal serum testosterone, even if they are infertile. However, in those with anorchia, in which both testes have undergone spermatic cord torsion, hormone replacement therapy with testosterone is necessary. This treatment begins at puberty and consists of application of transdermal testosterone gel or monthly testosterone injection therapy. Insertion of testicular prostheses is recommended also.

## History

Maternal, paternal, and familial risk factors for UDT should be ascertained, including hormonal exposure in utero and a family history of a UDT. Male children of men with a UDT have a 10 % of being affected, and the risk also is 10 % for male siblings. There is an increased risk of a UDT following in vitro fertilization. Birth history is important, as 30 % of premature males have a UDT.

Awareness of associated medical conditions is helpful, as undescended testes are common in boys with congenital heart disease, anorectal malformations, spina bifida, and many genetic syndromes. It is helpful to determine whether the testis was undescended at birth and whether it descended spontaneously. In boys with spontaneous testicular descent during infancy, reascent of the testis is common in older boys. In older boys with a UDT, a history of a retractile testis is common, and ascent of the scrotal testis is becoming recognized with increasing frequency. Past surgical history may reveal that the boy underwent inguinal hernia repair as an infant; approximately 1–2 % of these boys later develop a UDT because of scar formation around the spermatic cord, preventing normal growth of the spermatic cord. Finally, it is helpful to ask the parents whether they have observed the testes in the scrotum.

## Physical Examination

A thorough genitourinary exam is performed. The abdomen is examined for evidence of any surgical scars. The genitalia are examined for size and normal development. The position of the urethral meatus should be determined, as undescended testes are common in boys with hypospadias. In boys nearing puberty, assessment for a varicocele should be performed also, by examining the patient in a standing position.

For examination of the inguinal canal and scrotum, it is helpful to have the boy completely undressed, to help him relax. In a boy who is particularly anxious, distraction with reading material or a game can be helpful. The boy should be examined in the supine position with the lower extremities in a frog-leg position. The scrotum is examined for development and symmetry. A UDT often is associated with underdevelopment of the ipsilateral hemiscrotum. On the other hand, with a retractile testis, the scrotum typically is well rugated and similar in appearance to the opposite side.

If the testis is not in the scrotum, the examining fingers of the nondominant hand should be swept along the inguinal canal toward the scrotum, and the opposite (dominant) hand should be used to try to palpate the testis. Sometimes the testis will be palpable only by a "pop" under the fingers. The testis can be particularly difficult to palpate in a boy who is obese.

If the inguinal testis can be manipulated into the scrotum, the examiner should determine whether it stays in the scrotum. Signs suggesting that the testis is retractile include determining that the testis is similar in size to the opposite testis and that it stays in the scrotum. On the other hand, if it seems difficult to manipulate the testis into the scrotum, the spermatic cord is tight, or the testis seems smaller than the opposite testis, then it is probably a UDT.

If the testis is nonpalpable with these maneuvers, then traction should be applied to the ipsilateral hemiscrotum, because the UDT usually attached to the scrotum by the gubernaculum. In addition, the soap test should be used. Soap is applied to the inguinal area and to the examiner's hands and the physical exam is repeated. The soap reduces the friction between the hand and testis and will make it much easier to palpate the testis, if it is present. One "soft" sign that a testis is absent is contralateral testicular hypertrophy, but this finding is not 100 % diagnostic.

## Laboratory Tests

In most cases, no laboratory tests are necessary in a boy with a UDT. However, assessment for a disorder of sex development (aka intersex) should be performed in boys with subcoronal or more severe hypospadias and a UDT or bilateral nonpalpable testes. For example, bilateral nonpalpable gonads in a phenotypic male could be a sign of a virilized female with congenital adrenal hyperplasia (CAH). In addition, a disorder of sex development (e.g., mixed gonadal dysgenesis, true hermaphroditism, or male pseudohermaphroditism) is present in 15 % of phenotypic males with hypospadias and a palpable UDT and 50 % of phenotypic males and a nonpalpable testis. In these cases, a karyotype should be obtained.

## Imaging Tests

In boys with a nonpalpable testis, 50 % are abdominal or high in the inguinal canal, and 50 % are atrophic in the scrotum or inguinal canal secondary to spermatic cord torsion in utero. If an imaging test could identify boys with an atrophic testis with 100 % accuracy, then exploration would be unnecessary. Unfortunately, no imaging test provides this level of accuracy, and for this reason imaging is not recommended in most cases, because it rarely eliminates the need for surgical exploration and does not change the surgical approach.

Many primary care physicians obtain an ultrasound study (US) if the testis is nonpalpable to try to localize the testis. If the testis is abdominal, usually the US does not visualize the testis because of overlying bowel gas. If the testis is atrophic in the scrotum, the US will be negative. If the testis is inguinal, the US will localize the testis, but these testes should be palpable under normal circumstances. Consequently, US is unnecessary in most cases. The main situation in which US for a nonpalpable testis should be considered is in the obese patient, in whom an inguinal testis may be difficult to palpate.

Computerized tomography (CT) and magnetic resonance imaging (MRI) are much more accurate than US in identifying the UDT. However, neither test is 100 % accurate. In addition, CT exposes the child to significant radiation and children undergoing MRI generally require general anesthesia.

## Management of the Child with an UDT

### Hormonal Therapy

Hormonal treatment is used infrequently. The theory is that because testicular descent is under androgenic regulation, human chorionic gonadotropin (which stimulates Leydig cell production of testosterone) or luteinizing hormone-releasing hormone (LHRH) may stimulate testicular descent. Although hormonal treatment has been used in Europe, randomized controlled trials have not shown either of these hormonal preparations to be effective in stimulating testicular descent. There has been some preliminary evidence that an LHRH analog, buserelin, may be helpful in increasing germ cell number and normalizing testicular histologic features.

### Surgical Treatment

Most testes can be brought down to the scrotum with an orchiopexy (also known as orchidopexy), which involves an inguinal incision, mobilization

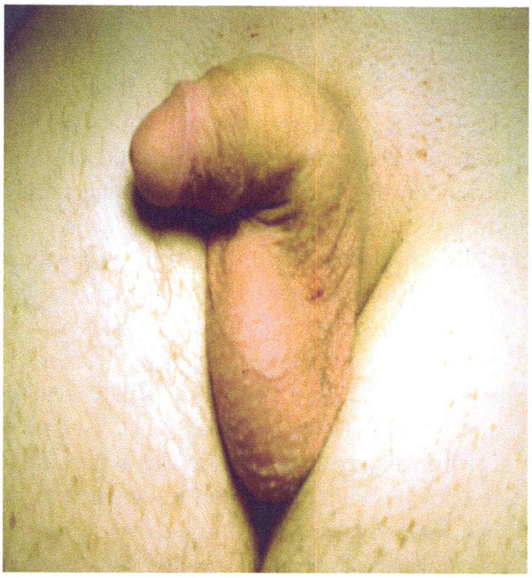

**Fig. 20.3** Adolescent male with absent left testis scheduled for placement of testicular prosthesis. Note right compensatory testicular hypertrophy

of the testis and spermatic cord, and correction of the indirect inguinal hernia. The procedure is typically performed on an outpatient basis and has a success rate of 98 %. Orchiopexy is performed as early as 6 months, to maximize the potential for future fertility. In some boys with a testis that is close to the scrotum, a prescrotal orchiopexy can be performed. In this procedure, the entire operation is performed through an incision along the edge of the scrotum. Often the associated inguinal hernia also can be corrected with this incision. Advantages of this approach over the inguinal approach include shorter operative time and less postoperative discomfort.

In boys with a nonpalpable testis, diagnostic laparoscopy is performed in most centers. This procedure allows safe and rapid assessment of whether the testis is intra-abdominal (Fig. 20.3). In most cases, orchiopexy of the intra-abdominal testis located immediately inside the internal inguinal ring is successful, but orchiectomy should be considered in more difficult cases or when the testis appears to be atrophic. A two-stage orchiopexy sometimes is needed in boys with a high abdominal testis. Boys with abdominal testes are managed with laparoscopic techniques at many institutions.

In adolescent boys with an absent testis, placement of a testicular prosthesis should be considered. Testicular prostheses are available for older children and adolescents when absence of the gonad in the scrotum may have an undesirable psychological effect. The US Food and Drug Administration (FDA) has approved a saline testicular implant. Solid silicone "carving block" implants also are used. Placement of testicular prostheses early in childhood is recommended for boys with anorchia (absence of both testes).

## When to Refer

A male newborn with an UDT may have spontaneous testicular descent until 3–4 months of age. Male infants and boys older than 4 months should be referred to a pediatric surgical specialist for orchiopexy. In addition, in boys with a suspected retractile testis, referral to a pediatric urologist should be considered.

## Guidelines on Cryptorchidism

The American Urological Association released guidelines on cryptorchidism in 2014. Their recommendations include:

### Diagnosis

*Guideline Statement* 1: Providers should obtain a gestational history at initial evaluation of boys with suspected cryptorchidism.

*Guideline Statement* 2: Primary care providers should palpate the testes for quality and position at each recommended well-child visit.

*Guideline Statement* 3: Providers should refer infants with a history of cryptorchidism (detected at birth) who do not have spontaneous testicular descent by 6 months (corrected for gestational age) to an appropriate surgical specialist for timely evaluation.

*Guideline Statement* 4: Providers should refer boys with the possibility of newly diagnosed (acquired) cryptorchidism after 6 months (corrected for gestational age) to an appropriate surgical specialist.

*Guideline Statement* 5: Providers must immediately consult an appropriate specialist for all phenotypic male newborns with bilateral, nonpalpable testes for evaluation of a possible disorder of sex development (DSD).

*Guideline Statement* 6: Providers should not perform ultrasound or other imaging modalities in the evaluation of boys with cryptorchidism before referral because these studies rarely assist in decision making.

*Guideline Statement* 7: Providers should assess the possibility of a DSD when there is increasing severity of hypospadias with cryptorchidism.

*Guideline Statement* 8: In boys with bilateral, nonpalpable testes who do not have CAH, providers should measure levels of Müllerian-inhibiting substance (MIS or anti-Müllerian hormone) and consider additional hormone testing, to evaluate for anorchia.

*Guideline Statement* 9: In boys with retractile testes, providers should monitor the position of the testes at least annually to monitor for secondary ascent.

## Treatment

*Guideline Statement* 10: Providers should not use hormonal therapy to induce testicular descent, as evidence shows low response rates and lack of evidence for long-term efficacy.

*Guideline Statement* 11: In the absence of spontaneous testicular descent by 6 months (corrected for gestational age), specialists should perform surgery within the next year.

*Guideline Statement* 12: In prepubertal boys with palpable, cryptorchid testes, surgical specialists should perform scrotal or inguinal orchidopexy.

*Guideline Statement* 13: In prepubertal boys with nonpalpable testes, surgical specialists should perform examination with the patient under anesthesia to reassess for palpability of the testes. If the testes are nonpalpable, surgical exploration and (if indicated) abdominal orchidopexy should be performed.

Guideline Statement 14: At the time of exploration for a nonpalpable testis in boys, surgical specialists should identify the status of the testicular vessels to help determine the next course of action.

Guideline Statement 15: In boys with a healthy contralateral testis, surgical specialists may perform an orchiectomy (removal of the UDT) if a boy has either very short testicular vessels and vas deferens, a dysmorphic or very hypoplastic testis, or postpubertal age.

*Guideline Statement* 16: Providers should counsel boys with a history of cryptorchidism and/or monorchidism and their parents regarding potential long-term risks and provide education on infertility and cancer risk.

If the child is younger than 6 months, he should be monitored across time for potential spontaneous descent of the testes, which may occur very frequently initially after birth but less likely closer to age 6 months and is rare or absent after age 6 months.

If the testis remains undescended and is palpable, open surgical repair is performed, either through an inguinal incision or a scrotal incision. If the testis is nonpalpable, the patient is examined under anesthesia. If a palpable nubbin is felt in the hemiscrotum and especially if the contralateral testis is hypertrophic, the surgeon can consider a primary scrotal approach to remove the vanishing testis.

If there are no palpable nubbins and the testis is not palpable, an open exploration with an abdominal orchiopexy is performed. If the testis is present, an open or laparoscopic procedure or a 1- or 2-stage Fowler-Stephens procedure is performed. If the vessels enter the internal ring, an inguinal exploration is performed to confirm a vanishing testis or inguinal testis.

Finally, if blind-ending vessels are seen in the abdomen, that should terminate the procedure.

## Recommended Reading

Agarwal PK, Elder JS, Diaz M. Retractile testis: is it really a normal variant? J Urol. 2006;175:1496–9.

American Urological Association. https://www.auanet.org/education/guidelines/cryptorchidism.cfm

Bergu B, Baker LM, Docimo SG. Cryptorchidism. In: Gearhart JP, Rink RC, Mouriquand PDE, editors. Pediatric urology. 2nd ed. Philadelphia: Elsevier; 2010. p. 563–76.

Elder JS. Disorders and anomalies of the scrotal contents. In: Kliegman RM, Stanton BF, St Geme III JW, Schor NF, Behrman RE, editors. Nelson textbook of pediatrics. 19th ed. Philadelphia: Elsevier (Saunders); 2011. p. 1858–64.

Kollin C, Stuckenborg JB, Nurmio M, et al. Boys with undescended testes: endocrine, volumetric and morphometric studies on testicular function before and after orchidopexy at nine months or three years of age. J Clin Endocrinol Metab. 2012;97:4588–95.

Wood HM, Elder JS. Cryptorchidism and testicular cancer: separating fact from fiction. J Urol. 2009;181:452–61.

# Testicular Torsion

# 21

Sherry S. Ross and H. Gil Rushton

Spermatic cord torsion, most commonly referred to as testicular torsion, was recognized early in human history. Greek mythology described young men struck by arrows of the gods resulting in an acute disease leading to testicular atrophy. These myths presumably explained the sudden pain and subsequent atrophy of testicular torsion [1]. In 1776, John Hunter, a London surgeon, described a case of testicular torsion in a young man [1]. However, Delasiauve is credited with the first case report of torsion of the spermatic cord, published in 1840 [1]. Then in 1857, Curling reported a case of testicular detorsion and fixation [1]. With such a long history of recognition and treatment of spermatic cord torsion, it would seem that testicular loss from this event would be virtually eliminated. However, more testes are lost than saved as we continue to look for better ways to educate parents and patients, to diagnose early testicular torsion, and to prevent testicular injury.

S.S. Ross, M.D. (✉)
University of North Carolina, Chapel Hill, NC, USA
e-mail: sherry.ross@dm.duke.edu

H. Gil Rushton, M.D., F.A.A.P.
Children's National Medical Center, Washington, DC, USA

## Scrotal Anatomy

Spermatic cord torsion most commonly occurs in males between the ages of 10 and 19, with a median of 15 years of age. The incidence of testicular torsion in this age group is approximately 8.6 cases per 100,000 [2]. To understand the etiology of testicular torsion, it is necessary to have an adequate understanding of scrotal anatomy. The scrotum consists of seven layers of tissue, including the skin, the dartos fascia, the external spermatic fascia, the cremasteric layer (fascia and muscle), and the most inner tunica vaginalis, which has a parietal and visceral layer which are normally adherent to one another. With normal testicular anatomy, the inner visceral layer of the tunica vaginalis is intimately attached to the spermatic cord and superior pole of the testicle (Fig. 21.1a). However, when the visceral layer attaches to the spermatic cord more proximally above the testis, a sac of free space is created which results in an abnormally free and mobile distal spermatic cord and testicle. This abnormality is referred to as the "bell-clapper" deformity (Fig. 21.1b). Because the testicle and distal spermatic cord hang freely within the tunica vaginalis, the testicle can twist one or multiple times. When twisting of the spermatic cord (vessels and vas deferens) occurs within the tunica vaginalis, it is referred to as

R. Rabinowitz et al. (eds.), *Pediatric Urology for the Primary Care Physician*, Current Clinical Urology,
DOI 10.1007/978-1-60327-243-8_21, © Springer Science+Business Media New York 2015

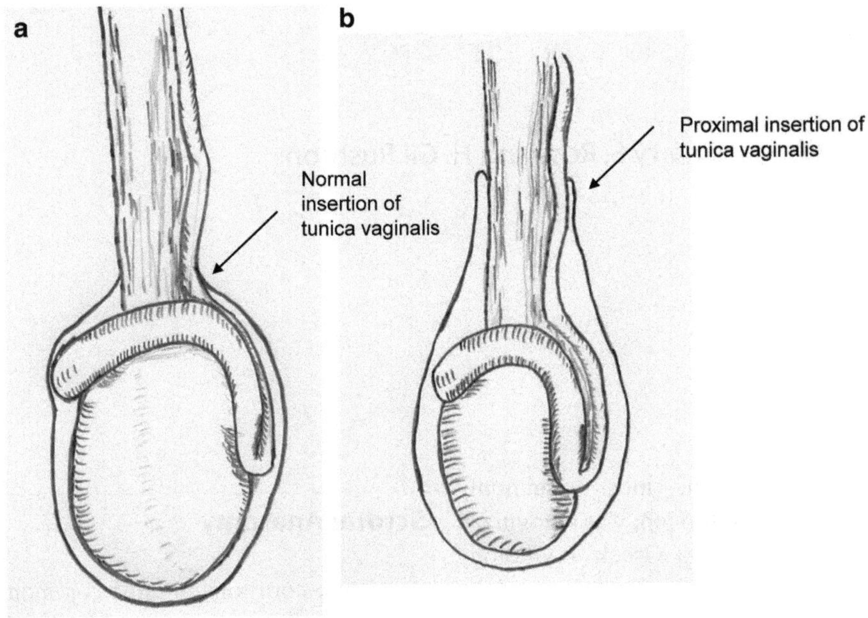


**Fig. 21.1** (**a**) Normal insertion of tunica vaginalis. (**b**) Bell-clapper deformity: note insertion of tunica vaginalis proximal to cord insertion site

"intravaginal" torsion. Occlusion of vascular structures prevents blood flow to and from the testis, resulting in pain and predisposing the testicular tissue to necrosis if blood flow is not restored promptly.

## Clinical Presentation

In the absence of trauma, the differential diagnosis for the acute scrotal pain includes spermatic cord torsion, torsion of the testicular appendage, epididymitis, hernia and occasionally, tumor. Accurate diagnosis can be difficult, and since time is of the utmost importance, knowledge of the signs and symptoms of testicular torsion is critical. While some boys may have gradual onset or limited pain, testicular torsion most often produces sudden onset of severe testicular pain. The pain may be localized to the scrotum or may be referred to the abdomen or inguinal area. Nausea and vomiting are present in about 60 % of boys with acute torsion [3]. The positive predictive value for nausea and vomiting associated with testicular pain is 96 % and 98 %, respectively [4].

Some boys may have a history of intermittent episodes of similar testicular pain consistent with torsion-spontaneous detorsion of the testis. In cases of suspected intermittent torsion, orchiopexy should be recommended. In this situation, the timing of surgery is more elective, unless the patient is experiencing an acute episode of pain.

## Physical Examination

The physical exam is important in the diagnosis of torsion of the spermatic cord. In the early period of testicular torsion, examination of the scrotum will often include a high-riding testicle, caused by twisting of the spermatic cord which results in shortening of the cord and elevation of the testicle. Twisting of the cord can also leave the testicle in a transverse orientation, referred to as a horizontal lie. Diffuse and exquisite tenderness is usually present. Scrotal wall edema and erythema are often present in the later phases of testicular torsion, and reactive hydroceles may prevent thorough evaluation of the testicle. An absent cremasteric reflex is common. The cremasteric reflex is elicited by gently stroking the ipsilateral inner thigh or lower abdomen prior to examination of the testicle itself. *A positive reflex, indicated by retraction of the testis superiorly as a result of contraction of the cremasteric muscle fiber, is highly predictive of the absence of torsion.* In contrast, a negative or absent cremasteric reflex is suspicious, but not diagnostic, of torsion.

## Consultation

When the clinical picture strongly suggests testicular torsion, diagnostic imaging should never delay emergent urological evaluation, particularly if the onset of pain occurred within the previous 6–8 h. Timing of intervention after torsion of the spermatic cord is of critical importance in the potential viability of the testicle. Studies have shown that irreversible ischemic damage may begin as soon as 4 h after torsion [5]. After 6–8 h of spermatic cord torsion, approximately 90 % of testicles will be nonviable, a rate that approaches 100 % after 24 h [6].

Additionally, the cord may make more than one 360° turn. The degree of spermatic cord torsion may play a role in the potential viability of the testicle after detorsion. Session et al. reported a greater degree of torsion in the testicles requiring orchiectomy (median of 549°) compared to the testicles that were salvaged (median of 360°), even though the range (180–1,080°) was the same in both groups [3].

## Manual Detorsion

Restoration of blood flow is the immediate goal in cases of spermatic cord torsion (Fig. 21.2). An attempt to manually detorse the testicle is generally recommended to more rapidly restore blood flow and provide pain relief. Classically, torsion of the cord is described as a medial turn or inward twist of the testicle. Thus, when manual detorsion is attempted, the testicle is first turned laterally in an outward direction, often referred to as the "open book" method. It is helpful to first pull downward on the testicle prior to attempting to detorse it. While most cases are the result of medial torsion of the cord, in up to 1/3 of cases the testicles will undergo torsion in a lateral direction [3]. Therefore, inward rotation of the torsed testis may be necessary in some cases. Although painful to perform, manual detorsion can provide almost immediate relief and promptly restore blood flow to the ischemic testis (Fig. 21.3a, b).

While manual detorsion may be successful, as indicated by immediate pain relief and a testicle lying vertically in a low-lying scrotal position, it does not eliminate the need for surgical exploration, as recurrent torsion is likely. However, the timing of surgery is somewhat more elective and can be deferred for 1 or 2 days if the patient is pain-free.

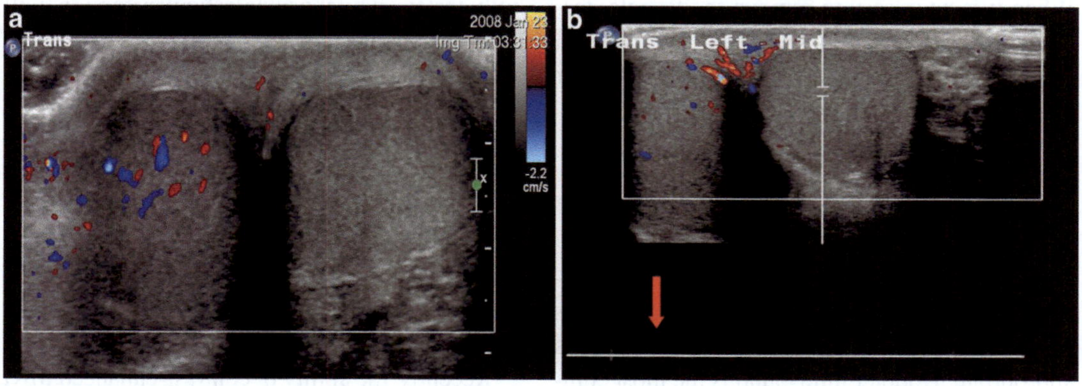


**Fig. 21.2** (**a**) Note absence of flow to left testicle as measured by Doppler ultrasound. (**b**) Attempts to measure arterial blood flow result in a flat wave form (*arrow*). This indicates absence of blood flow consistent with testicular torsion

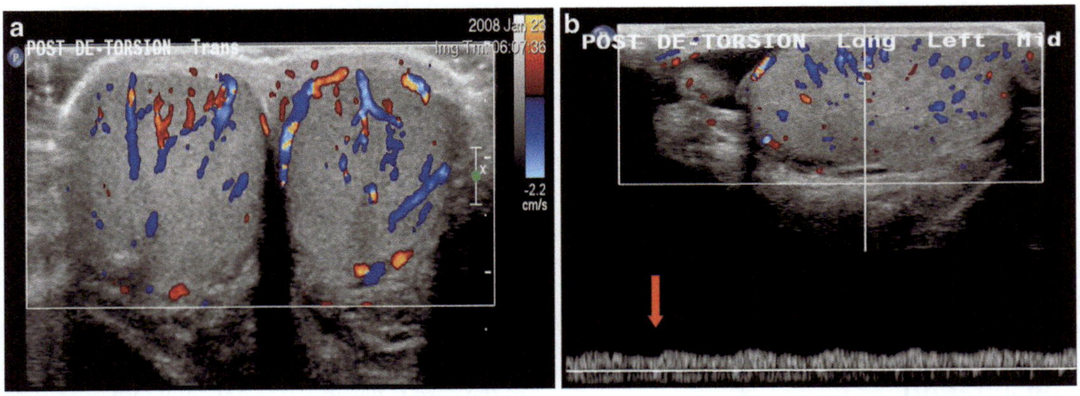


**Fig. 21.3** Post-detorsion of the testicle. (**a**) Note return of blood flow to left testicle as measured by Doppler ultrasound. (**b**) Attempts to measure arterial blood flow result in an arterial wave form (*arrow*). This indicates return of blood flow successful testicular detorsion

## Surgical Intervention

Urologic consultation and potential surgical exploration are indicated in any patient presenting with the described clinical scenario, even when manual detorsion is thought to have been successful. During surgical exploration, the affected testicle is examined for evidence of viability. If the testicle appears viable after a period of observation, the testicle is placed in the scrotum and stitched in multiple sites to the inner surface of the hemiscrotum to prevent future torsion. If the testicle appears necrotic, the organ is removed. The contralateral testicle is always fixated to the scrotum since the bell-clapper deformity is present bilaterally in the majority of cases. When it is necessary to remove the testicle, testicular prostheses are available once pubertal development is complete. While torsion after orchiopexy has been reported, it is very rare.

## Radiological Imaging

When clinical symptoms and physical exam findings are equivocal or when the onset of pain is greater than 24 h, radiological evaluation is appropriate. Doppler ultrasound is the most common modality currently used to evaluate for testicular torsion. However, the gray scale pattern of testicular torsion is nonspecific. Torsed testicles can have a homogenous, normal appearance in early torsion or a heterogeneous pattern in cases of hemorrhagic infarct. *Since gray scale findings are nonspecific, evaluation of testicular blood flow with Doppler ultrasound is essential in the examination for testicular torsion.* The absence of testicular blood flow on color Doppler ultrasound is 86 % sensitive, 100 % specific, and 97 % accurate in the diagnosis of torsion [7].

Nuclear imaging is an alternative modality to evaluate for testicular torsion. Testicular scintigraphy is performed by injecting intravenously 99 m Tc pertechnetate. Blood flow studies and fixed images are then obtained. A normal examination will reveal symmetric blood flow in both testes, while acute testicular torsion will result in unilateral decreased flow (Fig. 21.4a). Late-phase torsion is characteristically demonstrated by a central photopenic zone surrounded by a rim of increased reactive hypervascularity, the so-called "doughnut" sign (Fig. 21.4b). The presence of an intrascrotal hydrocele can result in a false-positive result, simulating late-phase torsion. Transillumination of the scrotal contents or sonography can help distinguish between a hydrocele and testicular torsion.

Recently, the ability of contrast-enhanced MRI in the diagnosis of testicular torsion was evaluated

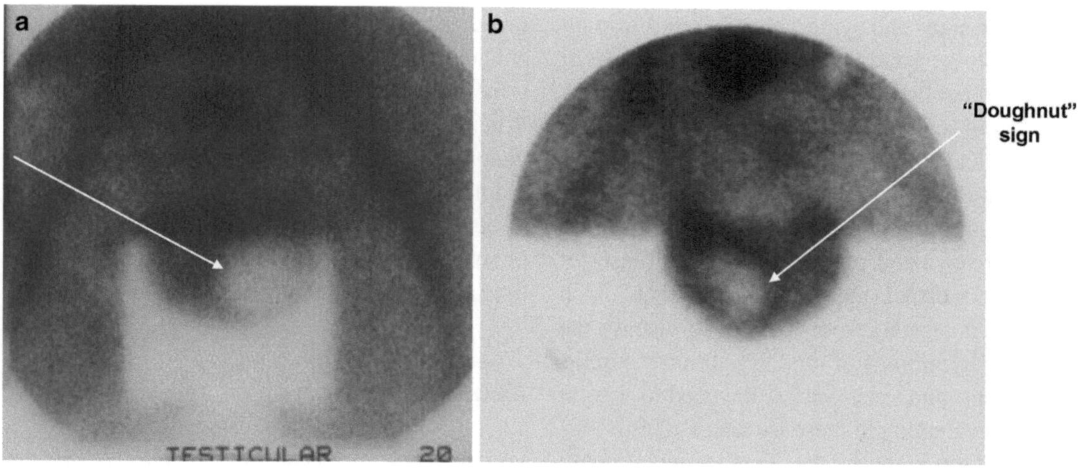


**Fig. 21.4** (**a**) *Acute torsion*: note poor uptake of radioisotope in the right testicle as indicated by the *arrow*. (**b**) *Late-phase torsion*: late-phase torsion is demonstrated by a central photopenic zone surrounded by a rim of increased reactive hypervascularity resulting in the "doughnut" sign

[8]. Failure of the testicle to enhance was diagnostic of torsion. While the sensitivity (93 %) and specificity (100 %) of MRI are promising, prospective trials are needed to verify these findings [8]. Additionally, MRI often requires sedation, is not as readily available as sonography, and continues to be expensive. *It should be strongly emphasized that, whenever the clinical presentation and evaluation is suggestive of acute torsion, manual or surgical detorsion should never be delayed in order to obtain imaging.*

## Fertility

In spite of timely intervention and restoration of blood flow, testicular atrophy may occur. In one study of 90 boys with follow-up after successful detorsion, 11 (27 %) had ≥15 % decrease in size of the affected testicle when compared to the contralateral side [3]. Animal studies have shown that significant changes occur, including spermatogenic disruption and germ cell apoptosis, after various intervals of testicular ischemia [9]. Some studies have even suggested that changes in blood flow to the testis and/or the development of autoantibodies may affect the contralateral testis and future fertility [10]. Other studies have suggested that congenital dysplasia of the testicle may already be present in some patients who are prone to testicular torsion [11]. While the association between testicular torsion and decreased fertility continues to be debated, it is known that there is a decrease in fertility potential in men who have only one testicle [7]. Therefore, prompt intervention is necessary to preserve as much testicular tissue as possible.

## Risk Factors for Orchiectomy

In 2005, Mansbach et al. evaluated risk factors for orchiectomy in boys presenting with spermatic cord torsion. After adjusting for various factors, age was the only significant predictor of orchiectomy. In fact, for every 1-year increase in age, the adjusted odds of having an orchiectomy increased by 1.08 (95 % CI, 1.03–1.13), or 8 % per year. For each 10-year increase in age, the odds of having an orchiectomy doubled ($1.08^{10} = 2.2$) [2]. The most likely explanation for these findings is that males within the age range when torsion is most likely to occur often do not seek early medical attention for problems with their genitalia. In a study by Nasrallah et al., 318 teenagers between the ages of 12 and 18 were surveyed to examine their knowledge and understanding of the necessity for genital examination and of the signs and symptoms of serious testicular pathology, including torsion. Up to 85 % of males did not believe that testicular swelling was a reason to seek medical attention, and 36 % felt that medical attention was unnecessary for testicular swelling and pain [8]. It is obvious that the medical community must focus more on the education of boys and parents prior to the onset of puberty to dispel these misconceptions. Each office visit offers an opportunity to discuss the signs and symptoms of torsion with both parents and patients and to emphasize the need for urgent medical evaluation in these instances. This is particularly important in the years leading up to puberty when torsion is more common.

## Differential for Scrotal Pain

*Torsion of a testicular appendix* can present with symptoms similar to testicular torsion. However, there are differences in the clinical presentation. Torsion of the appendix tends to occur at a younger age. Pain is typically not as severe, and nausea and vomiting are rarely present. The "blue dot" sign represents infarction of the appendix testis and is a bluish-black pea-sized area of discoloration which can often be seen through the thin prepubertal scrotal skin at the superior pole of the testis. When present, it is pathognomonic for torsion of the testicular appendix. The cremasteric reflex is usually present in boys with torsion of the appendix testis, and Doppler ultrasound reveals blood flow to the affected testicle.

*Epididymitis* can also present with symptoms similar to testicular torsion. However, pain usually develops more gradually compared with torsion. Tenderness is usually localized to the superior pole of the testis and is often associated with fever and pyuria. On physical examination, the scrotal skin is often thickened and erythematous, and a reactive hydrocele may be present. The cremasteric reflex is usually present in early stages of infection. However, in the later stages, the reflex may be absent or diminished. Doppler ultrasound will reveal increased blood flow to the affected testicle/epididymis. Urinalysis may reveal pyuria and urine culture is mandatory in prepubertal boys. When present, bacterial infection should raise suspicion in prepubertal boys of an ectopic ureter draining into the seminal vesicles. This is best screened for with renal/bladder sonography which, in suspicious cases, can be obtained at the same time as the scrotal ultrasound.

## Neonatal Torsion

Perinatal torsion most often occurs prenatally and accounts for approximately 10 % of all torsion cases. While the exact etiology remains unknown, it is thought that, prior to fusion of the outer parietal layer of the tunica vaginalis to the dartos tissues, the recently descended testicle is freely mobile within the scrotal sac. This potentially allows the entire spermatic cord and surrounding tissue to torse, which, unlike torsion in older boys, most often occurs proximal to the attachment of the tunica vaginalis to the testis and cord. Thus, this is termed "extravaginal" torsion. In contrast to adolescents with acute torsion, neonatal torsion most often presents with painless swelling and discoloration of the scrotum due to hemorrhagic necrosis of the testicle. The testicle is often firm and a hydrocele may be present. While sonography may be performed, findings are not as specific for neonatal testicular torsion, as it is often difficult to see testicular blood flow even in the normal neonatal testicle. Consequently, the physical examination is generally diagnostic.

Treatment of neonatal torsion is controversial. Advocates for immediate surgical exploration argue that the possible salvage of the torsed testicle and the opportunity for fixation of the contralateral testicle to prevent subsequent bilateral torsion are advantageous in these newborns. Unfortunately, salvage of the torsed testicle in neonates is exceptionally rare even with prompt diagnosis and urgent surgical exploration. Bilateral synchronous or asynchronous neonatal torsion does rarely occur. However, in these unfortunate cases the likelihood of salvage is poor. In 1 study of 30 cases of bilateral neonatal torsion, only 2 testicles were salvaged with immediate surgical intervention [12]. Based on reports such as this, many oppose surgical intervention quoting poor salvage rates and arguing that the risk of contralateral torsion is very low. Additionally, opponents of surgery feel that the risks of anesthesia in the young neonate outweigh the small potential advantages of emergency surgery, especially if expert pediatric anesthesia is unavailable.

In cases of unilateral neonatal torsion, the clinical condition of the newborn should be considered, and parents should be counseled concerning the anesthetic risks, the low rate of testicular salvage, and the rare but possible risk of synchronous or asynchronous torsion of the contralateral testis. In cases of bilateral torsion, these risks, in addition to the need for long-term medical follow-up and hormonal replacement therapy, should be discussed.

## Conclusions

Acute testicular torsion is a true urologic emergency. It is necessary for physicians to have a thorough knowledge of the clinical presentation and physical findings in boys with torsion of the spermatic cord. In cases of suspected torsion, urologic consultation should be prompt and should not be delayed by radiological evaluation. Since increasing age is the most important risk factor resulting in orchiectomy, the medical community must assume a more proactive role in the education of both parents and patients as we try to eliminate the unfortunate and preventable lost of the testicle.

## References


1. Noske H, Kraus SW, Altinkilic B, et al. Historical milestones regarding torsion of the scrotal organs. J Urol. 1996;159:13–6.
2. Mansbach J, Forbes P, Peters C. Testicular torsion and risk factors for orchiectomy. Arch Pediatr Adolesc Med. 2005;159:1167–71.
3. Sessions AE, Rabinowitz R, Hulbert W, et al. Testicular torsion: direction, degree, duration and disinformation. J Urol. 2003;169:663–5.
4. Jefferson RH, Perez LM, Joseph DB. Critical analysis of the clinical presentation of acute scrotum: a 9-year experience at a single institution. J Urol. 1997;158(3 Pt 2):1198–200.
5. Bartsch G, Frank S, Marberger H, Mikuz G. Testicular torsion: late results with special regard to fertility and endocrine function. J Urol. 1980;124:375–8.
6. Jayanthi VR. Adolescent urology. Adolesc Med Clin. 2004;15(3):521–34.
7. Ferreira U, Netto Junior NR, Esteves SC, et al. Comparative study of the fertility potential of men with only one testis. Scand J Urol Nephrol. 1991;25:255–9.
8. Nasrallah P, Nair G, Congeni J, et al. Testicular health awareness in pubertal males. J Urol. 2000;164:1115–7.
9. Turner TT, Brown KJ. Spermatic cord torsion: loss of spermatogenesis despite return of blood flow. Bio Reprod. 1993;49:401–7.
10. Williamson RC, Thomas WE. Sympathetic orchidopathia. Ann R Coll Surg Engl. 1984;66:264–6.
11. Dominguez C, Martinez Verduch M, Estornell F, et al. Histological study in contralateral testis of prepubertal children following unilateral testicular torsion. Eur Urol. 1994;26:160–3.
12. Cooper CD, Synder OB, Hawtrey CE. Bilateral neonatal testicular torsion. Clin Pediatr. 1997;36:653–6.

# Testis Tumor

# 22

Jonathan Ross

## Introduction

Pediatric testis tumors are relatively rare compared with testis tumors occurring postpubertally and with other pediatric urologic tumors, such as Wilms' tumor. The incidence of testis tumors in children is 0.5–2.0 per 100,000 children, accounting for only 1–2 % of all pediatric tumors. Testis tumors are classified by the putative cell of origin. Those arising from germ cells include yolk sac tumors (YSTs), teratomas, and epidermoid cysts. Stromal tumors include juvenile granulosa cell tumors, Leydig cell tumors, Sertoli cell tumors, and mixed or undifferentiated stromal tumors. Gonadoblastomas contain both germ cell and stromal elements. Secondary tumors rarely affect the testis, although testicular involvement with acute lymphoblastic/lymphocytic leukemia (ALL) is an important exception. By far the most common testis tumors in children are teratomas which are benign and YSTs which are malignant.

Until recently, because of their rarity, most information on prepubertal testis tumors was obtained from small series and case reports. The appropriate management of YSTs in children has been clarified by recent multicenter trials, including those by the Children's Oncology Group. There is little data regarding the behavior and management of testis tumors occurring in adolescents. The majority of testis tumors in the teen years are malignant mixed germ cell tumors, the same as seen in adults. These tumors have been extensively studied in the adult population, and it is assumed that the adolescent tumors are equivalent.

## Presentation and Evaluation

While testis tumors in children are rare, a prompt diagnosis is obviously important when they do occur, and primary care physicians will often be the first to see these patients. Testis tumors most commonly present as a testicular mass. The mass may be noted by the patient or detected on a routine physical examination. Approximately 10 % of patients have a hydrocele at presentation, which may be secondary to the tumor or coincidental. The presence of a hydrocele may delay the diagnosis of a testis tumor, and an ultrasonogram should be considered for any boy with a hydrocele in whom the testis cannot be palpated. Occasionally, patients will present with pain—presumably from an acute bleed into the tumor. Physical examination will usually reveal a hard mass in the testicular parenchyma. These masses must be distinguished from extratesticular lesions such as epididymal cysts (see Table 22.1).

J. Ross, M.D. (✉)
Department of Pediatric Urology, University Hospitals Rainbow Babies and Children's Hospital, 11100 Euclid Avenue RBC 2311, Cleveland, OH 44106, USA
e-mail: jonathan.ross@uhhospitals.org

R. Rabinowitz et al. (eds.), *Pediatric Urology for the Primary Care Physician*, Current Clinical Urology, DOI 10.1007/978-1-60327-243-8_22, © Springer Science+Business Media New York 2015

**Table 22.1** Differential diagnosis of a scrotal mass

| Lesion | Physical exam | Typical lesion appearance |
|---|---|---|
| Testicular tumor | Hard mass within the testis | Heterogeneous mass within the testis |
| Paratesticular tumor (rhabdomyosarcoma) | Usually very large hard irregular scrotal mass | Heterogeneous mass encasing the testis |
| Epididymal cyst | Smooth round mass usually in the head of the epididymis and separate from the testis | Round fluid-filled cyst in the epididymis separate from the testis |
| Hydrocele | Round smooth transilluminating mass filling the scrotum | Fluid surrounding normal testis |
| Hernia | Soft irregular mass filling inguinoscrotal region—may feel gas—usually reducible | Bowel loops in the scrotum with normal testicle |
| Testicular torsion | Extremely tender swollen high-riding testis with erythema of scrotal wall—reactive hydrocele may be present | Swollen testis with lack of blood flow |
| Torsion of the appendix testis | Moderately tender nodule at upper pole of the testis with erythema of the scrotum—reactive hydrocele may obscure findings | Normal testicular blood flow with swollen appendix—may not be distinguishable from epididymitis |
| Epididymitis | Tender epididymis with normal testis—inflammation may include the testis | Swelling and increased blood flow to the epididymis—may not be distinguishable from appendiceal torsion |

Once a testis tumor is suspected, a thorough physical examination is undertaken. Signs of androgenization or feminization should be sought. Metastatic disease is uncommon, and the primary sites—the retroperitoneum and lungs—are unlikely to result in symptoms or physical findings. In rare cases, metastases to the bone or central nervous system may occur. Symptoms or signs of involvement at these locations are important in guiding the radiographic evaluation.

The initial radiographic evaluation of children with a suspected testis tumor is limited. Because many prepubertal testis tumors are benign, any metastatic evaluation is usually deferred until tissue confirmation of the tumor's histology is obtained. However, when a malignancy is suspected (e.g., in children with an elevated alpha-fetoprotein (AFP) level or in adolescents), a computerized tomography scan (CT) of the abdomen may be obtained preoperatively. Imaging of the primary tumor is sometimes helpful. Ultrasonography is most often employed (see Fig. 22.1). It is able to distinguish testicular tumors from benign extratesticular lesions. The extent of testicular involvement can also be determined, which is helpful if testis-sparing surgery is being considered. The ultrasonographic appearance of specific testis tumors has been described. Unfortunately, ultrasound findings are too inconsistent to allow a definitive diagnosis of a specific tumor.

Tumor markers play an important role in the evaluation and follow-up of childhood testis tumors. AFP is the most important tumor marker. It is an albumin precursor synthesized by the yolk sac and fetal liver and gut. AFP is specific for YST. Levels are elevated in 80–90 % of children with a YST, and AFP has a biological half-life of approximately 5 days. An elevated level of AFP preoperatively in a child nearly always reflects the presence of a YST. An important caveat is that AFP levels are normally quite high in infancy (see Table 22.2). An "elevated" level in a boy less than 1 year of age does not rule out the possibility of a benign tumor, such as teratoma. The beta subunit of human chorionic gonadotropin (HCG) is an important marker in adolescent testis tumors, but this is rarely elevated in children because the histological types that lead to elevated HCG levels are rarely encountered in prepubertal testis tumors.

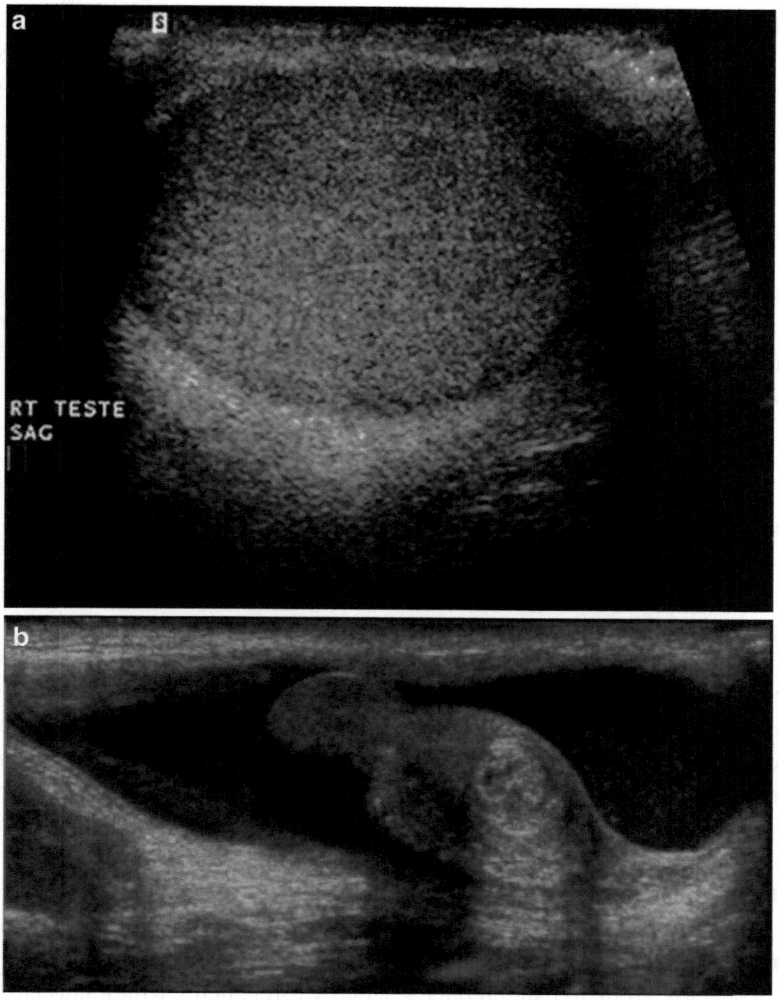


**Fig. 22.1** Ultrasonic findings of a testicular tumor in a boy presenting with a hydrocele. (**a**) A normal testis which has an ovoid shape and homogenous texture. (**b**) The affected testicle. A round hyperechoic mass is seen within the normal parenchyma surrounded by the fluid of the hydrocele

**Table 22.2** Alpha-fetoprotein (AFP) levels in normal infants (data from Wu JT, Book IL, Sudar K, Serum alpha-fetoprotein (AFP) levels in normal infants, Pediatr Res 1981; 15:50–52)

| Age | AFP level (ng/mL) | Standard deviation |
|---|---|---|
| Newborn (term) | 48,406 | ±34,718 |
| 1 month | 9,452 | ±12,610 |
| 2 months | 323 | ±278 |
| 3 months | 88 | ±87 |
| 4 months | 74 | ±56 |
| 5 months | 46.5 | ±19 |
| 6 months | 12.5 | ±9.8 |
| 7 months | 9.7 | ±7.1 |

## Management

Any child with an intratesticular mass should be referred promptly for surgical intervention. Testis tumors can be rapidly growing, and evaluation and treatment should be undertaken immediately. The standard approach to a testis tumor is an inguinal orchiectomy. Increasing consideration has been given to performing testis-sparing surgery for benign testicular tumors. This is particularly attractive in prepubertal patients because many, if not most, prepubertal tumors are benign.

The preoperative evaluation plays a significant role in patient selection for testis-sparing surgery. An elevated AFP level in a child over 1 year of age virtually always reflects the presence of a YST and precludes a testis-sparing approach. However, in older children with a normal AFP and in infants, the likelihood of a benign tumor is considerable. This is also true in boys presenting with androgenization. For these patients, if there is salvageable normal testicular parenchyma evident, an inguinal exploration with excisional biopsy of the lesion should be considered so that a testis-sparing approach may be performed if a benign histology is confirmed on frozen section analysis. This approach is rarely indicated in adolescents, for whom the majority of tumors are malignant. After orchiectomy, some children with testicular tumors require additional evaluation and therapy. The type of adjunctive management selected will depend on the histology of the primary tumor and the results of radiographic and biochemical studies. The intensity of follow-up also depends on the malignant potential of the primary tumor.

## Germ Cell Tumors

### Yolk Sac Tumor

YST accounts for nearly all malignant prepubertal testis tumors. The majority of patients with YST present under 2 years of age. Metastatic evaluation of YSTs includes a computed tomography (CT) scan of the abdomen and pelvis to rule out retroperitoneal lymph node or hepatic metastases and a chest X-ray or chest CT scan to rule out pulmonary metastases. Bone and brain metastases are rare. Therefore, bone scans and head CT scans are obtained only when there is clinical suspicion of metastases at these sites. Serum AFP level is also measured postoperatively. Its half-life is approximately 5 days, and a persistent elevation of AFP after orchiectomy suggests the presence of metastatic disease. However, AFP levels as high as 50,000 ng/mL can occur in normal infants, and levels greater than 50 ng/mL can occur in children up to 6 months of age. Therefore, serial measurements are particularly important in infants.

A tumor-node-metastasis (TNM) staging system exists for testis tumors, but its applicability to pediatric tumors is limited owing to the infrequent employment of retroperitoneal lymph node dissection (RPLND) in these patients. Several other systems have been proposed. The simplest system segregates patients into three stages. Stage I patients have tumor confined to the testis with a negative metastatic evaluation and a normalization of AFP postoperatively. Stage II patients have retroperitoneal disease detected by radiographic studies or RPLND and/or a persistent elevation of AFP postoperatively. Stage III patients have metastatic disease beyond the retroperitoneum. Approximately 80 % of children with YSTs have stage I tumors.

Historically, RPLND was the most common form of adjunctive therapy for the treatment of YSTs. With the widespread use of AFP to detect occult metastases and improvements in multiagent chemotherapy, the reliance on RPLND to diagnose and treat metastatic disease in prepubertal patients has waned. The operative morbidity of RPLND in children is significant, including wound complications, bowel obstruction, chylous ascites, and anejaculation as adults due to injury to the sympathetic nerves. Currently retroperitoneal surgery in prepubertal patients is limited to excisional biopsy of retroperitoneal masses in patients with a normal AFP and excisional biopsy of residual masses following chemotherapy—both rare events.

Chemotherapy is very effective in treating metastatic YST. The most commonly used regimens include cisplatin or carboplatin in combination with other agents such as etoposide and bleomycin. Because children with metastatic disease often have multiple sites of spread, chemotherapy is particularly appropriate for these patients. Radiation does not play a role in the standard treatment for metastatic YST. The selection of adjuvant therapy for YST depends on the stage of the tumor. The trend in managing stage I tumors is toward observation. The recurrence rate for patients with stage I tumor managed by observation is approximately 15 %, and virtually all of these patients can be salvaged with chemotherapy. Patients with stage I tumor are therefore generally observed closely without adjuvant therapy. Patients are evaluated on a regular basis with serum AFP level, CT of the abdomen and pelvis, and chest X-ray. Recurrent disease is usually treated with chemotherapy. If the patient remains free of disease for 2 years, then he is almost certainly cured, though annual follow-up is continued.

Patients with a negative metastatic evaluation, but a failure of the AFP to normalize, are generally treated with chemotherapy. It must be remembered that a "normal" AFP in infants may be quite high. Patients with positive lymph nodes on CT scan are also usually treated with chemotherapy. An RPLND is considered when retroperitoneal disease is not responding to chemotherapy or for a persistent mass after chemotherapy when the AFP level has normalized. Some of these residual masses will contain only necrotic tumor and calcifications. Chemotherapy is also the mainstay of treatment for patients with hematogenous metastases. Chemotherapy with second-line agents is used for patients failing to respond to standard agents. Surgical excision and radiation should also be considered for those with limited sites of metastatic disease who fail to respond to chemotherapy. Even in the face of metastatic disease, the prognosis for children with YST is excellent.

### Teratoma and Epidermoid Cyst

Teratoma is the most common benign prepubertal testis tumor. The median age of presentation is 13 months, with several patients presenting in the neonatal period. Histologically, teratomas consist of tissues representing the three germinal layers—endoderm, mesoderm, and ectoderm. The presence of cysts on ultrasonography suggests the diagnosis but is neither sensitive nor specific. Epidermoid cysts are benign tumors composed entirely of keratin-producing epithelium. They are distinguished from dermoid cysts, which contain skin and skin appendages, and from teratomas, which contain derivatives of other germ cell layers. On ultrasonography, most epidermoid cysts appear as discrete intratesticular masses with areas of increased echogenicity corresponding to the keratin debris or peripheral calcification. Other areas of decreased echogenicity may also be present corresponding to regions of the cyst not filled with debris. However, these findings are variable, and an epidermoid cyst may appear as a fairly homogeneous solid mass. The primary value of ultrasonography is in characterizing the mass as intratesticular and in excluding abnormalities elsewhere in the testis that would necessitate total orchiectomy. Teratomas and epidermoid cysts are universally benign in prepubertal children. Testis-sparing surgery is a reasonable consideration for these patients. In older children with teratoma, the normal testicular parenchyma must be carefully evaluated. If there is histological evidence of pubertal changes, then an orchiectomy is performed because teratomas are potentially malignant in postpubertal males. Epidermoid cysts are benign in children and adults and may be treated by simple tumor excision. For patients with epidermoid cyst and prepubertal patients with teratoma, no radiographic studies or follow-up for the development of metastatic disease is required. Because of the potential for malignancy, postpubertal patients with teratoma should be evaluated and followed on the same protocol as adults with other malignant germ cell tumors.

### Adolescent Germ Cell Tumors

Adolescent testis tumors are usually malignant, the most common histologies being embryonal cell or mixed germ cell. RPLND plays a larger role in these patients than in younger children with YSTs. Depending on the specific histology and the philosophy of the treating physicians, stage I germ cell tumors in young adults may be treated with observation, a brief course of chemotherapy or an RPLND. Patients with metastatic disease are usually treated with chemotherapy, though RPLND may have a role in patients with minimal retroperitoneal disease.

## Stromal Testis Tumors

Stromal testis tumors are rare in children, and there are no large series to guide their management. However, anecdotal reports and small series in the literature offer some experience on which to base therapy. Leydig cell tumors are universally benign in children. They usually present between 5 and 10 years of age with precocious puberty. Presenting symptoms include an early growth spurt, prominent external genitalia, erections, pubic and axillary hair, facial hair, acne, and deepening of the voice. Other causes of precocious puberty include central nervous system lesions, adrenocortical carcinoma, and congenital adrenal hyperplasia (CAH). In the presence of a testicular mass, a Leydig cell tumor is the most likely diagnosis. An elevated testosterone level with low or normal follicle-stimulating hormone and luteinizing hormone levels is consistent with a Leydig cell tumor. Normal levels of 17-hydroxyprogesterone exclude the diagnosis of CAH. Because virilization may present before a tumor is palpable, all boys with precocious puberty and no obvious cause should undergo an ultrasonogram of the testicles to rule out a small tumor. Leydig cell tumors may be treated by orchiectomy or testis-sparing excision. Persistence of androgenic effects may be due to a contralateral tumor, but this is rare in children. However, even after successful removal of a solitary tumor, androgenic changes are not completely reversible, and some children may proceed through premature puberty.

Sertoli cell tumors account for only 2 % of primary prepubertal testis tumors. Sertoli cell tumors are usually hormonally inactive in children, although they may occasionally cause gynecomastia or isosexual precocious puberty. Whereas all reported cases to date have been benign in children under 5 years of age, there have been a few cases of malignant Sertoli cell tumors in older children. Orchiectomy is sufficient treatment in infants, although a metastatic evaluation could be considered in infants with worrisome histological findings. Older children should undergo an abdominal CT scan and chest x-ray to rule out metastases. When metastatic disease is present, aggressive combination treatment including RPLND, chemotherapy, and radiation therapy should be considered.

The large cell calcifying Sertoli cell tumor is a clinically and histologically distinct entity with a higher incidence of multifocality and hormonal activity. Whereas standard Sertoli cell tumors are more common in adults, large cell calcifying Sertoli cell tumors are found predominantly in children and adolescents. Most present with a testicular mass. Approximately one fourth of patients have bilateral and multifocal tumors. The presence of calcifications results in a characteristic ultrasonographic appearance including multiple hyperechoic areas. Approximately one third of patients with large cell calcifying Sertoli cell tumor have an associated genetic syndrome and/or endocrine abnormality. The two syndromes most commonly associated with large cell calcifying Sertoli cell tumor are Peutz-Jeghers syndrome and Carney's syndrome. Peutz-Jeghers syndrome is an autosomal dominant disorder consisting of mucocutaneous pigmentation and hamartomatous intestinal polyposis. Features of Carney's syndrome include myxomas of the skin, soft tissue, and heart; myxoid lesions of the breast; lentigines of the face and lips; cutaneous blue nevi; Cushing's syndrome; pituitary adenoma; and schwannoma. Awareness of this familial syndrome is important because patients and their first-degree relatives are at risk for the potentially lethal associated entities. Whereas they are occasionally malignant in adults, large cell calcifying Sertoli cell tumors have been universally benign in patients under 25 years of age. Orchiectomy is sufficient treatment for children.

Juvenile granulosa cell tumor is a stromal tumor bearing a light microscopic resemblance to ovarian juvenile granulosa cell tumor. Granulosa cell tumors occur almost exclusively in the first year of life, most in the first 6 months. Structural abnormalities of the Y chromosome and mosaicism are common in boys with juvenile granulosa cell tumor. Several cases have been described in association with ambiguous genitalia. These tumors are hormonally inactive and benign. Although these children should undergo chromosomal analysis, no treatment or metastatic evaluation is required beyond orchiectomy or tumor enucleation.

## Gonadoblastoma

Gonadoblastomas contain both germ cells and stromal cells. Gonadoblastomas occur more frequently in postpubertal patients, but they may be seen in childhood. Gonadoblastoma occurs almost exclusively in dysgenetic gonads, usually in association with an intersex disorder. Gonadoblastoma is more likely to occur in dysgenetic gonads occurring in patients with a Y chromosome or evidence of some Y chromatin. Gonadoblastomas occur in 3 % of patients with true hermaphroditism and 10–30 % of patients with mixed gonadal dysgenesis or pure gonadal dysgenesis and an XY karyotype. They also occur commonly in the dysgenetic testis syndrome.

Gonadoblastomas are usually asymptomatic—often detected incidentally when dysgenetic gonads are removed. However, virilization has been associated with some of these tumors. Forty percent of gonadoblastomas are bilateral. Whereas gonadoblastomas are benign, overgrowth of the germinal components leading to a dysgerminoma (also known as seminoma) occurs in as many as 50 % of cases. Approximately 10 % develop overtly malignant tumors. While most invasive tumors associated with intersex occur in young adulthood, there are several reports in children as well.

Gonadoblastomas are treated by orchiectomy. Indeed, any dysgenetic gonad in a child with a Y chromosome should be removed prophylactically in infancy or early childhood. Tumors are much less likely in patients who lack a Y chromosome such as those with Turner's syndrome or XX patients with pure gonadal dysgenesis. When malignant degeneration is present, a metastatic evaluation and appropriate follow-up are indicated. Fortunately, these tumors are radiosensitive and have a favorable prognosis.

## Hyperplastic Nodules in Congenital Adrenal Hyperplasia

Adrenal rest tissue can be found along the spermatic cord and in the testicular hilum of newborns. This tissue generally regresses in infancy but may persist in boys with CAH. Stimulation of the tissue by high levels of adrenocorticotropic hormone can lead to multiple, usually bilateral nodular growths in the testes. Some patients with milder unrecognized forms of CAH may present with testicular masses. In such patients who present with precocious puberty, the testicular masses could be misinterpreted as Leydig cell tumors. The nodules of CAH are very similar histologically to Leydig cell tumors, potentially perpetuating the error even after excision. Therefore, any child presenting with precocious puberty and a testicular mass(es) should undergo an endocrinologic evaluation, including measurement of serum 17-hydroxyprogesterone, to distinguish these two entities.

The hyperplastic nodules of CAH are benign. Many, but not all of these nodules, will resolve or significantly reduce in size in response to steroid replacement or an increase in steroid therapy. If this occurs, the patient may safely be followed with serial examinations and/or ultrasonography. Because any testicle may develop a true testicular tumor, a biopsy should be performed on any nodules that fail to respond to adjustments in steroid replacement.

## Leukemia

Secondary malignancies of the testicle are rare. The most important is ALL. Only 2 % of boys with ALL will have overt clinical evidence of testicular involvement at diagnosis. This is usually reflected in firm diffuse enlargement of one or both testicles and portends a poorer prognosis. Subclinical (i.e., microscopic) involvement of the testes is present in approximately 20 % of patients with ALL at the time of diagnosis. However, most patients with microscopic testicular involvement achieve a complete remission following modern standard chemotherapy. Conversely, some patients without microscopic evidence of testicular involvement at diagnosis will ultimately relapse in the testicles. Therefore, pretreatment testicular biopsy is unnecessary because it does not predict those patients who are prone to have persistent or relapsing disease at that site.

Relapse in the testicles after chemotherapy used to occur in approximately 10 % of patients. The testis may represent a protected site from chemotherapy, more prone to relapse. However, with modern ALL chemotherapy, testicular relapse occurs in less than 1 % of cases. Postchemotherapy biopsy in the absence of physical findings (to rule out occult persistence of tumor in the testes) is therefore no longer routine. Those few patients with testicular enlargement persisting or occurring after chemotherapy should undergo biopsy to confirm testicular ALL. Most of these patients will be found to have relapsed at other sites as well and require additional intensive systemic chemotherapy to prevent ultimate clinical hematological relapse. Radiation to the testicles is also required. In the rare cases of unilateral testicular relapse, consideration is given to orchiectomy. This could allow lower doses of radiation to the remaining testicle and, ultimately, better endocrine function than would occur with higher doses of radiation to both testicles if the affected testicle were left in place. In any case, most patients with testicular relapse after chemotherapy can be salvaged and attain long-term survival. Relapse during chemotherapy portends a more dire outcome.

## Recommended Reading

Coppes MJ, Rackley R, Kay R. Primary testicular and paratesticular tumors of childhood. Med Pediatr Oncol. 1994;22:329.

Cortez JC, Kaplan GW. Gonadal stromal tumors, gonadoblastomas, epidermoid cysts, and secondary tumors of the testis in children. Urol Clin North Am. 1993;20:15.

Ross JH, Rybicki L, Kay R. Clinical behavior and a contemporary management algorithm for prepubertal testis tumors: a summary of the Prepubertal Testis Tumor Registry. J Urol. 2002;168:1675.

Schlatter M, Rescorla F, Giller R, et al. Excellent outcome in patients with stage I germ cell tumors of the testes: a study of the Children's Cancer Group/Pediatric Oncology Group. J Pediatr Surg. 2003;38:319.

# Adolescent Varicocele

# 23

Thomas Tailly and Guy Bogaert

## Definition

The word varicocele is derived from the Latin word for vein, varix, and the Greek word for mass, kele. This mass of veins is actually a varicose condition of the veins of the pampiniform plexus.

The varicocele as a medical entity and its treatment was described in a book for the very first time by Cornelius Celsus (c. 25 BC–c. 50 AD) in his "De Medicina": The veins are swollen and twisted over the testicle, which becomes smaller than its fellow in as much as its nutrition has become defective. He already differentiated between three different levels of dilated veins with separate surgical procedures for each.

## Epidemiology

Varicoceles in paediatric urology occur on average in 4–7 % of paediatric population. The incidence however is clearly age-dependent. Before the age of 10, less than 1 % of boys will present with a varicocele. From then on the incidence increases with age to reach a 15 % incidence in boys of about 14–15 years old. This is comparable to the adult population. It appears in approximately 15 % of males at clinical examination.

About 90 % of varicoceles occur unilaterally left-sided. Right-sided varicoceles are usually noted as part of a bilateral varicocele but almost never as a unilateral finding [1].

Varicoceles vary in size and can be classified in three groups. Dubin and Amelar classified varicoceles in three size groups according to findings at clinical examination (Table 23.1) [2].

Hirsh et al. classified varicoceles according to the degree of reflux identified by colour Doppler ultrasound scan (Table 23.2) [3].

## Aetiology

The exact aetiology of varicocele is still uncertain, but several hypotheses exist on its probable cause which is thought to be the anatomy of testicular vascularisation.

### Anatomy

The testicular blood supply consists of three arteries: testicular, vasal and cremasteric artery with their concomitant veins. These arteries and veins are supported by various collaterals. The proximal part of the pampiniform plexus is drained via the testicular vein. The distal part of the pampiniform plexus is drained via the anterior scrotal vein into the femoral vein.

T. Tailly, M.D. • G. Bogaert, M.D., Ph.D. (✉)
Department of Urology, University Hospitals Gasthuisberg, Leuven, Belgium
e-mail: guy.bogaert@uzleuven.be

R. Rabinowitz et al. (eds.), *Pediatric Urology for the Primary Care Physician*, Current Clinical Urology,
DOI 10.1007/978-1-60327-243-8_23, © Springer Science+Business Media New York 2015

The anatomical differences between left and right venous return at the level of the testicular vein are used to explain the presence of dilated veins of the pampiniform plexus mainly on the left side (Fig. 23.1a, b).

**Table 23.1** Classification of varicoceles in three size groups according to findings at clinical examination

| |
|---|
| Grade 1: only palpable on Valsalva manoeuvre |
| Grade 2: palpable but not visible without Valsalva manoeuvre when standing upright |
| Grade 3: visible without Valsalva manoeuvre when standing upright |

**Table 23.2** Classification of varicoceles according to the degree of reflux identified by colour Doppler ultrasound scan

| |
|---|
| Grade 1: no spontaneous venous reflux but inducible reflux with Valsalva manoeuvre |
| • Pattern 1: only very little reflux at the beginning of the Valsalva |
| • Pattern 2: reflux during the full length of the Valsalva |
| Grade 2: intermittent spontaneous venous reflux |
| Grade 3: continuous spontaneous venous reflux |

On the right side, the testicular vein drains straight into the vena cava in a sharp angle. On the left side, on the other hand, the testicular vein drains into the left renal vein in an almost 90° angle.

Another possible cause would be the so-called nutcracker syndrome. This hypothesis claims that the presence of varicocele is caused by impingement of the left renal vein between the superior mesenteric artery and abdominal aorta, proximal to the point where the testicular vein enters the renal vein [4].

The study of Graif et al. comparing flow velocity of left and right testicular vein supports these theories. They showed that a decrease in the aorto-mesenteric distance and angle was significantly correlated to lower flow velocity of the left renal vein and an increase in testicular vein diameter [5].

The absence of venous valves in the testicular vein [6] and the increased arterial blood flow to the testis at puberty exceeding the venous capacity are some of many other postulated plausible causes of the varicocele.

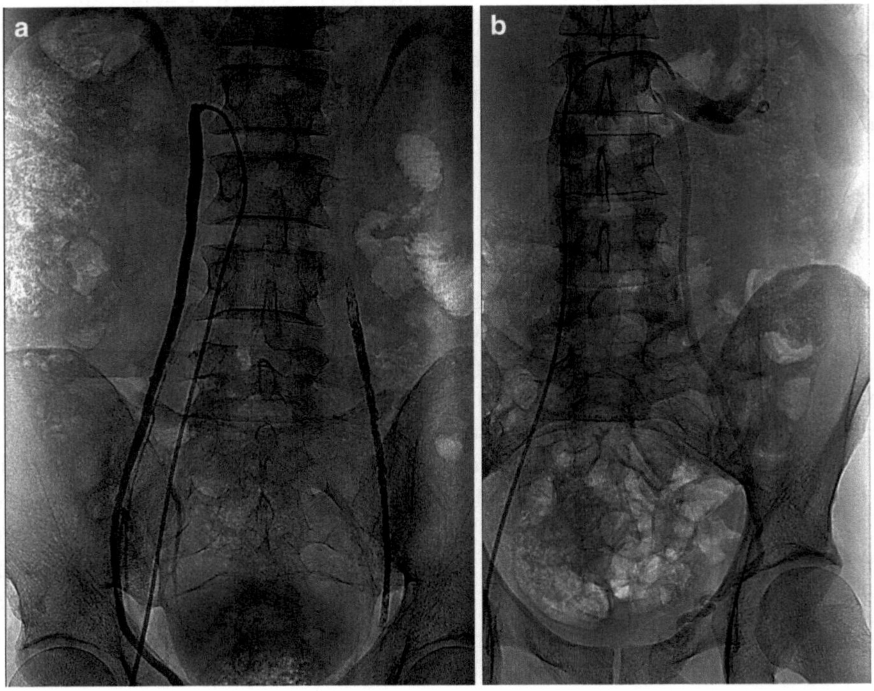


**Fig. 23.1** (**a**) Right testicular vein. (**b**) Left testicular vein draining into the left renal vein. Courtesy of S. Heye MD, Department of Radiology, University Hospitals Leuven

## Genetics

Raman et al. demonstrated a genetic susceptibility for varicocele. They showed that over half of first-degree relatives of varicocele patients are also found to have a certain grade of varicocele on physical examination, with the highest frequency (>70 %) among brothers [7].

## Secondary Causes

In case of a unilateral right varicocele or a varicocele in a prepubertal boy, secondary causes of varicocele should be considered and further diagnostics may be necessary. The most important secondary factors are obstruction of renal or testicular vein by tumour or tumour thrombus, retroperitoneal tumours or adenopathies, retroperitoneal fibrosis and liver cirrhosis. Therefore, an abdominal ultrasound should be performed to exclude any secondary factors [8] (Fig. 23.2a, b).

## Predisposing and Associated Factors

Several studies have shown that certain somatometric characteristics have been identified as "risk factors" for developing a varicocele. All these papers report similar results, pointing out that age, height and penile length are positively correlated with varicocele whereas BMI, pubic hair distribution and left testicular volume were negatively correlated with varicocele [9, 10].

A high BMI seemed to be a protective factor for varicocele. This can probably be explained by the presence of more adipose tissue between the superior mesenteric artery and aorta preventing the nutcracker effect to occur. Tsao et al. indeed showed that the prevalence and severity of varicoceles inversely correlated with obesity. These findings were statistically significant and support the explanation that obesity may result in a decreased nutcracker effect [11].

Height was also a predictive factor for finding varicocele. Again this factor can be attributed to anatomic factors. Taller boys have a larger column of hydrostatic pressure on the pampiniform plexus. Also the angle between superior mesenteric artery and aorta is smaller resulting in more nutcracker effect.

Testicular volume, pubic hair and penile length are indicators of different stages of pubertal development. Therefore, the accelerated pubertal development with growth spurt and increased androgen secretion may explain these correlations with varicocele.

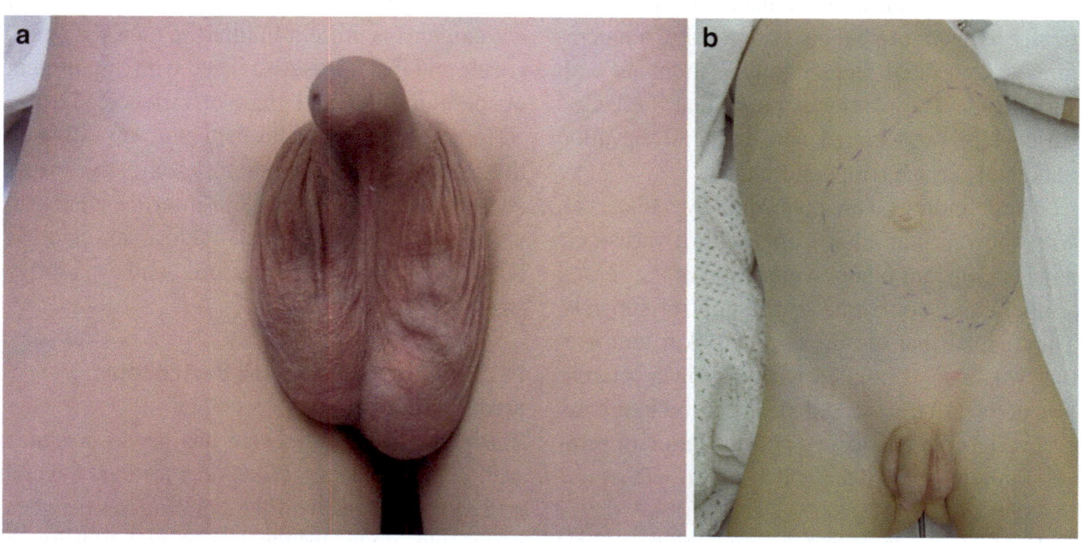


**Fig. 23.2** (**a**) Prepubertal varicocele grade 3. (**b**) Large Wilms tumour causing varicocele

# Effects of Varicocele

## Pathophysiology

The importance of varicocele lies in its possible negative effect on fertility. Several pathophysiologic hypotheses on why varicocele has such a detrimental effect on fertility have been postulated.

### The Hypothermia Hypothesis

Testes are located extracorporeally in all mammals. The surrounding temperature of testicular tissue has to be lower than body temperature for optimal spermatogenesis.

According to several studies, 31 °C is the ideal temperature for DNA synthesis in the human testis, and a rise in testicular temperature towards 37 °C causes an impairment of DNA synthesis. RNA synthesis and protein synthesis reach their maximum at about 34 °C and are also temperature-dependent. The slight variation of the testicular temperature may cause spermatogenic dysfunction because of delicate temperature sensitivity of the testicular DNA synthesis [12, 13].

Another Japanese group has confirmed these findings after studying in vitro DNA polymerase at different incubation temperatures. DNA polymerase activity was significantly reduced when incubated at 37 °C compared to incubation at 31 °C [14].

Goldstein and Eid found that not only intratesticular temperature but also scrotal skin temperature was elevated significantly in humans with varicocele. They demonstrated that unilateral varicocele is associated with bilateral elevation of scrotal surface temperature [15].

These findings were confirmed by Salisz et al. who showed that adolescents with a varicocele had a significant bilateral elevation of the scrotal temperatures compared to the control subjects. They added that elevated scrotal skin temperature was also correlated with a growth retardation of the left testis and that successful treatment of a varicocele results in a normalisation of scrotal skin temperature and catch-up growth of testis volume [16].

Dahl et al. described a countercurrent heat exchange mechanism half a century ago where, in normal circumstances, the testicular temperature is kept lower than body temperature. The non-varicose pampiniform plexus surrounds the testicular artery and cools down the arterial blood as it enters the testicles [17].

In patients with varicocele this effect is minimised to absent, probably due to lower flow velocity in the pampiniform plexus, causing elevated scrotal temperatures.

It seems obvious therefore that a rise in temperature in the testicular tissue due to varicocele can cause impaired spermatogenesis due to inhibition of DNA polymerase. This was also suggested on histological level as Hienz et al. noted that hyperthermic injury was consistent with the reduction in spermatogonal numbers observed in testis biopsy samples from patients with a varicocele [18].

### The Oxidative Stress Hypothesis

Oxidative stress, or the negative effect of reactive oxygen radicals, has also been suggested to play a role in infertility in men with varicocele. Sikka et al. showed that in a normal situation, there is a balance between these oxygen radicals and antioxidants to prevent spermatozoa to get damaged. Ageing, environmental toxicants and, more importantly, any form of genitourinary inflammation or stress can cause an imbalance between these oxygen radicals and antioxidants, resulting in possible spermatozoa damage [19].

Abd-Elmoaty et al. confirmed that this imbalance of high level of oxidants vs. low level of antioxidants is present in infertile men with varicocele and that this is associated with impairment of sperm motility and grade of varicocele [20].

In a recent study, Shiraishi et al. investigated the role of scrotal temperature, oxidative stress and apoptosis in the testis in infertile men with varicocele. They showed a close association between scrotal temperature and oxidative stress [21].

### Factors Correlated with Varicocele and Infertility

The presence of varicocele has been correlated with several adverse effects on a testicle. Several articles have described the correlations between varicocele grade, testicular size and fertility or semen quality. We try to summarise the most important correlations.

The definition for fertile sperm by the WHO (World Health Organization) is an ejaculate of at least 2 mL with at least 20 million sperm per mL and 50 % progressive motility [22].

Adolescents and adults have 15 % prevalence for varicocele. About 35–50 % of men with primary infertility and 70–80 % of men with secondary infertility present with clinical varicoceles. This increased incidence suggests not only that varicocele is an important factor in male infertility but also that varicocele causes a progressive effect on testicular function [23, 24].

On the other hand, only 15–20 % of males with a varicocele require treatment for infertility, suggesting that most men with a varicocele have no fertility problems [1].

According to a large multicenter study by the WHO, varicocele is clearly associated with testicular dysfunction and male infertility. A palpable varicocele was detected in 25.4 % of men with altered semen quality but in only 11.7 % of normozoospermic men. The study determined an association between varicocele and a decrease in ipsilateral testicular volume, semen quality and Leydig cell dysfunction [25].

### Varicocele Grade and Fertility

Controversial data exist on the effect of varicocele grade on semen quality. Recently, Al-Ali et al. showed that oligozoospermia was present twice as much in patients with grade 3 varicocele compared to patients with varicocele grade 1 or 2. They also stated that sperm density significantly decreased with increasing grade of varicocele [26].

These results correlate with the previously published results of Steckel et al. who stated that men with grade 3 varicocele had lower sperm counts and poorer fertility indexes compared to men with grades 1 and 2 varicocele [27].

However, Diamond et al. and Shiraishi et al. reported no significant difference between varicocele grade and semen quality [21, 28].

### Testicular Size and Fertility

Does size matter? Measurement of testicular size in adolescents with varicocele is of diagnostic and prognostic importance. As semen parameters do not belong in assessing a varicocele in an adolescent, the effect of varicocele on testicular size and the correlation between size and semen quality is very important. Whether or not testicular size should influence the decision to treat has become clear in the literature.

Previous studies have revealed that 10 % size variance between testes without associated abnormalities such as presence of a varicocele is to be considered as normal [29].

Diamond et al. showed that sonographically derived volume differentials greater than 10 % between normal and affected testes in Tanner V adolescents correlate with a significantly decreased sperm concentration and total motile sperm count [28].

Sigman and Jarow showed a statistically higher incidence of hypotrophy in grade 3 varicoceles (73 %) compared to grade 1 and 2 varicoceles (49 % and 55 %, respectively). There was also a significant difference in total motile sperm count between men with or without testicular hypotrophy. There appeared to be a trend of decreasing sperm count with increasing difference in testicular size, although this was not statistically significant [30].

Haans and Laven et al. also stated that left testicular growth failure in patients with varicocele relative to controls correlated with lower total sperm number, but they did not find a correlation with sperm concentration [31, 32].

In contrast, Guarino et al. found no predictive value of testicular volume measurement with regard to semen analysis in Tanner V adolescents. This study however showed no statistical difference in testicular volume difference in patients with vs. without varicocele [33].

Skoog et al. explained that a volume difference between the two testes becomes clear in adolescents with varicocele during the rapid growth of the testes during puberty. They also stated that the loss of testicular volume is accompanied by a decrease in the sperm count and advocated the early diagnosis of the disease, as this is important for the prevention of sperm impairment and infertility [1].

Summarising previous statements, we can assume that the presence of a varicocele in adolescents might predispose the adolescent for future infertility and that testicular size or rather size differential is an indicator for decrease in semen quality.

This would mean that according to differential testicular volume, adolescents can be categorised in higher- or lower-risk groups regarding future fertility.

### Treatment Effect of Varicocelectomy

*Fertility*: Although many individual studies report improvement of fertility after varicocele repair, there are still conflicting opinions as to whether a varicocele repair improves fertility.

The Cochrane meta-analysis of 2009 suggests there is no benefit in a couple's chance of conceiving after varicocele treatment [34]. We should bear in mind though that men with varicoceles and normal semen parameters preoperatively were also included in the results of the meta-analysis.

Ficarra on the other hand reviewed randomised clinical trials for varicocele treatment on patients with varicoceles with impaired semen quality and proved that treatment had a beneficial effect on pregnancy with an increase in pregnancy rates of 36.4 % in contrast to only 20 % increase in the control group [35].

These results are comparable to Marmar's, whose meta-analysis on treatment for infertile men with varicocele and impaired semen quality showed to be in favour of treatment [36].

Agarwal et al. showed in a recent meta-analytical research that surgical varicocelectomy significantly improves semen parameters in infertile men with palpable varicocele and abnormal semen parameters [37].

Steckel et al. and Jarow et al. both demonstrated that varicocele repair in grade 3 varicoceles was correlated with a higher improvement of semen quality, compared to grade 1 and 2 varicocele repair [27, 38].

Cayan et al. on the other hand showed a statistically significant improvement in sperm concentration, total motile sperm and testosterone levels after varicocele treatment, regardless of varicocele grade [39].

The most important message here is that treatment of varicocele has a positive effect on sperm quality. Whether or not the grade of varicocele is of importance in regaining fertility is probably of lesser importance.

*Testicular size*: Cayan et al. showed that preoperatively soft testis regained firmness after surgery and noted a catch-up growth after treatment. Although this effect is no longer statistically significant when treatment occurs after the age of 14, these adolescents still show a significant improvement of semen parameters postoperatively regardless of testicular volume [39].

In the controlled prospective study by Laven et al., adolescents with varicoceles that were treated had an increase in left testicular volume and sperm concentrations, whereas those with untreated varicoceles did not show these improvements [32].

Skoog et al. suggested that the rapid and noticeable improvements of testicular size in the adolescent are due to the fact that the testes are still in the process of developing and may be able to undergo "catch-up growth" and gain function [1].

Salisz et al. showed that varicocele treatment not only results in improved fertility and catch-up growth of testicular size but also in normalisation of scrotal skin temperature [16].

## Importance of Varicocele in General Medicine

As the effect of a varicocele on fertility has been clearly argumented, it is obvious that varicocele is an important entity to recognise, whether you are a family practitioner, paediatrician or urologist.

Results of a survey on practice patterns of paediatricians on varicoceles showed that a significant percentage of paediatricians does not routinely perform physical exam for varicoceles or examines for varicoceles appropriately. Eighty-five percent of paediatricians did refer the patient to a urological practice when a varicocele was diagnosed [40].

In Belgium, during primary school and high school, children are obligated to visit a so-called school doctor, which examines the children for the most common ailments and disabilities, like hearing, sight, IQ, etcetera. Boys are also routinely checked for puberty grade according to Tanner, testicular volume and presence or absence of varicocele at physical examination. When a varicocele is present, the children are usually referred to their family practitioner or paediatrician.

It is therefore important for a family practitioner to be able to recognise the varicocele entity, the grade of varicocele and to estimate whether or not there might be a volume differential between left and right testicle. A family practitioner should be aware of the risks of varicocele and if necessary should make the call to refer the patient to a urological practice for further examination and, if necessary, treatment.

## How to Evaluate a Varicocele

Clinical evaluation is most important in evaluating a varicocele. Blood tests have no diagnostic value, neither do urine tests. Ultrasound may be helpful for evaluating the testicular volume and perhaps vascularisation.

Additional radiologic imaging is not necessary to search for subclinical varicocele, because only a varicocele detected by physical examination should be considered potentially significant [41].

In contrast to adult varicocele, methods to assess reproductive function such as semen analysis, testis biopsy and fine needle aspiration with flow cytometry are not recommended for the adolescent with a varicocele.

Physical examination of adolescent males in search of a varicocele should be done in a temperature-controlled room, with warm hands, with the patient first in the supine and afterwards in the upright position. Attention should go out to the palpability and visibility of possible varicocele with or without Valsalva and whether or not it disappears when lying down. Varicocele as found at clinical examination should be categorised according to Dubin and Amelar as mentioned above [2].

Pubertal phase and testicular development can be scored according to Marshall and Tanner [42]. The Tanner method of describing the stages of pubertal development is widely accepted, objective and clinically useful.

Testicular size can be measured at clinical examination with an orchidometer (Prader, Takihara or Seager). Measurement of the contralateral testis is important to evaluate for volume differential (*right testicular volume – left testicular volume)/right testicular volume* × 100 = %.

In clinical examination of a varicocele patient, testicular volume and volume difference should be measured as it is previously shown that testicular volume clearly correlates with sperm quality. Whether this difference should be mentioned in millilitres or percentages is of little importance.

As previously stated, a 10 % size variance between testes without associated abnormalities is to be considered as normal [29].

A volume difference of less than 2 mL can be due to the measurement technique alone. Skoog et al. showed that testicular size variation of greater than 2 mL by ultrasound constitutes significant growth arrest [1].

Cayan et al. stated that the testicular volumes measured with ultrasound and the Prader orchidometer were statistically significantly consistent, and this correlation remained highly consistent regardless of age or testicular volume on both sides of the subjects [43]. Diamond et al. also reported a strong linear relationship between testicular volume measurements using orchidometer and ultrasound. They would however suggest to use ultrasound for assessing volume differentials as orchidometers are too insensitive for these estimates [44].

Recently, Walker and Kogan questioned the necessity of scrotal ultrasound in detecting a 20 % size difference in testicular volume in patients with varicocele. They calculated that it would cost 5,597 $US for office-based and 12,226 $US for hospital-based ultrasound to prevent 1 missed testicular size difference of 20 % [45].

It is improbable that a clinically significant size difference would be missed at consecutive clinical examinations. Therefore, ultrasound should not be part of the routine examination in varicocele patients.

## Referral and Indications for Treatment of Varicocele

### When to Refer

As it has become clear that testicular volume correlates with sperm quality, even in adolescents, patients with varicocele and difference in testicular volume of more than 10 % should be referred to a urological practice.

Treatment of varicocele is always an elective procedure. As varicocele is never an acute finding, there is no urgent or emergent setting for this pathology.

### When to Treat?

In this chapter we've discussed so far what a varicocele is, what effects it can have on testicular size and fertility and that treatment of a varicocele in patients with volume differential of more than 10 % or infertility can result in catch-up growth of the left testicle and increase of sperm quality.

It should therefore be clear that when these factors are present in adolescent males with varicocele, treatment is most certainly justified. When none of these factors are present, surgery should only be indicated when the patients suffer from pain or scrotal inconvenience due to this varicocele.

The report on varicocele and infertility by the Practice Committee of the American Society for Reproductive Medicine clearly states the indications for treatment of a varicocele in adolescents and adults [46].

The current American Urological Association recommendations advise offering of varicocelectomy to all adult men, seeking or not seeking conception, with any clinically palpable varicocele and abnormal semen parameters (Table 23.3).

According to the above-mentioned guidelines, men consulting for fertility problems with a borderline spermiogram and clinically present varicocele would not always be considered for varicocele treatment. Mori et al. suggest to revise these guidelines as borderline spermiograms are likely to evolve to infertile spermiograms, as varicocele has been shown to have a progressive effect on fertility [47].

**Table 23.3** Indications for treatment of a varicocele in adults

| |
|---|
| When the male partner of a couple attempting to conceive has a varicocele, treatment of the varicocele should be considered when all of the following conditions are met: |
| 1. The varicocele is palpable on physical examination of the scrotum. |
| 2. The couple has known infertility. |
| 3. The female partner has normal fertility or a potentially treatable cause of infertility |
| 4. The male partner has abnormal semen parameters or abnormal results from sperm function tests |
| Varicocele treatment for infertility is not indicated in patients with either normal semen quality or a subclinical varicocele. An adult male who is not currently attempting to achieve conception, but has a palpable varicocele, abnormal semen analyses and a desire for future fertility, also is a candidate for varicocele repair. Young adult males with varicoceles who have normal semen parameters may be at risk for progressive testicular dysfunction and should be offered monitoring with semen analyses every 1–2 years in order to detect the earliest sign of reduced spermatogenesis |

A deterioration in semen quality usually only becomes clear in subfertile men, when trying to conceive with their partner. As the prevalence of varicocele in adolescents and adults is about the same, the varicocele is probably present for certain years before subfertility becomes apparent. Even though grade 3 varicoceles might be correlated with a higher percentage in impaired semen quality, lower grade varicoceles probably have had a cumulative effect on the testicle/semen by adulthood.

As only 15–20 % of adults with varicocele will present themselves for infertility treatment, it is clear that not all adolescents presenting with varicocele require prophylactic surgical treatment (Table 23.4).

Skoog et al. nicely summarised their findings on why to treat a varicocele [1]. The recommendations are similar to those published in the report on varicocele and infertility (Table 23.5). These indications are widely accepted and are also used in Europe.

**Table 23.4** Indications for treatment of a varicocele in adolescents

| |
|---|
| Adolescent males who have unilateral or bilateral varicoceles and objective evidence of *reduced testicular size* ipsilateral to the varicocele also should be considered candidates for varicocele repair. If objective evidence of reduced testis size is not present, then adolescents with varicoceles should be followed with annual objective measurements of testis size and/or semen analyses in order to detect the earliest sign of varicocele-related testicular injury. Varicocele repair should be offered on detection of testicular or semen abnormality |

**Table 23.5** Indications for treatment of varicocele

| | |
|---|---|
| 1. | A greater than 2 mL difference in testicular volume as noted on serial ultrasonographic examinations |
| 2. | A two standard deviation decrease in testicular size when compared with normal testicular growth curves |
| 3. | Scrotal pain |
| 4. | Large or bilateral varicoceles |

## How to Manage Varicocele

### Aims of Intervention

Treatment of adult varicocele aims to improve the rate of pregnancy in couples in which the male partner has varicocele and the woman has no residual identified fertility problems. It also aims to reduce pain and discomfort associated with varicocele, with minimal adverse effects.

The main goal of treatment of adolescent varicocele is preservation of fertility or prevention of infertility. Therefore, the ideal technique for varicocele repair should include preservation of optimal testicular function, elimination of the varicocele and as low as possible complication rates.

In search of the ideal treatment for varicocele, different methods and approaches have been suggested. After studying the different methods used to date, Cayan et al. stated that the best treatment modality for varicocele in infertile men should include higher seminal improvement and spontaneous pregnancy rates with lower rates of complications such as recurrence or persistence, hydrocele formation, and testicular atrophy [48]. Therefore, the ideal technique should aim for ligation of all internal and external spermatic veins with preservation of spermatic arteries and lymphatics.

### Treatment Modalities

#### Ivanissevich Technique of Ligation

This technique performs high ligation of the spermatic veins, close to the iliac crest.

#### Bernardi Technique of Ligation

Ligation of the internal spermatic vein close to the internal (deep) inguinal ring is done.

#### Palomo Technique of Ligation

The retroperitoneal internal spermatic vein and artery are ligated at the level of the anterior superior iliac spine. Thanks to the high ligation, there is no injury to the cremasteric arteries, which ensure the testicular blood supply after ligation of the spermatic artery [49].

Ivanissevich, Bernardi and Palomo procedures are usually performed under general anaesthesia on an outpatient basis. Occasionally, the surgery is performed with a local anaesthetic.

#### Subinguinal Varicocele Ligation

The spermatic vein(s) are ligated just below the external inguinal ring, and this technique may be useful in men with a history of inguinal surgery. A subinguinal approach is more difficult than a high inguinal ligation and is performed under local anaesthetic.

#### Embolisation Catheterisation of the Left Spermatic Vein Through the Left Renal Vein

Selective spermatic venography visualises venous anatomy. The spermatic vein can then be embolised by various methods, including coils, detachable balloons, sclerosant agents or a combination of either. Transcatheter embolisation is performed on an outpatient basis under intravenous sedation and analgesia.

## Antegrade Sclerotherapy

A small incision is made at the root of the penis. The selected vein is ligated and a small catheter is placed beyond the ligature to infuse sclerosing agent. This sclerosing agent produces endothelial destruction, resulting in occlusion of the spermatic vein. Tauber and Johnsen were the first to describe this procedure [50].

Most commonly seen complications are residual varicocele and hydrocele. Hydroceles occur in 0–10 % after varicocele treatment, depending on the technique used. Hydroceles occur due to lymphatic damage at the time of venous ligation.

Cayan et al. recently published a meta-analysis on defining the best suitable technique for treating clinically significant varicoceles in infertile men with abnormal semen analysis [48]. They compared Palomo approach, microsurgical inguinal or subinguinal technique, laparoscopic varicocelectomy, radiologic embolisation and Ivanissevich approach. Results showed that microsurgical repair was by far the best option for treatment, with a higher spontaneous pregnancy rate (42 %), very low recurrence rate (1 %) and low complication rate (0.44 %). Thirteen percent of radiologic embolisation interventions were unsuccessful. In this meta-analysis, patients who underwent laparoscopic treatment had major complications in almost 8 %.

When comparing Cayan's and Skoog's review on treatment technique, they described quite similar results for treatment failure, residual or recurrent varicocele and complication rates [1, 48]. Of the compared treatment modalities, microsurgical treatment seems to have the best results. Palomo treatment and laparoscopic approaches show to have a high recurrence and complication rate, therefore being the least suited treatment options for varicocele.

Sadly enough neither Skoog nor Cayan included any results of antegrade sclerotherapy in their analysis in search of the most suitable technique for varicocele treatment, although results with this treatment modality are very good.

Galfano et al. even proposed this to be the first choice in treatment of varicocele because of the safety and efficacy of the treatment and the low persistence and complication rate after treatment [51].

Also from an economical point of view, antegrade sclerotherapy is the first choice of treatment as it is far less expensive than any other alternative [52].

## References

1. Skoog SJ, Roberts KP, Goldstein M, Pryor JL. The adolescent varicocele: what's new with an old problem in young patients? Pediatrics. 1997;100:112.
2. Dubin L, Amelar RD. Varicocele size and results of varicocelectomy in selected subfertile men with varicocele. Fertil Steril. 1970;21:606–9.
3. Hirsh AV, Cameron KM, Tyler JP, et al. The Doppler assessment of varicoceles and internal spermatic vein reflux in infertile men. Br J Urol. 1980;52:50–6.
4. El Sadr AR, Mina A. Anatomical and surgical aspects in the operative management of varicoceles. Urol Cutaneous Rev. 1950;54:257–62.
5. Graif M, Hauser R, Hirshebein A, et al. Varicocele and the testicular-renal venous route: hemodynamic Doppler sonographic investigation. J Ultrasound Med. 2000;19(9):627–31.
6. Wishahi MM. Anatomy of the venous drainage of the human testis: testicular vein cast, microdissection and radiographic demonstration. A new anatomical concept. Eur Urol. 1991;20(2):154–60.
7. Raman J, Walmsley K, Goldstein M. Inheritance of varicocele. Urology. 2005;65:1186–9.
8. Mohammed A, Chinegwundoh F. Testicular varicocele: an overview. Urol Int. 2009;82(4):373–9. Epub 2009 Jun 8.
9. Prabakaran S, Kumanov P, Tomova A, et al. Adolescent varicocele: association with somatometric parameters. Urol Int. 2006;77(2):114–7.
10. Kumanov P, Robeva RN, Tomova A. Adolescent varicocele: who is at risk? Pediatrics. 2008;121(1):e53–7.
11. Tsao CW, Hsu CY, Chou YC, Wu ST, et al. The relationship between varicoceles and obesity in a young adult population. Int J Androl. 2009;32(4):385–90. Epub 2008 Oct 21.
12. Nakamura M, Namiki M, Okuyama A, et al. Optimal temperature for synthesis of DNA, RNA, and protein by human testis in vitro. Arch Androl. 1988;20(1):41–4.
13. Okuyama A, Koh E, Kondoh N, et al. In vitro temperature sensitivity of DNA, RNA, and protein syntheses throughout puberty in human testis. Arch Androl. 1991;26(1):7–13.
14. Fujisawa M, Hayashi A, Okada H, et al. Enzymes involved in DNA synthesis in the testes are regulated by temperature in vitro. Eur Urol. 1997;31(2):237–42.
15. Goldstein M, Eid JF. Elevation of intratesticular and scrotal skin surface temperature in men with varicocele. J Urol. 1989;142(3):743–5.

16. Salisz JA, Kass EJ, Steinert BW. The significance of elevated scrotal temperature in an adolescent with a varicocele. Adv Exp Med Biol. 1991;286:245–51.
17. Dahl EV, Herrick JF. A vascular mechanism for maintaining testicular temperature by counter-current exchange. Surg Gynecol Obstet. 1959;108:697–705.
18. Hienz HA, Voggenthaler J, Weissbach L. Histological findings in testes with varicocele during childhood and their therapeutic consequences. Eur J Pediatr. 1980;133:139–46.
19. Sikka SC. Oxidative stress and role of antioxidants in normal and abnormal sperm function. Front Biosci. 1996;1:e78–86.
20. Abd-Elmoaty MA, Saleh R, Sharma R, Agarwal A. Increased levels of oxidants and reduced antioxidants in semen of infertile men with varicocele. Fertil Steril. 2010;94(4):1531–4.
21. Shiraishi K, Takihara H, Matsuyama H. Elevated scrotal temperature, but not varicocele grade, reflects testicular oxidative stress-mediated apoptosis. World J Urol. 2010;28(3):359–64.
22. World Health Organization. Laboratory manual for the examination of human semen and sperm-cervical mucus interaction. 4th ed. New York: Cambridge University Press; 1999.
23. Gorelick JI, Goldstein M. Loss of fertility in men with varicocele. Fertil Steril. 1993;59(3):613–6.
24. Witt MA, Lipshultz LI. Varicocele: a progressive or static lesion? Urology. 1993;42:541–3.
25. World Health Organization. The influence of varicocele on parameters of fertility in a large group of men presenting to infertility clinics. Fertil Steril. 1992;57:1289–93.
26. Mohamad Al-Ali B, Marszalek M, Shamloul R, et al. Clinical parameters and semen analysis in 716 Austrian patients with varicocele. Urology. 2010;75(5):1069–73.
27. Steckel J, Dicker AP, Goldstein M. Relationship between varicocele size and response to varicocelectomy. J Urol. 1993;149:769–71.
28. Diamond DA, Zurakowski D, Bauer SB, et al. Relationship of varicocele grade and testicular hypotrophy to semen parameters in adolescents. J Urol. 2007;178(4 Pt 2):1584–8. Epub 2007 Aug 16.
29. Zachmann M, Prader A, Kind HP, et al. Testicular volume during adolescence. Crosssectional and longitudinal studies. Helv Paediatr Acta. 1974;29:61.
30. Sigman M, Jarow JP. Ipsilateral testicular hypotrophy is associated with decreased sperm counts in infertile men with varicoceles. J Urol. 1997;158:605.
31. Haans LCF, Laven JSE, Mali WPTM, et al. Testis volumes, semen quality, and hormonal patterns in adolescents with and without a varicocele. Fertil Steril. 1991;56:731.
32. Laven JSE, Haans LCF, Mali WPTM, et al. Effects of varicocele treatment in adolescents: a randomized study. Fertil Steril. 1992;58:756.
33. Guarino N, Tadini B, Bianchi M. The adolescent varicocele: the crucial role of hormonal tests in selecting patients with testicular dysfunction. J Pediatr Surg. 2003;38:120.
34. Evers JH, Collins J, Clarke J. Surgery or embolisation for varicoceles in subfertile men. Cochrane Database Syst Rev. 2009;(1):CD000479.
35. Ficarra V, Cerruto MA, Liguori G, et al. Treatment of varicocele in subfertile men: the Cochrane review—a contrary opinion. Eur Urol. 2006;49(2):258–63. Epub 2006 Jan 4.
36. Marmar JL, Agarwal A, Prabakaran S, et al. Reassessing the value of varicocelectomy as a treatment for male subfertility with a new meta-analysis. Fertil Steril. 2007;88(3):639–48. Epub 2007 Apr 16.
37. Agarwal A, Deepinder F, Cocuzza M, et al. Efficacy of varicocelectomy in improving semen parameters: new meta-analytic approach. Urology. 2007;70:532–8.
38. Jarow JP, Ogle SR, Eskew LA. Seminal improvement following repair of ultrasound detected subclinical varicoceles. J Urol. 1996;155:1287–90.
39. Cayan S, Akbay E, Bozlu M. The effect of varicocele repair on testicular volume in children and adolescents with varicocele. J Urol. 2002;168(2):731–4.
40. Kubal A, Nagler HM, Zahalsky M, Budak M. The adolescent varicocele: diagnostic and treatment patterns of pediatricians. A public health concern? J Urol. 2004;171(1):411–3.
41. Jarow JP, Sharlip ID, Belker AM, et al. Best practice policies for male infertility. J Urol. 2002;167:2138–44.
42. Marshall WA, Tanner JM. Variations in the pattern of pubertal changes in boys. Arch Dis Child. 1970;45:13.
43. Cayan S, Akbay E, Bozlu M, et al. The comparison of physical examination, orchidometry, and color Doppler ultrasonography in the diagnosis of pediatric varicocele and the measurement of testicular volume. J Urol. 2001;165(Suppl):148, abstract 606.
44. Diamond DA, Paltiel HJ, DiCanzio J, et al. Comparative assessment of pediatric testicular volume: orchidometer versus ultrasound. J Urol. 2000;164(part 2):1111.
45. Walker AR, Kogan BA. Cost-benefit analysis of scrotal ultrasound in treatment of adolescents with varicocele. J Urol. 2010;183(5):2008–11.
46. Practice Committee of American Society for Reproductive Medicine. Report on varicocele and infertility. Fertil Steril. 2008;90(5 Suppl):S247–9.
47. Mori MM, Bertolla RP, Fraietta R, et al. Does varicocele grade determine extent of alteration to spermatogenesis in adolescents? Fertil Steril. 2008;90(5):1769–73.
48. Cayan S, Shavakhabov S, Kadioğlu A. Treatment of palpable varicocele in infertile men: a meta-analysis to define the best technique. J Androl. 2009;30(1):33–40. Epub 2008 Sep 4.
49. Palomo A. Radical cure of varicocele by a new technique: preliminary report. J Urol. 1949;61:604–7.

50. Tauber R, Johnsen N. Antegrade scrotal sclerotherapy for the treatment of varicocele: technique and late results. J Urol. 1994;151(2):386–90.
51. Galfano A, Novara G, Iafrate M, et al. Surgical outcomes after modified antegrade scrotal sclerotherapy: a prospective analysis of 700 consecutive patients with idiopathic varicocele. J Urol. 2008;179(5): 1933–7. Epub 2008 Mar 18.
52. Ficarra V, Zanon G, D'Amico A, et al. Percutaneous, laparoscopic, and surgical treatment of idiopathic varicocele: analysis of costs. Arch Ital Urol Androl. 1998;70(2):57–64.

# Phimosis

# 24

Robert D. Schwarz and Shubha De

Phimosis is defined in the concise Oxford English Dictionary as "a congenital narrowing of the opening of the foreskin so that it cannot be retracted." The term derives from the Greek word meaning "muzzling," which carries connotations of "covering, protecting, and preventing expression." Baby boys are normally born with phimotic foreskins and it is unusual for a baby without other penile pathology to have a freely retractable prepuce (Fig. 24.1). Uncircumcised boys gradually develop such that glanular adhesions separate and the preputial meatus grows allowing for skin retraction. The age by which the maturation is complete varies but may be well into adolescence. One British study of 12-year-old boys with unretractable foreskins found that all but a few were easily retractable by age 16 years. Those data suggest that it would be unwise to tell parents that their son's foreskin should be retractable by a certain age or else they would have to have surgery. The medical indications for surgery, rather,' should relate to specific risks, pathology, or morbidity.

R.D. Schwarz, M.D., F.R.C.S.C. (✉)
Division of Urology, Department of Surgery, Dalhousie University, 5850/5980 University Avenue, P.O. Box 9700, Halifax, NS, Canada, BK3 6R8
e-mail: robert.schwarz@iwk.nshealth.ca

S. De, M.D.
Cleveland Clinic Foundation, Cleveland, OH, USA

## Should the Foreskin Be Pushed?

Many parents are eager that their son's foreskin should develop as soon as possible, and they want to hasten its growth. There are widely held beliefs that retracting the skin forcefully will hasten its development. On the contrary, vigorous retraction not only does not help the skin's growth, but can result in microscopic tears and trauma which may lead to increased collagen and scarring, and as a result may *retard* the growth and development of the skin.

Vigorous retraction can also sensitize the child so that he expects a painful manipulation any time he is bathed or examined. That induced sensitivity can develop to a point that the parents interpret it as pain and may request surgery.

## Paraphimosis

Occasionally vigorous retraction of the skin will bring the preputial meatus back over the glans where it can form a tight ring proximal to the coronal sulcus (Fig. 24.2). From that point the child and his parents cannot bring the skin forward over the glans to its normal position. By the time you see the boy, there is an edematous ring of skin between the corona of the glans and the tight circumferential preputial meatus. In order to reduce the paraphimosis, we recommend appropriate analgesia/sedation with or without a local

R. Rabinowitz et al. (eds.), *Pediatric Urology for the Primary Care Physician*, Current Clinical Urology,
DOI 10.1007/978-1-60327-243-8_24, © Springer Science+Business Media New York 2015

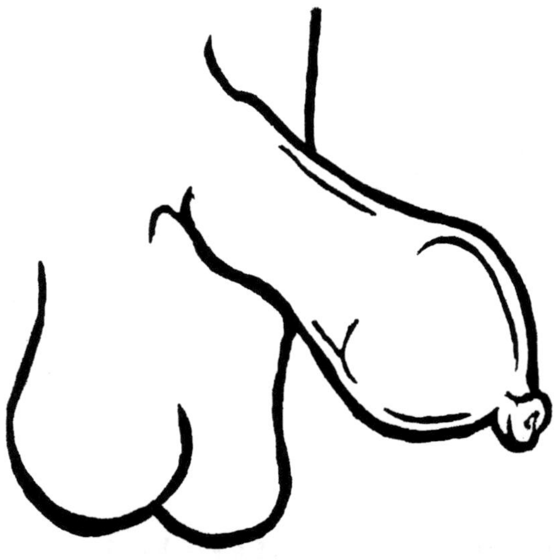

**Fig. 24.1** Line drawing of a normal physiologic phimosis

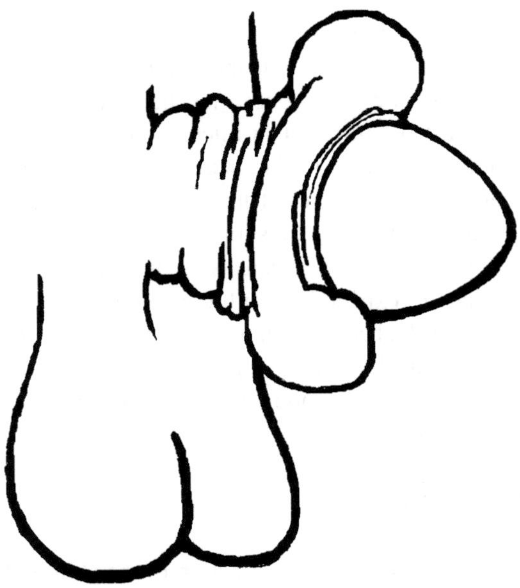

**Fig. 24.2** Paraphimosis—a line drawing showing paraphimosis. The edematous ring is proximal on the shaft to the glans and coronal sulcus. The constricting band will be just proximal to the edematous ring

anesthesia dorsal nerve block. Then one can grasp the tight ring and pull it forward while slipping the glans backward. I find that if you use the index and middle fingers of both hands on the tight preputial ring to pull forward and both thumbs to push the glans backward, it is usually a quick and easy procedure. The child is immediately relieved and he and his parents have learned not to retract without replacing the skin. We have seen paraphimosis occur following medical catheterization where the staff failed to return the skin to its normal position.

## What About Cleaning the Penis?

Many parents are concerned about cleaning the penis, especially under the foreskin. The skin of the glans and inner surface of the foreskin are rich in sensory nerves. Think of rubbing soap in your eyes or mouth. Not only is it unnecessary but also it is very irritating. For babies and young children, a bath in warm water without manipulation is all that is needed to rinse the skin of the penis.

## Smegma and Balanitis

There are normal adhesions between the inner epithelium of the foreskin and the glans. As the skin matures, the adhesions separate to allow for mobility between the layers. Before that maturation, sometimes there can be an entrapped collection of smegma at the level of the coronal sulcus proximal to the adhesions. Examining the boy, you can often see a yellowish lump on the side of the penile shaft. It is not usually inflamed or tender. Smegma is made up of desquamated epithelial cells and oily skin secretions. There also can be a nonpathogenic mycobacterium and other skin bacteria, but smegma by itself is not pathogenic. When the adhesions separate, the smegma will extrude. Sometimes it can be quite irritating as it makes its way out. Again, warm water soaks will soften the sticky, cheesy material and allow it to extrude more easily.

Balanitis, short for balanoposthitis, refers to acute inflammation of the preputial sac. Although this is not a rare medical problem, little has been published in the literature to define the cause or best management, so we are left treating these boys based on our best experience (weak evidence). Most boys we see are prepubertal. They present with an acute painful red swelling. They do not have systemic findings (fever or constitutional changes). Valid voided urine specimens are impossible and generally the kids don't have UTIs, nor do they usually require any antibiotics. Most often the boys will get better within a day or two coincident with local hygiene care. We usually advise multiple warm baths. We think that helps "clean out" any irritant in the preputial hood, but there is not good evidence to support any management strategy. Those boys who we review later have universally returned to their pre-morbid condition.

When does the morbidity of recurrent balanitis demand surgical intervention? Because it is a morbidity indication, judgment and balance of risks become the critical decision-making tools and one has to listen to the concerns of the child as well as his parents. Most boys with two or three episodes over a year or 2 will hope that they have gone through their last episode and will not feel the necessity of surgery. Rarely, recurrent balanitis is said to be a presenting symptom of diabetes.

## Ballooning

Often a child and parents will observe the preputial sac fill and become distended when the child is voiding. This does not bother the child. Sometimes it can make it difficult for him to direct his urinary stream especially when the urine flow is starting. With time and maturation, the issue of the ballooning resolves (Fig. 24.3).

Rarely the preputial sac can become so distended as to result in "mega-prepuce." There is no strict measurement difference between ballooning and mega-prepuce. Ballooning may reach a golf ball size while mega-prepuce is usually greater than 5 cm in diameter. The Law of Laplace relates wall tension of a sphere to internal pressure. With children who have mega-prepuce, the relation between wall tension and pressure is such that these kids should be considered for surgery.

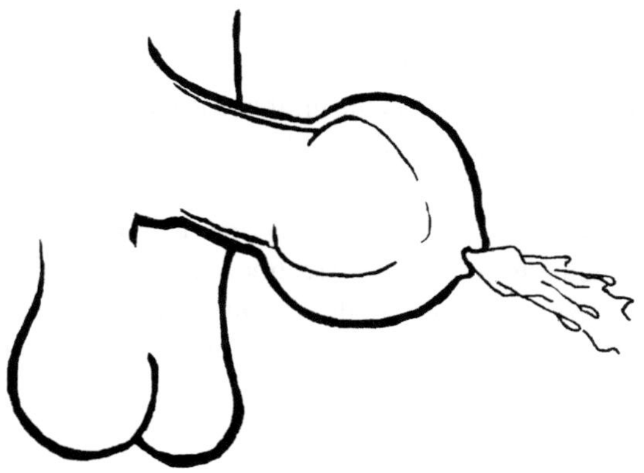

**Fig. 24.3** Ballooning—line drawing of preputial ballooning during voiding

## BXO and Other Dermatological Pathologies

BXO (balanitis xerotica obliterans) is an idiopathic condition usually involving the preputial meatus and sometimes is more extensive involving the glans or the urethral meatus. On exam one can observe a thick, rigid, white ring around the preputial meatus. There may be radial hypervascularity peripheral to the involved tissue. The lesion area feels thickened and leathery. The child may indicate that the foreskin was previously retractable but no longer can get back. It may crack and bleed.

Histologically BXO looks like lichen sclerosus et atrophicus with a thickened dermis and thin epidermis. There is controversy whether this lesion is premalignant. The evidence is weak. Some authors suggest early BXO may respond to steroid cream and we have seen one or two kids resolve after using topical steroids. The problem is that we have relied on clinical diagnosis alone. Other medical treatments have not performed better than placebo.

It used to be felt that BXO was rare in children, but many recent studies have shown that a large proportion of children requiring medically indicated circumcision show features of BXO. Usually circumcision resolves BXO unless the condition involves the urethral meatus in which case meatotomy or meatoplasty may be required. The foreskin is often used as skin graft donor site in the construction of the urethra for hypospadias or urethral structure disease. BXO has been reported in the graft and usually requires complete reconstruction of the grafted region.

Almost every other type of skin condition has been reported to occur on the foreskin from eczema to poison ivy. Treatment usually focuses on the underlying condition. One can think of the foreskin as a protective covering for the glans and the urethra.

## The Circumcision Controversy

No discussion of phimosis would be complete without considering the risk/benefit analysis of neonatal circumcision. Scientific data cannot give us an absolute answer. Unfortunately it is a debate colored more by emotion and preconceptions than good outcomes data, and even the valid outcomes studies will provide data to each side of the debate. There is a nice review of both sides in a recent CUAJ (Table 24.1) [1, 2].

The data that supports routine neonatal circumcision include urinary infections, penile cancer, STDs, and avoiding future foreskin urinary or sexual problems (see above). It has long been observed that uncircumcised babies are at greater risk of UTIs than babies who had been circumcised. The pathogenesis seems to be related to colonization of the preputial sac with uropathic coliforms and the probably hematogenous spread to the kidneys. It is unclear how great the renal risk is for those babies who are affected by bacteriuria. Many of the babies with bacteriuria were found through screening studies. Different studies have estimated different changes in rates of bacteriuria following circumcision. Does the renal risk following neonatal UTI in uncircumcised babies justify circumcising everyone? The numbers are not really known. The reduction of renal risk must be balanced by the morbidity and expense of neonatal circumcision for all.

Penile cancer has also been associated with the covered glans and it seems the younger the baby is when circumcised, the lower the risk. The greatest risk of penile cancer occurs in the developing world and equatorial climates. In the western world where health care and hygiene are the norm, the rates of penile cancer, even in uncircumcised populations, are low enough to lose the clear advantage of universal circumcision.

Recently several papers have addressed the reduction in STDs especially HIV/AIDS associated with circumcision. From a public health perspective this is especially valid in sub-Saharan Africa and among other particularly vulnerable populations. In the developed world where one hopes safe sexual practices prevail, the benefit is lost. A recent Cochrane review failed to support the benefit of circumcision related to HIV/AIDS.

Avoiding future problems or preventative surgical intervention is a strong argument for many parents. They will have heard stories of relatives, friends, or neighbors who had problems with their foreskin. They will often ask that their babies are circumcised as infants, "when they don't feel it," rather than later when it carries morbidity. There is good data showing that neonates experience significant pain with circumcision and although the memory isn't recalled specifically, it does effect the child's future interaction with health care workers and other behaviors. The question of preventative surgery is also

**Table 24.1** Circumcision controversy

| Pro circumcision | Neutral | Against circumcision |
|---|---|---|
| Prevention of: | • Cosmetic | • Risks-surgery in neonate |
| • Penile cancer | • Sexual pleasure/function | – Bleeding |
| • UTI in babies | • Prevention of | – Infection/sepsis |
| • STDs (?) | • Future morbidity | – Tissue loss |
| | • Religious/cultural | • Trauma and pain |
| | | • Meatitis and meatal stenosis |
| | | • Buried penis |

interesting. In the same vein, we would have to consider a prophylactic appendectomy, or tonsillectomy and cholecystectomy. Clearly the families would agree that those surgeries would be unreasonable.

There are a number of discussion points which are often brought up but which are really neutral from a scientific point of view. There are the religious or cultural imperatives with which we cannot and should not argue. Other families will want their baby circumcised for cosmetic reasons or so their son will "look like dad." Beauty is in the eye of the beholder. From the child's point of view, he is more likely to want to look like his schoolmates than his father. Finally, there is the question of sexual function and sexual pleasure. Again that is next to impossible to measure; however, there are proponents on each side of the debate who try to argue their cause on the basis of sexual issues.

We must not forget that circumcision is a surgical procedure and as such carries some risks. Babies do experience pain (see above). There can be bleeding, infection, and tissue loss, and children who have had neonatal circumcisions are at much greater risk of developing meatitis and meatal stenosis. Significant bleeding, infection, or tissue loss is fortunately quite rare but can be devastating. Children have died following neonatal circumcision and there have been babies who have lost most of their penis following circumcision. One remembers the famous Joan-John case. Rare as these disasters are, you only need to see one to have it impact your judgment.

In summary, there are arguments to be made on both sides of the circumcision debate. The controversy has been going on since Greco-Roman times and will likely continue long after you and I. We look forward to seeing greater scientific data added. In the mean time, we make the best decisions we can and advise families without emotion or bias. There are some legitimate medical indications for circumcision—specifically BXO and recurrent balanitis with morbidity. Phimosis itself is not an indication for circumcision except for mega-prepuce or the postadolescent boy with sexual difficulties. Of course, hypospadias is an absolute contraindication to circumcision. Nova Scotia has one of the lowest circumcision rates in North America, closer to that of northern Europe than the US rates. Our view is "if it ain't broke, don't fix it." We do not feel the data require us to proceed with prophylactic intervention. The American Academy of Pediatrics has made a number of policy statements on the subject. The most recent of which [3, 4] covers many of the same issues and leaves the final surgical decision to the process of informed consent.

## References

1. MacNeily AE. Routine circumcision: the opposing view. Can Urol Assoc J. 2007;1:395–7.
2. Houle A-E. Circumcision for all: the pro side. Can Urol Assoc J. 2007;1:398–400.
3. Report of the taskforce on circumcision. AAP Task Force on circumcision. Pediatrics 1989;84(4):388–91.
4. Circumcision policy statement. American Academy of Pediatrics. Task Force on circumcision. Pediatrics. 1999;103(3):686–93.

# Paraphimosis

# 25

Daniel Lewinshtein and Anne-Marie Houle

## Introduction

Paraphimosis is diagnosed when the foreskin in an uncircumcised male becomes stuck behind the corona and forms a tight band of constricting tissue, which prevents its return to the natural position (Fig. 25.1). It is one of the rare urologic emergencies that may challenge the general physician [1] and must be treated as such. Phimosis, a non-urgent medical condition where the foreskin cannot be retracted, must be distinguished from paraphimosis (Fig. 25.2).

Attentiveness to returning the foreskin to its original position following physical examination or urologic procedure will prevent most cases of paraphimosis. If, however, paraphimosis is suspected, rapid evaluation with the help of a urologic consultation when needed is indicated. If left untreated, paraphimosis can have grave consequences, and thus urgent treatment is always warranted.

D. Lewinshtein, M.D.
Department of Urology, Montréal University, Quebec, QC, Canada

A.-M. Houle, M.D., F.R.C.S.C., M.B.A. (✉)
Surgery Department, CHU Sainte-Justine, Montréal University, Chemin de la Côte Sainte-Catherine, Montréal, QC, Canada
e-mail: anne-marie_houle@ssss.gouv.qc.ca

## Etiology

The most common and preventable cause of paraphimosis is human error. Paraphimosis generally occurs after self-retraction for any reason, parental foreskin manipulation, penile examination, urethral catheterization, cystoscopy, or any other urologic procedure requiring foreskin manipulation. Typically, the foreskin is pulled back and inadvertently, the child, the parent, or the medical professional forgets to return the retracted foreskin to its original position, thereby causing the paraphimosis. With regard to the pediatric population, commonly the child or his parent is overly zealous in his or her attempt to retract a phimotic foreskin, which results in a paraphimosis. Parents should be warned to progressively try to retract phimotic foreskins in order to prevent the aforementioned complication. Furthermore, parents should be advised to avoid causing the foreskin to crack or bleed while attempting foreskin retraction. Other more infrequent causes of paraphimosis include cases occurring after glans piercing with metal rings [2] and cases occurring after penile erections [3].

## Pathophysiology

A tight constricting band of tissue forms when the foreskin rests in the proximal position behind the corona for a lengthened period of time. Consequently, this constricting ring reduces

R. Rabinowitz et al. (eds.), *Pediatric Urology for the Primary Care Physician*, Current Clinical Urology,
DOI 10.1007/978-1-60327-243-8_25, © Springer Science+Business Media New York 2015

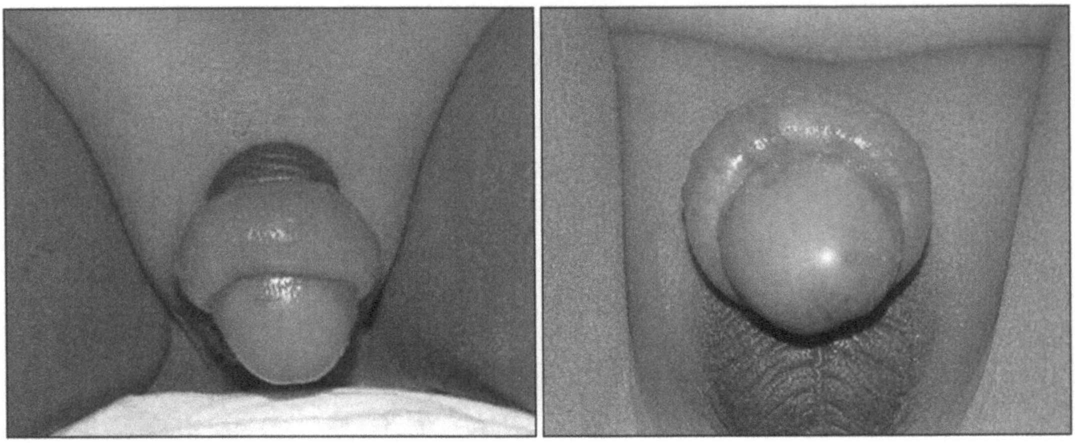

**Fig. 25.1** Paraphimosis in a child. Reprinted with permission from Resident and Staff Physician. Pediatric photo quiz. 2007;53(6)

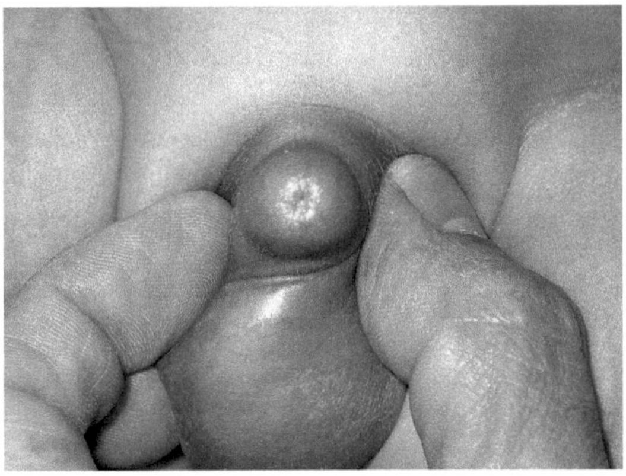

**Fig. 25.2** Phimosis in a child

blood and lymphatic flow to and from the prepuce and the glans penis. The glans and prepuce become swollen and edematous secondary to venous and lymphatic stasis and local ischemia, and a vicious cycle ensues with further inflammation with prolonged retraction. Penile gangrene and necrosis with retraction for days to weeks have been reported in the literature [4].

## History and Physical Examination

The patient should be questioned on self-retraction for any reason. The duration, severity, and quality of the pain associated with the paraphimosis should be sought. However, in some cases pain is not present. This is apparent in patients with reduced peripheral sensation such as diabetics and paraplegics with indwelling catheters. Furthermore, a detailed history of recent penile examination, catheter placement, or endoscopic surgery of urogenital tract should be elicited. Circumcision or partial circumcision status should be obtained from the patient since inspection alone can be difficult secondary to the changes in skin color and texture. Infrequently, infants and young children may present with obstructive voiding symptoms and even acute urinary obstruction when the paraphimosis is severe [5].

The physical examination should focus on the presence or absence of foreskin, the color of the glans, the amount of constriction, and the turgor of the glans. Visual inspection usually reveals an enlarged and congested glans penis with a collar of swollen foreskin behind the corona. The rest of the penis including the shaft is usually unremarkable. The color of the glans should be evaluated. A pink or red glans with adequate capillary refill implies proper blood supply, while a gray or black area may indicate the initiation of necrosis. Palpation of the glans can help to differentiate viable from nonviable tissue. A soft and pliable glans is normal, while a firm and fixed glans is representative of ischemic tissue.

Paraphimosis often occurs in patients with indwelling catheters, and their presence can often impede the successful reduction of the paraphimosis. Their removal is recommended if initial reduction is impossible; however, it is paramount to elicit the reason for their initial placement so that their replacement can occur after successful reduction.

The rest of the genitourinary examination should be completed including scrotal, rectal, and renal examination.

## Treatment

The goals of treatment are to reduce penile edema and the complete reduction of the paraphimosis. The efficacy of treatment options is based on anecdotal reports and a few small cohort retrospective studies, as no randomized trials exist. The treatments range from noninvasive to surgical procedures. Patients generally require narcotics, sedatives, topical anesthesia, or a penile nerve block before an attempt at reduction due to the extreme pain associated with the procedure [6]. When performing the reduction in children, a topical anesthetic such as 2 % lidocaine gel or EMLA cream (2.5 % prilocaine/2.5 % lidocaine) applied 30 min before the reduction attempt is the preferred method.

## Manual Reduction

Glans edema may be reduced with constant circumferential manual pressure around the distal penis. The classic technique consists of placing both thumbs on the glans and letting the other fingers wrap around the prepuce. A steady pressure is applied to the glans while countertraction is applied to the foreskin while attempting to bring down the prepuce. If successful, the constricting band will be brought down distal to the glans with the rest of the foreskin (Fig. 25.3).

If an initial reduction does not work, intermittent ice packs may be applied to the penis after it has been wrapped with gauze or other appropriate dressing until swelling and inflammation have decreased enough for manual reduction [7]. Furthermore, a compressive elastic dressing may be placed around the penis for 5–7 min to further reduce edema if initial measures are unsuccessful [8].

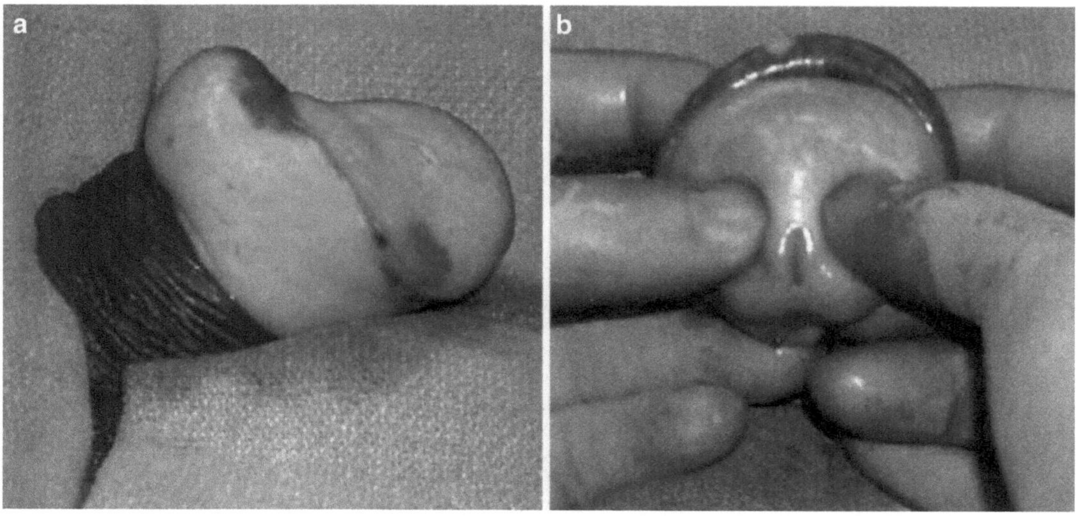


**Fig. 25.3** Manual reduction of a paraphimosis. Reprinted with permission from "Paraphimosis: Current Treatment Options," December 15, 2000, American Family Physician. Copyright © 2000 American Academy of Family Physicians. All Rights Reserved

## Medical Treatment

If an initial attempt at simple manual reduction is unsuccessful, the following medical treatments may be used as adjuncts to manual reduction, which serve to increase the probability of success. Some authors have advocated the use of fine granulated sugar to reduce glans and foreskin swelling [9]. Theoretically, the granulated sugar should induce an osmotic gradient across the skin and cause fluid to be extracted from the swollen tissues. The sugar is spread liberally over the surface of edematous tissues and left in place for 2 h and then manual reduction is reattempted.

Other authors have championed the use of hyaluronidase [10]. This is the enzyme responsible for the breakdown of hyaluronic acid. Theorists suggest that by breaking down the viscous hyaluronic acid, tissue resistance is decreased and diffusion is enhanced between tissue planes. In practical terms, 1 $cm^3$ of hyaluronidase (150 U/$cm^3$ Wydase; Wyeth-Ayerst Laboratories, Philadelphia, PA) is injected into the edematous tissue at one or more sites. Resolution of edema is almost immediate, at which point reduction can be reattempted.

## Minimally Invasive Techniques

If conservative therapy fails, prompt urologic consultation is warranted so that surgical treatment can be attempted. The urologist's artillery includes several minimally invasive techniques including foreskin puncture and glans aspiration.

The puncture technique may be used in which multiple punctures are made with a large gauge needle in the edematous foreskin to permit rapid and effective drainage of the trapped fluid [11].

Others have performed blood aspiration of the glans penis [12]. Simply, a tourniquet is applied proximal to the constricting foreskin and a 20-gauge needle is inserted into the glans parallel to the urethra and 3–12 mL of blood is aspirated (Fig. 25.4). The extraction of corporeal blood reduces swelling and reduction may be subsequently attempted.

Finally, another treatment for refractory paraphimosis is the application of four Babcock clamps directly to the constrictive ring, which is used to gently reduce the constrictive ring (Fig. 25.5). The proponents of this method suggest that it works 100 % of the time [13].

## Surgical Treatment

An emergency dorsal slit is the procedure of choice if all other forms of treatment fail to reduce the foreskin. The procedure should be performed by a physician with experience and under local anesthesia for adults and under general anesthesia or deep sedation in the pediatric population.

Briefly, the penis and foreskin are cleaned and draped. The constricting band is crushed dorsally

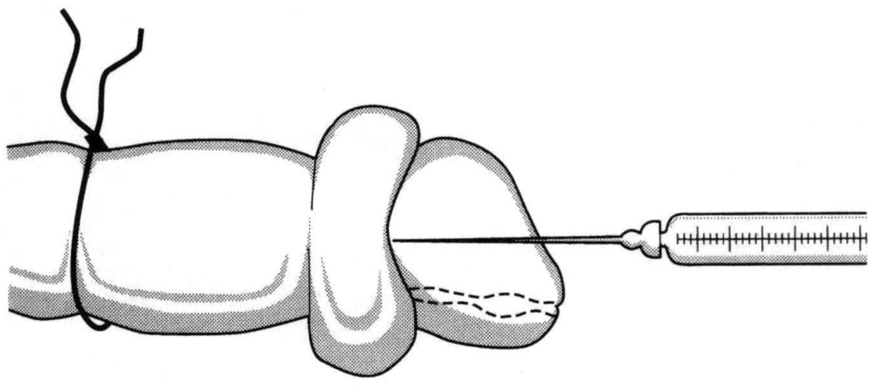

**Fig. 25.4** Position of tourniquet and needle to perform blood aspiration of the glans penis to reduce a paraphimosis. From Reduction of paraphimosis: A technique based on pathophysiology. V. Raveenthiran. British Journal of Surgery 1996, 83, 1247. Permission is granted by John Wiley & Sons Ltd on behalf of the BJSS Ltd

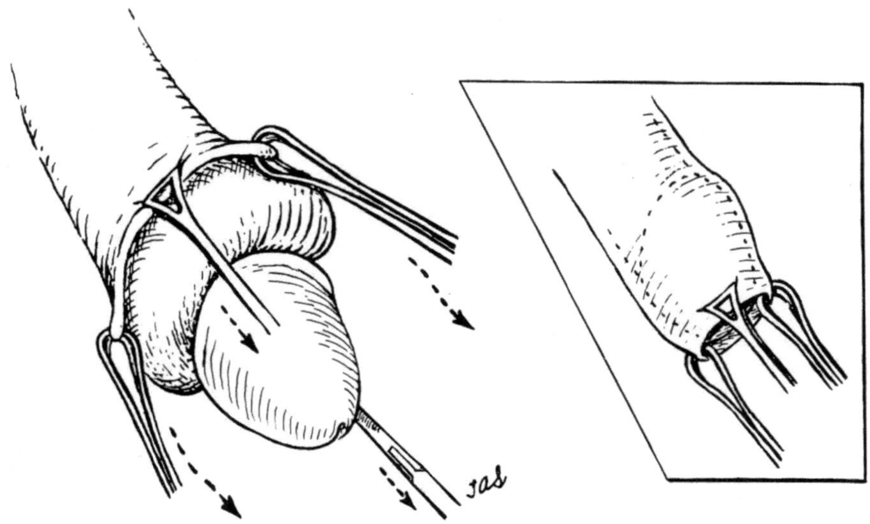

**Fig. 25.5** Placement of Babcock clamps to reduce a paraphimosis. From Reduction of paraphimosis. Roy W. Skoglund, JR and Warren H. Chapman. The Journal of Urology. Copyright © 1970 by The Williams & Wilkins Co

with application of a straight hemostat for 30 s. Next, a dorsal slit in the constricting band is made sharply with a scalpel where the hemostat was placed. The prepuce with constricting band is then reduced distally. The incision is re-approximated perpendicular to the incision with absorbable 4-0 suture.

Definitive treatment for paraphimosis, circumcision, should be performed at a later date for all cases of paraphimosis to prevent recurrence.

## Conclusion

Paraphimosis is a urologic emergency that the general physician may encounter. The primary care physician should know how to recognize and treat this condition which must be done promptly. Initial conservative therapy is usually successful and should be attempted by the general practitioner. However, if initial attempts are unsuccessful, more invasive therapies are needed and should be guided via urologic consultation. Ultimately, circumcision is recommended as definitive therapy at a later time to prevent recurrence.

## References


1. Olson C. Emergency treatment of paraphimosis. Can Fam Physician. 1998;44:1253–4, 1257.
2. Jones SA, Flynn RJ. An unusual (and somewhat piercing) cause of paraphimosis. Br J Urol. 1996;78:803–4.
3. Higgins SP. Painful swelling of the prepuce occurring during penile erection. Genitourin Med. 1996;72:426.
4. Hollowood AD, Sibley GN. Non-painful paraphimosis causing partial amputation. Br J Urol. 1997;80:958.
5. Ochsner MG. Acute urinary retention. Compr Ther. 1986;12:26–31.
6. Krauss DJ. Reduction of paraphimosis. Urology. 1985;25:337.
7. Nielson JB, Sorensen SS, Hojsgaard A. Paraphimosis treated with the ice glove method. Ugeskr Laeger. 1982;144:2228–9.
8. Ganti SU, Sayegh N, Addonizio JC. Simple method for reduction of paraphimosis. Urology. 1985;25:77.
9. Kerwat R, et al. Reduction of paraphimosis with granulated sugar. BJU Int. 1998;82:755.
10. Devries CR, et al. Reduction of paraphimosis with hyaluronidase. Urology. 1996;48:464–5.
11. Hamdy FC, Hastie KJ. Treatment for paraphimosis: the puncture technique. Br J Surg. 1990;77:1186.
12. Raveenthiran V. Reduction of paraphimosis: a technique based on pathophysiology. Br J Surg. 1996;83:1247.
13. Skoglund RW, Chapman WH. Reduction of paraphimosis. J Urol. 1970;104:137.

# Meatal Stenosis

# 26

Brent W. Snow

## Introduction

Narrowing of the urethral meatus at the tip of the glans penis is called meatal stenosis. Almost always this is acquired and seldom congenital except when associated with hypospadias. It is thought that meatal stenosis is a result of recurrent meatitis or meatal inflammation that occurs after circumcision, generally within the diaper (ammoniacal dermatitis) [1]. It is uncertain why this narrowing happens in a few boys and not all. The foreskin seems to protect the urethral meatus enough in uncircumcised boys that this seldom, if ever, occurs. It is suggested that the recurrent inflammation denudes the edges of the meatus and then they adhere ventrally progressing dorsally along the meatus leaving the meatus small or even pinpoint in appearance.

Other causes of meatal stenosis include stricture after prior hypospadias repair, narrowing after prolonged urethral catheter drainage, trauma to the glans penis, or balanitis xerotica obliterans. These can be differentiated from meatal stenosis generally by history. The balanitis xerotica obliterans usually produces a circumferential whitish coloration around the meatus that is inelastic, quite fibrotic and may be difficult to treat [2].

B.W. Snow, M.D. (✉)
Department of Surgery/Urology, Primary Children's Hospital, University of Utah School of Medicine, 100 North Capecchi Drive, Suite 2200, Salt Lake City, UT 84113, USA
e-mail: Brent.snow@hsc.utah.edu

## Diagnosis

Meatal stenosis is found in most patients because their parents notice their abnormal urinary stream or their physicians visually inspect their meatus. There may be symptoms of dysuria or blood spotting in the underwear due to the urinary stream splitting the fused tissues. Some patients have a significant amount of urinary leakage after urination because the urethra cannot drain properly and residual urine dribbles out slowly after cessation of the urinary stream.

Meatal stenosis does not generally lead to any significant urinary pathology, although older medical literature suggested that chronic obstruction of the meatus throughout childhood could cause bladder trabeculation and other problems. These findings are not attributed to meatal stenosis today. Urine tests or radiographic imaging is not required for meatal stenosis.

## Physical Exam

The physical exam of meatal stenosis is a visual inspection. The average newborn meatus is approximately 8 French and so the newborn meatus in most boys should easily accept the 5-French feeding tubes. As patients become older, between 1 and 6 years of age, the urethral meatus should accept an 8-French feeding tube. It is difficult to judge the meatus size on inspection because many times, the small meatus

R. Rabinowitz et al. (eds.), *Pediatric Urology for the Primary Care Physician*, Current Clinical Urology,
DOI 10.1007/978-1-60327-243-8_26, © Springer Science+Business Media New York 2015

stretches easily to accommodate a normal urinary stream and then returns to a smaller size after urination. The best way to make the diagnosis is to watch the patient urinate and see if the urinary stream is fine, forceful, and deflected dorsally. In practice, many boys with meatal stenosis have learned to aim their penis towards their feet so that the dorsally deflected urinary stream will go into the toilet. Some boys have not come to this realization and can make quite a mess in the bathroom.

Meatal stenosis is uncommonly diagnosed in patients who are not yet toilet trained because the urinary stream is seldom seen and cannot be evaluated in the office. Most of the time, the condition becomes evident during the toilet-training process; therefore, boys typically come to the attention of their primary care physicians in the preschool years.

## Treatment

Treatment of meatal stenosis may depend on the severity and the amount of obvious inflammation that is present. If the caliber of the urinary stream is only modestly reduced and the meatus has some obvious erythema with inflammation, then anti-inflammatory steroidal ointments are recommended, generally being applied twice a day for 4–6 weeks.

The most common treatment of meatal stenosis is a meatotomy. This is a simple procedure where a hemostat is placed in the narrow meatal opening and the meatal web on the ventral aspect of the glans penis is crushed with the hemostat one-half to two-thirds the distance to the coronal margin. After waiting 1–2 min, the hemostat can be removed and the crushed web can be incised with fine scissors down the middle of the crushed web, leaving the crimped edges on either side for appropriate hemostasis.

## Anesthesia Choices

Meatotomy requires some type of anesthesia. In the past, local anesthesia such as lidocaine with epinephrine was injected directly into the meatal web with a fine needle providing sufficient anesthesia for the procedure. However boys need to be restrained for this injection because of its distinctly uncomfortable nature.

Some patients are best treated with general anesthesia because of the age of the patient; they may not understand the explanation of the procedure that is being performed. If there is a psychological concern for the patient, it is best to have them asleep under anesthesia, rather than to have them be anxious and worried about a procedure on their genitalia in the doctor's office. On occasion parental anxiety is an indication for general anesthesia.

Most recently, topical anesthetic creams have been the mainstay of meatotomy procedures [3]. A generous amount of the topical anesthetic cream is placed on the entire glans penis and covered with a bio-occlusive dressing. Depending upon the topical anesthetic, 30 to >60 min is waited and then the bio-occlusive dressing and the topical anesthetic cream are removed. The glans penis itself generally has an edematous appearance to it after the cream has been in place for that length of time. The patient is prepped and draped sterilely and generally the parents can be in the procedure room to comfort the patient. In our office setting, we generally have the parents hold a large picture book over the child's chest to divert their attention and keep the procedure out of sight. The ventral web is then crushed with a hemostat and after waiting a few minutes, the incision is made. Once this has been completed, topical antibiotic ointment is placed on the edges of the meatus while showing the parents how to do this. Patient tolerance is really quite good. Occasionally they can feel some pressure when the meatal web is clamped, but usually that is all the discomfort that may occur. For a particularly anxious patient, midazolam has been used in a supplemental fashion to the anesthetic cream with good results. Less than 10 % of our patients have required this supplementation.

## Prevention of Recurrence

Prevention of restenosis is the primary focus after the meatotomy and the parents are encouraged to apply antibiotic ointment to the meatus several times a day for the next several weeks. Patients generally have some dysuria with urination for a day or two and are encouraged to take acetaminophen or ibuprofen for the 2 days after the procedure. There may be a small amount of blood in the underwear, but this resolves promptly. Patients are encouraged to drink lots of fluids after the procedure since this dilutes the urine and makes its passage more comfortable.

In our own office experience, we reported 226 patients with successful office meatotomies using local anesthetic cream with two recurrences and 23 of these patients having supplemental midazolam [4]. This has been a very successful procedure in our hands and we recommend it to others.

## Referral

The question of when to refer meatal stenosis comes up regularly. Once it has been documented that the stream is narrow and dorsally deflected, meatal stenosis does not resolve on its own. A meatotomy should be recommended unless there is ongoing active inflammation at the meatus, in which case steroid ointments may be helpful. The meatotomy procedure can be performed in a primary care physicians' office. It is helpful to remember that most insurance companies require pre-authorization for this "surgical procedure" so it generally cannot be done the same day as the diagnosis without causing an undue financial burden upon the parents. Referral of patients with meatal stenosis is generally initiated when the primary care physician chooses not to perform the meatotomy in their own office.

## References

1. Brown MR, Cartwright PC, Snow BW. Common problems in pediatric urology and gynecology. Pediatr Clin North Am. 1997;44(5):1091–115.
2. Snow BW, Cartwright PC. Office pediatric urology. In: Docimo SG, Canning D, Khoury A, editors. Clinical pediatric urology. 5th ed. Philadelphia: Informa Healthcare; 2007.
3. Steward DJ. Eutectic mixture of local anesthetics (EMLA): what is it? What does it do? J Pediatr. 1993;122(5 Pt 2):S21–3. Review.
4. Cartwright PC, Snow BW, McNees DC. Urethral meatotomy in the office using topical EMLA cream for anesthesia. J Urol. 1996;156(2 Pt 2):857–8; discussion 858–9.

# Balanitis

# 27

Bartley G. Cilento Jr.

## Introduction

Balanitis is nomenclature for inflammation of the glans penis. Posthitis refers to inflammation of the foreskin alone. Balanoposthitis refers to inflammation of both the glans penis and foreskin.

## Relevance

Balanoposthitis is relatively common occurring in approximately 4 % of uncircumcised boys. In the United States the regional rate of neonatal circumcision varies considerably with the highest in the Northeast/Midwest and the lowest in the Southwest. The national circumcision average is approximately 65 %. In 2007 birth rate was 4,317,119. Assuming 50 % are boys in whom 35 % of boys are uncircumcised (755,495) and 4 % incidence of balanoposthitis, this would result in approximately 30,219 cases per year. In most instances this condition occurs due to bacterial overgrowth. Bacterial overgrowth is facilitated by accumulated smegma or retain urine due to the presence of physiologic or pathologic phimosis. Recurrent episodes occur but are uncommon. Once the foreskin becomes retractable and routine hygiene is instituted the occurrence of balanoposthitis is unusual. Other less common causes of balanoposthitis include contact dermatitis, mechanical irritation, or trauma. Removal or avoidance of the causative irritant is curative.

B.G. Cilento Jr., M.D., M.P.H., F.A.A.P., F.A.C.S. (✉)
Department of Urology, Boston Children's Hospital, Longwood Avenue, Hunnewell, 3rd Floor, Boston, MA 02115, USA
e-mail: bartley.cilento@childrens.harvard.edu

## History

Balanoposthitis is characterized by redness of the foreskin and glans penis. There is often associated swelling due to the inflammatory process which can be dramatic. In severe cases, there can be a purulent discharge or urinary retention mostly due to volitional holding caused by severe dysuria. In rare instances, penile shaft cellulitis can occur and is an indication for oral or intravenous antibiotics. Ulceration, bleeding, and discoloration of the foreskin and glans can occur but are mild and uncommon.

## Physical Exam

The appearance of the foreskin varies depending on the degree of infection. In mild infections, the foreskin will appear swollen and there may be some mucopurulent discharge from the opening of the foreskin. In more severe cases, the foreskin will be swollen and erythematous with significant purulent discharge. Retraction of the

R. Rabinowitz et al. (eds.), *Pediatric Urology for the Primary Care Physician*, Current Clinical Urology,
DOI 10.1007/978-1-60327-243-8_27, © Springer Science+Business Media New York 2015

foreskin may not be possible due to the swelling or discomfort. In the most severe cases, there may be cellulolytic changes of the shaft of the penis. This would be an indication for admission and intravenous antibiotics.

## Evaluation

In nearly all cases, history and physical examination are all that is necessary in the evaluation of children with balanoposthitis. Other clinical circumstances or factors will dictate whether imaging is advisable or necessary.

## Imaging Studies

Urinary retention is usually volitional secondary to the dysuria caused by the inflammation. In cases of urinary retention, a renal/bladder ultrasound may be done to assess the degree of bladder distention or hydroureteronephrosis. Transient bladder decompression with a Foley catheter may be necessary but rarely is needed.

## Timing of Referral

Acute cases of balanoposthitis are rarely an acute surgical problem; therefore, surgical consultation can be accomplished after the acute infection has been treated. Patients with recurrent episodes of balanoposthitis or severe cases should be referred to a pediatric urologist for consideration of a circumcision. Single episodes of mild or moderate balanoposthitis do not need urologic consultation unless the patient or parents desire a circumcision.

## Management

Mild cases of balanoposthitis can be treated with conservative measures such as 2–3 warm baths with soapy water daily. Epsom salts can also be used. These warm bathes provide symptom relief of the discomfort and may facilitate voiding in those patients with dysuria and volitional holding. Patients should also be given oral analgesics to help relieve the discomfort associated with the soft tissue inflammation. Antibiotics (oral or intravenous) are reserved for: (1) severe cases, (2) presence of penile cellulitis, or (3) episodes unresponsive to conservative treatment.

Once the acute infection has been treated, patients with physiologic or pathologic phimosis may be treated with a topical steroid cream such as betamethasone valerate 0.1 % ointment to help relieve the phimosis. I suggest that the ointment is applied twice a day for 6 weeks. However the type of steroid varies as does the application duration (range 4–8 weeks). The results vary amongst the published series but range from 43 to 86 % [1–3]. The durability of the results is variable [1–3].

## References


1. Ghysel C, Vander Eeckt K, Bogaert GA. Long-term efficiency of skin stretching and a topical corticoid cream application for unretractable foreskin and phimosis in prepubertal boys. Urol Int. 2009;82(1):81–8.
2. Letendre J, Barrieras D, Franc-Guimond J, Adbo A, Houle AM. Topical triamcinolone for persistent phimosis. J Urol. 2009;182(4 Suppl):1759–63.
3. Esposito C, Centonze A, Alicchio F, Savanelli A, Settimi A. Topic steroid application versus circumcision in pediatric patients with phimosis: a prospective randomized placebo controlled clinical trial. World J Urol. 2008;26(2):187–90.

# 28 Urethrorrhagia

Patrick C. Cartwright

## Introduction

The term urethrorrhagia is used to describe bleeding from the urethra. It is largely a pediatric problem and commonly presents with blood spotting in the underwear between episodes of voiding or terminal hematuria. By definition, urethrorrhagia is "gross hematuria," but the distinctive finding of passing blood from the urethral meatus without voiding indicates that the source of bleeding is within the urethra at some point distal to the bladder neck. Any gross bleeding from a source above this will result in total hematuria, with the entire voided specimen being discolored (red or brown). Urethrorrhagia may also present during voiding with initial bloody appearance of the urine, but clear urine during the midstream. (Only 60 % of patients with observed urethrorrhagia will dipstick positive for blood on standard midstream urinalysis.) The other important complaint that will be associated in some cases is that of dysuria. Once the distinctive presentation is recognized, the differential diagnosis and resultant evaluation of urethrorrhagia prove to be quite different from the standard evaluation of gross hematuria in a child. It is important for both pediatricians and urologists to recognize this difference and, thereby, avoid imaging and lab evaluation that are unlikely to be helpful.

Urethrorrhagia may occur in both boys and girls, but is very predominantly a male problem. In girls, the recognized etiologies would include: urethral or bladder neck tumor (rhabdomyosarcoma), urethral stone, foreign body (sometimes vaginal), external or catheter trauma, sexual abuse, urethritis, prolapsing ureterocele, or urethral prolapse. Examination of the perineum is clearly important and any confirmation of urethral bleeding or abnormal exam finding in a female child warrants further evaluation. For boys, the list of potential causes includes: urethral tumor (rhabdomyosarcoma), benign urethral polyp, external trauma, self-instrumentation, catheterization, urethral foreign body or stone, urethral stricture, urethritis (including bacterial, viral, sexually transmitted disease (STD), chemical, nonspecific), meatitis, meatal stenosis, voiding dysfunction, and an idiopathic category. The idiopathic category is very important in boys as by far most patients will fall into this designation. Idiopathic urethrorrhagia will be discussed later in this chapter. There are more unusual causes (rectourethral fistula, persistent utricle) that should be considered in boys with other anatomic abnormalities, such as proximal hypospadias and imperforate anus. For any boy with urethrorrhagia and a history of a congenital malformation affecting pelvic structures or the genitalia, pediatric urologic consultation should be sought.

P.C. Cartwright, M.D. (✉)
Division of Urology, Department of Surgery, Primary Children's Medical Center, University of Utah School of Medicine, University of Utah, 100 North Mario Capecchi, Suite 2200, Salt Lake City, UT 84113, USA
e-mail: Patrick.cartwright@hsc.utah.edu

R. Rabinowitz et al. (eds.), *Pediatric Urology for the Primary Care Physician*, Current Clinical Urology, DOI 10.1007/978-1-60327-243-8_28, © Springer Science+Business Media New York 2015

Important aspects of the history with urethrorrhagia include: onset, duration, worsening over time, similar episodes in the past, hesitancy or straining to void (worrisome finding), dysuria, recent trauma/instrumentation, history of stones, location of any pain, and strength and direction of urinary stream. On exam, it is important to examine the meatus and penis directly and to palpate the entire course of the urethra. Suprapubic exam is essential to assess for mass or distended bladder and rectal exam to assess the prostatic urethra and bladder neck area may be required in specific patients. It can also be very helpful to watch the child void and to catch urine for analysis. Urinary infection and hypercalciuria should be ruled out with culture and spot urinary calcium/creatinine ratio. The associated symptoms, findings, or observations may point to one potential diagnosis over the others.

## Causes of Urethrorrhagia

The following categories include the more unusual diagnoses causing urethrorrhagia and particular findings associated with each of them.

### Meatal Inflammation

The edges of the meatus may adhere side to side. Some boys will have recurring problems with this for unknown. Direct inspection of the meatus will reveal lightly adherent edges and redness. With voiding, there is often initial dysuria and splaying of the stream, but as the meatal edges pop apart, the stream normalizes. These irritated meatal edges may intermittently bleed. Treatment is with topical steroid (hydrocortisone 1 % or betamethasone 0.05 % BID) for 4 weeks. If persistent after two courses of treatment, then observation over time may be most appropriate.

### Meatal Stenosis

Boys in diapers may develop narrowing of the meatus from chronic irritation. This causes the ventral portion of the meatus to fuse and thus leaves a pinpoint opening. When they toilet train later, these boys often have dorsal deflection of the stream and will have to aim at their feet in order to hit the bowl. Some boys will have associated dysuria and blood spotting of the underwear. Direct inspection of the meatus and observation during voiding will make this diagnosis; it is important to try and gently separate the meatus with lateral traction on each side to accurately diagnose stenosis. Urethral meatotomy is warranted and can be performed under either local anesthesia in the office or under light general anesthetic, depending on the age and personality of the child.

### Foreign Body or Stone

Exam along the course of the urethra will yield a mass or tenderness. Dysuria and WBC/RBC in urine are found. Urethroscopy is likely to be needed for extraction.

### Bacterial Urethritis

Urethral discharge or bleeding in a sexually active pubertal male suggests this diagnosis. White blood cells are found on the urinalysis. Treatment involves swab culture and selecting appropriate antibiotic.

### Tumor (Rhabdomyosarcoma of Bladder Neck or Prostate)

These rarely cause spotting in the underwear as the major finding but rather present with progressive obstructive voiding with occasional bleeding. A red flag in the child with urethrorrhagia is

**straining with urination**; this finding warrants prompt evaluation for obstruction. These patients may also have other systemic symptoms such as fatigue and weight loss.

## Benign Urethral Polyp

These are congenital, may intermittently bleed or obstruct, and more commonly present early in childhood. Polyps are usually located in the prostatic urethra and pain or dysuria is not common. Treatment is cystoscopic resection.

## Trauma/Stricture

Acute trauma (straddle injury, traumatic catheterization) can cause urethral bleeding for several weeks. Urethral bleeding at the time of trauma warrants a retrograde urethrogram. Traumatic injury may lead to stricture formation which may slow the stream and cause straining to void if the lumen narrows substantially. Milder strictures may only cause persistent bleeding and/or dysuria. Evaluation when there is concern for stricture is generally with a retrograde urethrogram.

## Idiopathic Urethrorrhagia

Much more commonly in boys, the etiology for urethrorrhagia is obscure and has often been viewed as idiopathic. If the diagnoses above have been considered and none seem likely, then idiopathic urethrorrhagia remains as the diagnosis. This may account for as many as 90 % of cases in boys. The mean age of onset for these cases is reported to be 7–9 years of age. The mean duration of symptoms is long—reported as 6–10 months; however, there is considerable variability running from weeks to years. One study reported complete resolution rates of 46 % at 6 months and 71 % at 1 year [1]. The vast majority of patients proved to have no long-term sequelae and the process appeared self-limited.

## Evaluation

Additional studies have shown that early evaluation when there are not specific concerning features (noted previously) is of little value. Utilizing routine cystoscopy at the time of presentation has very minimal yield other than finding variable degrees of urethral (usually bulbar) wall inflammation in 50 % of cases. Biopsies of these areas routinely show mild chronic inflammation with some rudimentary analysis in the past revealing viral inclusions within epithelial cells, suggesting a viral etiology (felt to be adenovirus) [2]. On occasion, there will be a shaggy, whitish patch in the bulbar urethra representing squamous metaplasia at the site of more persistent inflammation (cause unknown) [3]. Overall, cystoscopy and imaging are not recommended in evaluating idiopathic urethrorrhagia unless there are associated worrisome features (as above). The patient with particularly severe or persistent dysuria associated with urethrorrhagia may cause sufficient concern to warrant retrograde urethrography or cystoscopy. Many patients in this subgroup will have a finding of circumferential urethral inflammation within the bulbar urethra. Again, the etiology of this is unclear, but in follow-up it does appear that this subgroup of patients is prone to stricture. No specific effective therapy for these boys has been reported [4].

## Management

One recent study suggests that patients with dysfunctional elimination problems (bowel and bladder) may be predisposed to urethral bleeding due to high and turbulent flow through the urethra secondary to uncoordinated voiding attempts [5]. The conceptual concern is that this would cause recurring mild trauma to the lining of the urethra and resultant oozing of blood. This group reported a high incidence of voiding dysfunction in their patients with urethrorrhagia; others have not confirmed this. They also reported a quicker resolution of symptoms for those patients treated with anticholinergics, timed voiding, behavior modification, and laxatives. It would seem reasonable to treat boys in this manner if there are distinct symptoms of poor voiding habits such as: delaying, urgency, penile clutching, daytime wetting, and suprapubic discomfort.

The best course of management for most boys with "idiopathic urethrorrhagia" is continued observation and reassurance of the child and family. It is reasonable for a primary care provider to manage these patients without referral if there are no concerning features associated. Unless all concerns have resolved, reassessment and examination in 6 months is appropriate. Oral steroids and anti-inflammatory medications seem to have little impact on the course of the problem. Further imaging evaluation or cystoscopy is reserved for the patient with symptoms that persist past 12 months or who has progressive symptoms or dysuria that is significant enough to interfere with daily activities. This evaluation would generally involve ultrasound with the bladder full and empty and, in most cases, retrograde urethrogram. If there are concerns that show up on these studies or they are inconclusive, cystoscopic inspection will be required. If an obvious area of prominent, chronically inflamed mucosa is recognized cystoscopically (especially if there is squamous metaplasia), then submucosal injection of steroid can be considered but efficacy is unproven. As well, patients who have persistent urethrorrhagia (>12 months) may be at risk for urethral stricture formation from persistent inflammation. Cystoscopic inspection will reveal any stricture and allow incision.

## Conclusion

It is prudent to be aware of the generally benign course that idiopathic urethrorrhagia takes. That awareness will allow primary care providers and urologists alike to avoid the costly and time-consuming work-up for "gross hematuria" that is directed at finding mass lesions or nephritis, and focus on the real list of possibilities. Unusual symptoms that suggest a specific cause (vs. idiopathic) for urethrorrhagia should lead the primary care provider to consider early referral for urological consultation. Symptoms of obstructed voiding associated with urethrorrhagia should represent a red flag and do warrant early radiographic or cystoscopic assessment as intervention is more often required in this subgroup.

## References

1. Walker BR, Ellison ED, Snow BW, Cartwright PC. The natural history of idiopathic urethrorrhagia in boys. J Urol. 2001;166(1):231–2.
2. Kaplan GW, Brock WA. Idiopathic urethrorrhagia in boys. J Urol. 1982;128(5):1001–3.
3. Docimo SG, Silver RI, Gonzalez R, Müller SC, Jeffs RD. Idiopathic anterior urethritis in prepubertal and pubertal boys: pathology and clues to etiology. Urology. 1999;51(1):99–102.
4. Poch MA, Handel LN, Caesar RE, Decter RM, Caldamone AA. The association of urethrorrhagia and urethral stricture disease. J Pediatr Urol. 2007; 3:218–22.
5. Herz D, Weiser A, Collette T, Reda E, Levitt S, Franco I. Dysfunctional elimination syndrome as an etiology of idiopathic urethritis in childhood. J Urol. 2005; 173(6):2132–7.

# Urethral Stricture

# 29

Stacy T. Tanaka and John W. Brock III

## Introduction

Urethral strictures result from scarring in and around the urethra. Strictures can decrease the caliber of the urethral lumen and eventually obstruct urinary outflow. Other anomalies of the urethra which can cause obstruction that are not considered strictures include posterior urethral valves, anterior urethral valves, and meatal stenosis.

## Classification by Location

Urethral strictures occur primarily in boys compared to girls because of the longer length of the male urethra. Strictures can occur anywhere along the length of the urethra. The male urethra is divided into the posterior and anterior urethra, and strictures are often classified as posterior or anterior urethral strictures. The posterior urethra includes the sections of urethra that traverse the prostate and the urogenital diaphragm. The anterior urethra includes the bulbar urethra which is distal to the urinary sphincter and the penile urethra which runs along the ventral surface of the penile shaft to the tip of the penis.

## Classification by Etiology

Urethral strictures in children result from three main etiologies: traumatic, inflammatory/infectious, and congenital. Because symptoms can occur weeks to years after the inciting event, true etiology can be difficult to determine.

### Traumatic

Most pediatric urethral strictures result from iatrogenic trauma. Urethral strictures are a recognized complication of surgical reconstruction of congenital anomalies of the penis and urethra. Boys who have undergone previous hypospadias repair represent the largest group of pediatric patients with iatrogenic strictures. Other procedures that can cause urethral stricture are traumatic urethral catheterization and cystourethroscopy.

External trauma to the pelvis or perineum can also cause urethral injury. As these injuries heal, strictures can develop. An unstable pelvic fracture can disrupt the posterior urethra. A straddle injury such as falling on a crossbar of a bicycle can damage the anterior urethra by compressing it against the pubic bone.

S.T. Tanaka, M.D. (✉)
Division of Pediatric Urology, Monroe Carell Jr. Vanderbilt Children's Hospital, 4102 Doctor's Office Tower, 2200 Children's Way, Nashville, TN 37232-9820, USA
e-mail: stacy.tanaka@vanderbilt.edu

J.W. Brock III, M.D., F.A.A.P., F.A.C.S.
Division of Pediatric Urologic Surgery at Monroe Carell Children's Hospital at Vanderbilt, Nashville, TN, USA

R. Rabinowitz et al. (eds.), *Pediatric Urology for the Primary Care Physician*, Current Clinical Urology, DOI 10.1007/978-1-60327-243-8_29, © Springer Science+Business Media New York 2015

## Inflammatory/Infectious

Inflammatory or infectious urethritis is a less common cause of urethral stricture in children. Nontraumatic urethral catheterization can cause urethral inflammation and subsequent stricture formation. Accordingly, in cases where indwelling catheterization is required, duration of catheterization should be minimized. Sexually transmitted diseases can also cause inflammation and subsequent stricture. Before appropriate antibiotic treatment, gonococcal urethritis was a common cause of urethral stricture in older men. Although an unlikely etiology for pediatric urethral stricture, gonococcal urethral stricture may be considered in sexually active patients.

## Congenital

A minority of patients are found to have urethral strictures in the absence of prior urethral instrumentation, trauma, or inflammation. Without an identifiable etiology, these patients are assumed to have a congenital stricture.

# Importance in Primary Care

Although pediatric urethral stricture is uncommon, it is important for the primary care physician to differentiate a potential urethral stricture from more benign urinary complaints. Early referral to a pediatric urologist will avoid the potential complications of an untreated urethral stricture. Progressive scarring can obliterate the urethral lumen necessitating urgent placement of a suprapubic catheter to drain urine from the bladder. Additionally, even in the absence of frank urinary retention, partial urethral obstruction can possibly cause hydronephrosis and progressive renal damage.

The primary care physician can also decrease urethral stricture disease by preventing injury to the urethra. Providing anticipatory guidance for bicycle and motor vehicle safety protects the urethra from external trauma. Minimizing indwelling urethral catheterization decreases the risk of iatrogenic trauma. When catheterization is necessary, the smallest possible, well-lubricated catheter should be used. Urologic consultation should be obtained for any difficult catheterization.

# History

Boys with urethral strictures can present with a wide variety of nonspecific urinary symptoms that can occur weeks to years after the inciting event. Most patients describe symptoms associated with the inability to empty their bladders efficiently: weak or dribbling urinary stream, hesitancy, and straining to urinate. Urinary tract infection may also initiate an imaging workup that demonstrates a urethral stricture. Boys can also present with hematuria, dysuria, urinary frequency, and day and/or night wetting. Wetting after a previous dry period is more suspicious for an anatomic abnormality.

Because most urethral strictures have a traumatic etiology, reviewing risk factors in the past medical history is paramount. These risk factors include:

- History of previous urethral stricture
- History of pelvic fracture or straddle injury
- Prior traumatic urethral catheterization
- Prior urethral surgery including endoscopy, hypospadias repair, or genital reconstruction

# Physical Exam

The physical exam is usually normal in boys with urethral stricture. An abdominal exam may demonstrate a palpably distended bladder or an abdominal mass consistent with hydronephrosis. Observation of the voided urinary stream often shows a slowed or weakened stream.

# How to Evaluate

The following diagnostic studies may be used during the workup for a potential urethral stricture. Diagnosis is confirmed with urethrography and endoscopic examination of the urethra.

## Urinalysis

Urinalysis can evaluate hematuria and/or pyuria that may be associated with a urethral stricture.

## Urine Culture

Urine culture can confirm urinary tract infection that may be associated with a urethral stricture.

## Renal and Bladder Ultrasound

Renal and bladder ultrasound is often obtained in patients with urethral strictures because of urinary tract infection or hematuria on presentation. Although renal and bladder ultrasound cannot directly demonstrate a urethral stricture, it may show changes in the bladder and kidneys suggestive of outflow obstruction. Urethral obstruction can cause bladder wall thickening. A large post-void residual, the amount of urine that remains in the bladder after voiding, may be present. If the urethral obstruction is severe, unilateral or bilateral hydronephrosis may be present.

## Voiding Cystourethrogram and Retrograde Urethrogram

Voiding cystourethrogram (VCUG) and retrograde urethrogram (RUG) are radiologic studies which can be used to image the urethra. These studies can confirm the presence of a urethral stricture. In addition, the information provided about the length and location of the stricture can be critical for preoperative planning.

During the VCUG, a small urethral catheter is placed, and the bladder is filled with contrast dye. The child is then asked to void. Fluoroscopic images during voiding can demonstrate or rule out abnormal urethral anatomy. Occasionally, VCUG does not sufficiently demonstrate the distal extent of the stricture. To aid with preoperative planning, an RUG is sometimes necessary. During an RUG, a small catheter is placed at the urethral opening. Contrast is instilled through the catheter into the urethra, and the urethra is imaged by fluoroscopy.

## Uroflowmetry

Uroflowmetry is a noninvasive test performed in the urologist's office that measures urine flow rate as a function of time. Most individuals with a urethral stricture will have a decreased flow rate. Uroflowmetry is useful in older children who can cooperate with the study. After waiting to have a full bladder, the patient is asked to urinate in a specialized toilet which measures the speed of urine flow.

## Cystourethroscopy

Cystourethroscopy allows direct visualization of the urethral stricture by telescopic examination of the entire urethra and bladder. Children require general anesthesia for this procedure. The stricture can often be treated during the same anesthetic session.

## When to Refer

Because the treatment of urethral stricture is surgical, patients with potential urethral strictures should be referred to a pediatric urologist. The presence of the following signs and symptoms should increase a clinician's suspicion for a urethral stricture or other anatomic abnormality:

- Weak or slowed urinary stream
- Abnormal urinary symptoms with history of genital reconstructive surgery such as hypospadias repair, previous urethral stricture, pelvic fracture, straddle injury, or traumatic urethral catheterization
- Abnormal VCUG or renal/bladder ultrasound findings

The majority of potential urethral stricture patients can be referred to a pediatric urologist on a nonurgent basis. Urgent referral is required if the urethral stricture has precipitated acute urinary retention.

## Management

Urethral strictures are a surgical disease. Surgical treatment of the urethral stricture can involve dilatation of the stricture, endoscopic incision of stricture with laser or knife, or open excision of stricture with urethral reconstruction. The choice of treatment depends on length, location, and etiology of the stricture. Because urethral strictures can recur, continued attention to the urinary symptoms of these boys is warranted.

## Suggested Reading

Noe HN. Complications and management of childhood urethral stricture disease. Urol Clin North Am. 1983;10:531–5366.

Scherz HC, Kaplan GW. Etiology, diagnosis, and management of urethral strictures in children. Urol Clin North Am. 1990;17:389–94.

# HyposPadias

# 30

Warren Snodgrass

## Introduction

Hypospadias defines a congenital anomaly of the penis in which the urethral meatus opens proximal to the normal location. Most commonly, the meatus is located on the proximal glans or in the region of the coronal margin, but it can be found on the penile shaft, within the scrotum, or on the perineum. Typically, boys also have an incomplete dorsal foreskin and may exhibit ventral bending of the penis. Within the spectrum of related anomalies are boys with the urethral meatus properly located on the glans who have an incomplete foreskin and may also have ventral curvature, so-called *chordee without hypospadias*.

## Etiology and Epidemiology

Hypospadias is considered an arrest in normal penile development occurring between the 9th and 20th weeks of gestation. Since elongation of the genital tubercle and fusion of the urethral folds are hormone-dependent events, disruption of normal masculinization is considered an underlying cause of hypospadias, although postnatal testing only rarely reveals detectable defects in testosterone production, 5 alpha-reductase II activity, or the androgen receptor [1].

Hypospadias is the 2nd most common anomaly in boys, found in approximately 1:150. The incidence increases in association with low birth weight, twins, and maternal age over 35 years. The likelihood that a boy will have hypospadias increases to approximately 10 % if his father or sibling is affected.

Although hypospadias can occur in association with syndromes, in most cases, it is an isolated anomaly.

## Presentation

Hypospadias usually is visibly apparent during the newborn examination (Fig. 30.1) and sometimes is suspected on prenatal ultrasonography. The most obvious finding is the incomplete foreskin. Some practitioners refer to the appearance as a "natural circumcision" since the glans is visible, but the term is misleading and should not be used. When a dorsal foreskin is detected, examination next determines location of the meatus. The diagnosis is "chordee without hypospadias" when the meatus is in a normal position and hypospadias when it is found proximally. The glans also is incompletely fused in the ventral midline when the meatus is proximal.

A subset of hypospadias termed the megameatus intact prepuce variant occurs with a normally

W. Snodgrass, M.D. (✉)
Department of Urology, Pediatric Urology Section, Children's Medical Center and The University of Texas Southwestern Medical Center, 2350 Stemmons Freeway Suite F4300, Dallas, TX 75207, USA
e-mail: warren.snodgrass@childrens.com

R. Rabinowitz et al. (eds.), *Pediatric Urology for the Primary Care Physician*, Current Clinical Urology,
DOI 10.1007/978-1-60327-243-8_30, 

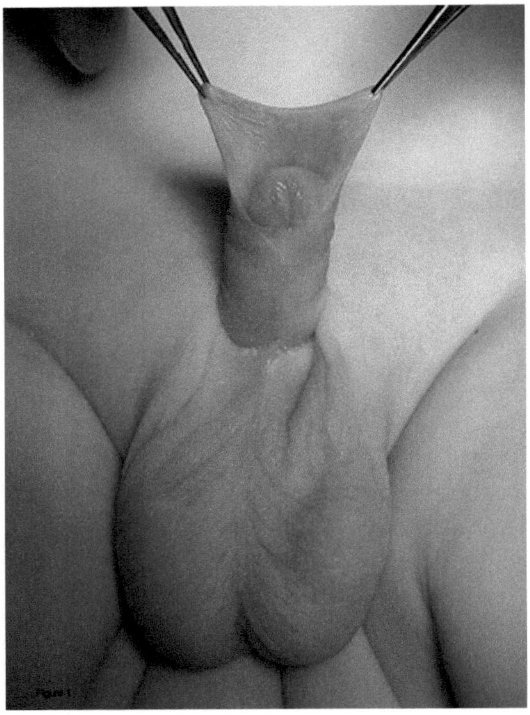

**Fig. 30.1** Hypospadias is visible during newborn examination

formed foreskin (Fig. 30.2) and so may not be detected until newborn circumcision is performed or the foreskin becomes retractable later in life.

Physical examination should also note position of the testes, and the finding of both a penile anomaly and undescended testis indicates a possible disorder of sexual differentiation. Other findings may include a deep cleft in the midline of the scrotum and/or transposition of the scrotum alongside and even above the penile shaft in proximal hypospadias.

Some practitioners confuse a penoscrotal to perineal hypospadias with intersex disorders, but the diagnosis of disordered sexual differentiation is limited to cases with associated gonadal anomalies.

## Evaluation

The diagnosis is established by physical examination. Radiologic testing of the urinary tract is not necessary, even with proximal hypospadias,

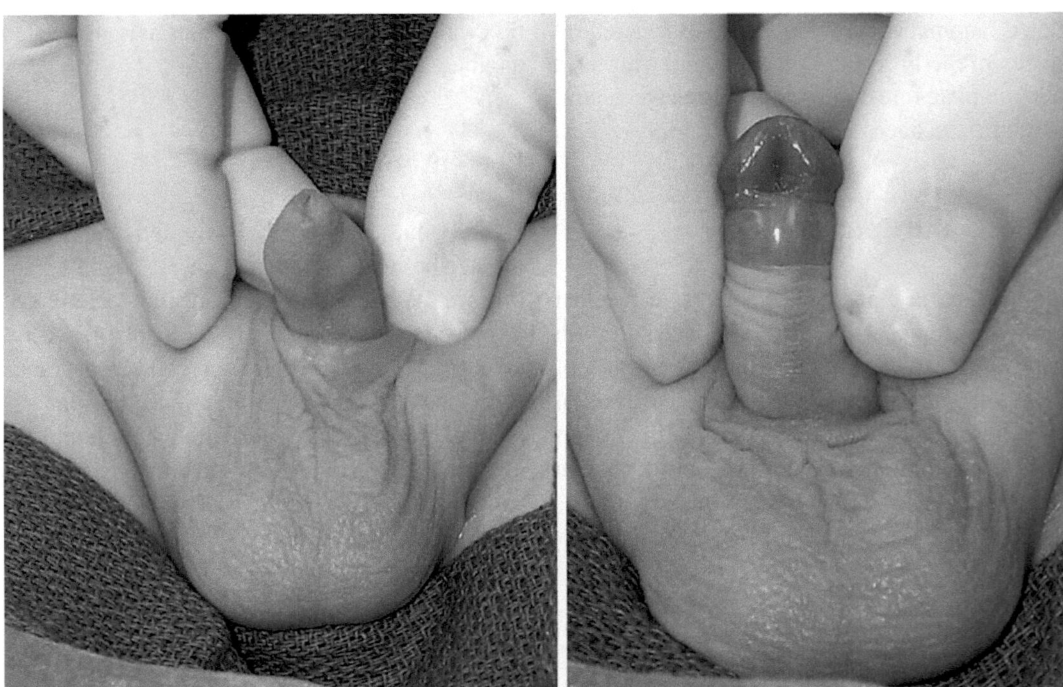

**Fig. 30.2** Megameatus intact prepuce (MIP) hypospadias variant

since renal development occurs at 4 weeks whereas penile formation happens later beginning at 9 weeks.

A karyotype should be obtained in newborns with both an undescended testis and hypospadias. Incidence varies from approximately 15 % if the testis is palpable to nearly 50 % for proximal hypospadias with a nonpalpable testis [2]. Possible findings include mixed gonadal dysgenesis and true hermaphroditism, while bilateral nonpalpable testes should raise suspicion of female pseudohermaphroditism due to adrenal hyperplasia regardless of the extent of penile development. Otherwise, neither chromosome analysis nor endocrine studies are needed in infants with isolated hypospadias.

## Reasons for Correction

Most often, hypospadias presents with a meatus on the proximal glans or at the corona. These patients will not have impaired fertility from the abnormal opening, but are likely to have difficulty aiming their urinary stream if left uncorrected. Normal voiding depends upon fusion of the glans over the urethra to direct the stream forward and focus it without lateral spaying. In addition, often a transverse web of skin is found just distal to the abnormal meatus that can defect the stream downward.

The dorsal foreskin also calls attention to the anomaly, not only in the newborn nursery but also in the locker room as boys mature. Hypospadias repair includes either circumcision or reconstruction of the foreskin to resemble a natural penis.

Ventral curvature is found in approximately 15 % of boys with distal forms of hypospadias and in over 50 % of those with the meatus on the proximal penile shaft or in the scrotum or perineum. Bending in distal cases most often is not so severe to cause difficulties with intercourse but in proximal hypospadias may preclude penetration.

Proximal cases additionally may have deep midline clefts in the scrotum and/or transposition of the scrotum higher than usual alongside the penile shaft. These findings combine with downward curvature of the penis to create a feminized appearance to the external genitalia.

Given these concerns and modern outcomes of surgical correction, repair is recommended for all but the most distal cases. A meatus that is located on the proximal glans but has 2 mm or more glans fusion ventrally does not present either a cosmetic or functional defect. If detected following circumcision, no additional repair is needed, but surgery to perform circumcision or foreskin reconstruction would still be advised for a dorsal prepuce.

## Timing of Surgery

A 1996 position paper from the American Academy of Pediatrics suggested the optimal time for elective genital surgery including hypospadias repair is between 6 and 18 months, to avoid intervention after the time genital awareness begins. Anesthetic considerations delay elective day surgery until after 2 months in full-term, healthy infants. During this time, the normal postnatal testosterone surge stimulates penile growth to a size that remains constant in relation to overall body size until puberty. Today, many pediatric urologists proceed with correction anytime after 3 months of age in full-term, healthy boys. Referral can be done soon after birth, in part to allay family concerns about the condition since few parents are aware that hypospadias exists.

Preoperative hormonal stimulation with either injectable or topical testosterone may be recommended when the glans appears small, almost exclusively in those with proximal hypospadias.

## Outcomes of Surgery

Today, the majority of operations are performed in infants in a single-stage, outpatient repair. Although several hundred techniques have been described since hypospadias repair began in the late 1800s, only a few are in common use today [3]. Most pediatric urologists repair distal cases by tubularizing the urethral plate (Fig. 30.3),

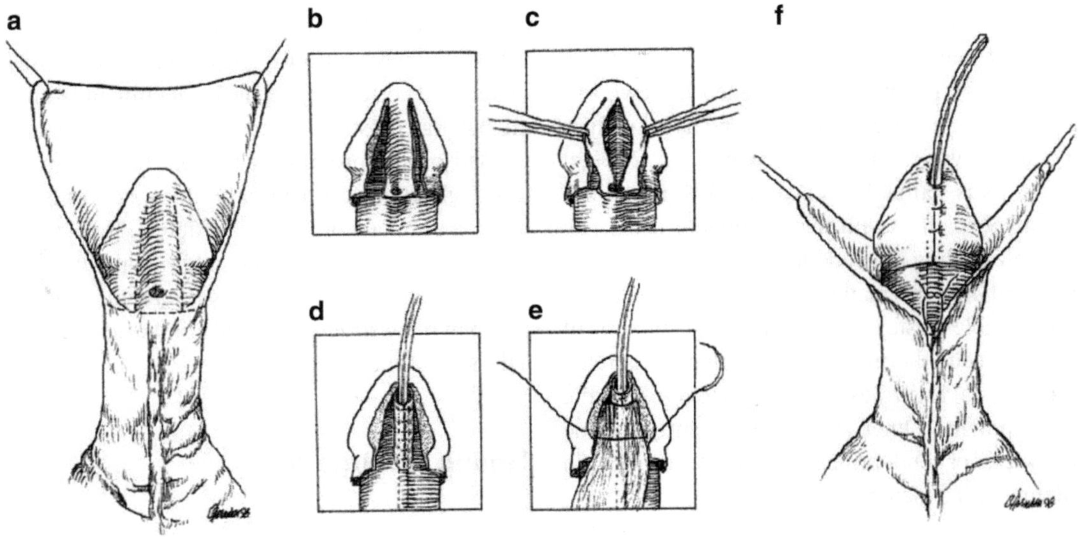


**Fig. 30.3** Tubularized, incised plate hypospadias repair. (**a**) *Horizontal dotted line* indicating circumscribing incision approximately 2 mm proximal to the meatus. *Vertical dotted lines* indicate the junction of the urethral plate to the glans wings. (**b**) Urethral plate is separated from the glans wings, which are then mobilized laterally. (**c**) The key step of the operation is a deep, midline incision into the urethral plate extending from within the meatus to its distal margin, but not continuing into the glans apex. (**d**) The plate is tubularized over a small stent leaving a generous, oval meatus. (**e**) The neourethra is covered by a dartos flap, and then glansplasty begins at the coronal margin. (**f**) Glans wings, mucosal collar, and ventral shaft skin are closed

midline tissues extending from the meatus to the tip of the glans where the urethral opening should have developed. Skin flaps from the penile shaft or foreskin are not used as often now as in the past for distal cases, but preputial flaps remain an option for proximal hypospadias (Fig. 30.4). Two-stage repairs today are unusual, reserved in primary cases for proximal hypospadias with severe ventral curvature or for those reoperations in which the previously created neourethra needs to be replaced.

Following surgery, urinary diversion is most commonly maintained with a urethral catheter for approximately 7–14 days, depending upon the severity of the defect. In infants and young boys, this stent can be placed into diapers for drainage without a collection bag. Oral antibiotics are routinely prescribed during catheterization, and in older patients, anticholinergics may also be recommended to reduce bladder irritability.

The expected outcome from modern hypospadias surgery is a penis that looks normal or nearly so (Fig. 30.5). Tubularization procedures create a natural-appearing meatus and glans, and modifications added to flap procedures seek to duplicate this success. Parents can choose either circumcision or foreskin reconstruction in nearly all distal and many proximal cases. While some reports suggest a higher complication rate when preputioplasty is done, we found no difference in expected outcomes with foreskin reconstruction [4]. A recent study [5] used standardized questionnaires to compare parents' impressions of cosmetic outcomes following hypospadias repair using a tubularization procedure versus circumcision in otherwise normal penises, finding no differences.

There are very limited data concerning functional results of modern hypospadias surgeries. Innovation seeking to improve surgical techniques

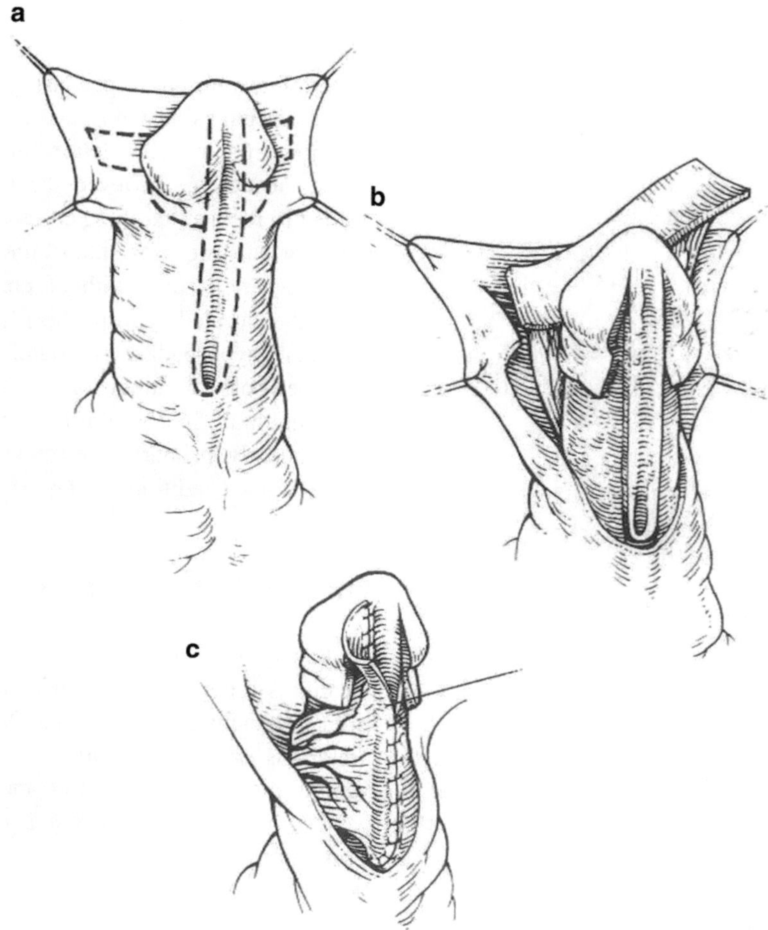

**Fig. 30.4** Onlay preputial flap. (**a**, **b**) A rectangular flap of appropriate length and a width of approximately 8–10 mm is cut from the inner prepuce, maintaining its blood supply. (**c**) The flap is rotated ventrally and sutured to the urethral plate. The pedicle of the flap is used to cover the neourethral suture lines

generally has outpaced long-term follow-up, and infants undergoing the initial repairs of some modern techniques have not yet have completed puberty. One report [6] of teens and adults operated as children using skin flaps found most satisfied with their repairs, although minor complaints of spraying stream and post-void dribbling were common. Similarly, those who had experienced ejaculation reported they had to milk semen from the urethra. While there are no reports describing outcomes of straightening procedures after puberty, there are also no reports raising concern that recurrent curvature commonly develops.

A number of complications are possible after hypospadias urethroplasty. The most common is urethrocutaneous fistulas, which are usually small leaks found along the neourethra, often near the coronal of the glans. Meatal stenosis may result in a pinpoint stream and straining to void. Part or the entire repair can dehisce. After skin flap procedures, ballooning of the reconstructed urethra can occur during urination, with post-void dribbling. Urethral strictures may develop, most often at the juncture of a tubularized skin flap to the native urethra. Unless symptomatic obstruction requires intervention sooner,

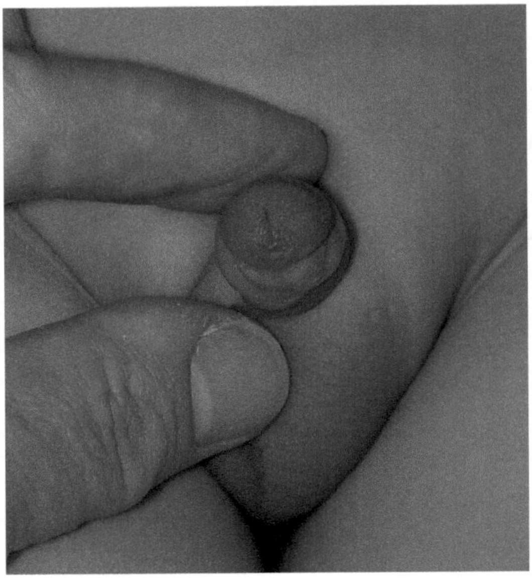

**Fig. 30.5** Postoperative appearance following tubularized incised plate repair

it is routine to postpone further intervention to correct these problems for at least 6 months to allow tissues a period of recovery.

## Circumcision in Newborns with Hypospadias

A common teaching is that circumcision must be avoided in newborns with hypospadias because the skin will be needed for urethroplasty. However, today, skin flap urethroplasty is much less common that in the past, and the reason to avoid newborn circumcision in most babies with hypospadias or chordee without hypospadias is that the Plastibell rings and Gomco clamps used to perform the procedures do not function properly when the foreskin is asymmetric and deficient ventrally. Accordingly, it remains best practice to defer circumcision until definitive repair of the hypospadias or other penile anomaly.

A subset of patients with hypospadias is born with a normal-appearing penis and complete foreskin. Knowledge that a urethral defect may be concealed beneath the foreskin has raised anxiety among practitioners who perform newborn circumcisions, resulting in aborted procedures when hypospadias is suspected. Consequently, some infants present to pediatric urologists with partial circumcision who have no hypospadias, but now require completion of circumcision under anesthesia. However, the foreskin is not needed to reconstruct these cases, and so infants with normal foreskins should undergo circumcision when desired without concern for the unusual concealed hypospadias [7].

When hypospadias is found unexpectedly after newborn circumcision, parents may suspect urethral injury during the procedure. Consequently, primary care providers should be aware of this condition to allay concerns.

## Chordee Without Hypospadias

A dorsal foreskin with a normally positioned meatus is a common anomaly within the spectrum that includes hypospadias. Most often, the urethra is otherwise healthy and any apparent ventral curvature results from the relative deficiency of ventral prepuce and shaft skin. Correction involves either circumcision or foreskin reconstruction performed after 3 months of age as discussed above.

Chordee without hypospadias less often indicates a more significant penile defect with ventral curvature that requires straightening procedures or rarely a hypoplastic urethra that must be reconstructed.

The term “chordee” originally was used to describe fibrous scar-like bands thought to cause ventral curvature in hypospadias, although histologic studies of ventral tissues failed to demonstrate these fibrous bands. Additionally, “chordee” has been used synonymously for “curvature,” as in the diagnosis of chordee without hypospadias. However, the use of the same word to indicate either curvature or tissues thought to cause curvature leads to confusion, especially in families who encounter the term on the Internet, and so with the exception of the ICD-9 code 752.62 terminology of “chordee without hypospadias,” the use of the word should be discouraged.

## References

1. Thomas DF. Hypospadiology: science and surgery. BJU Int. 2004;93:470–3.
2. Kaefer M, Diamond D, Hendren WH, et al. The incidence of intersexuality in children with cryptorchidism and hypospadias: stratification based on gonadal palpability and meatal position. J Urol. 1999;162:1003–6.
3. Manzoni G, Bracka A, Palminteri E, et al. Hypospadias surgery: when, what and by whom? BJU Int. 2004;94:1188–95.
4. Snodgrass WT, Koyle MA, Baskin LS, et al. Foreskin preservation in penile surgery. J Urol. 2006;176:711–4.
5. Snodgrass W, Ziada A, Yucel S, et al. Comparison of outcomes of tubularized incised plate hypospadias repair and circumcision: a questionnaire-based survey of parents and surgeons. J Pediatr Urol. 2008;4(4):250–4.
6. Lam PN, Greenfield SP, Williot P. 2-stage repair in infancy for severe hypospadias with chordee: long-term results after puberty. J Urol. 2005;174:1567–72.
7. Snodgrass WT, Khavari R. Prior circumcision does not complicate repair of hypospadias with an intact prepuce. J Urol. 2006;176:296–8.

# Chordee

# 31

Israel Franco and Jordan Gitlin

## Introduction

Chordee refers to an abnormal bend or angulation of the penis. In the simplest manner, this can be thought of as a chord pulling the penis up, down, or to the side. This is most noticeable with erections. The cause of the chordee or bend may be due to skin abnormalities, urethral abnormalities (hypospadias or epispadias), or anatomic abnormalities of the erectile bodies of the penis. To help understand this completely, further insight into penile anatomy is warranted.

## Anatomy

The penis is made up of three distinct structures or cylinders. There are two outer cylinders called the corporal bodies. These are the erectile bodies, and they are bound by a thin, but very strong outer wrapping called the tunica albuginea. The central cylinder contains the urethra, and glans (head of the penis), and is surrounded by softer, spongy tissue known as the corpus spongiosum. With an erection, the two outer cylinders fill with blood and become rigid. If the two erectile bodies are not equal, the shorter corpora, or the shorter side of the corpora will pull the penis in that direction with an erection.

The anatomic descriptive position for the penis is the erect state. Therefore, the urethra, which is on the undersurface of the penis, is in ventral position when erect. Ventral chordee would refer to a bend downwards, towards the scrotum (Fig. 31.1). Dorsal chordee refers to a bend towards the abdomen, or upper body. The nerves of the penis are on the dorsal or top aspect of the penis, over the corporal bodies, and these structures are all covered by skin.

## History of Chordee

According to a history of hypospadias by E. Durham Smith [1], the major significance of chordee was initially appreciated by Galen in the second century A.D., with the next report in the fourth century by Oribasius who reported that chordee interferes with intercourse. In the 16th century, there is a report of a Maltese woman requesting an annulment of marriage because of her husband's "deformity." Apparent evaluation by two physicians in courtroom describes an "inept male member that was short and curved, becoming more pronounced with rigidity." The marriage was thus annulled because "impotence as a bodily defect justifies annulment."

I. Franco, M.D., F.A.C.S., F.A.A.P. (✉)
Director of pediatric urology at Maria Fareri Children's Hospital, New York Medical College, Valhalla, NY 10595, USA
e-mail: Ifranco@pedsurology.com

J. Gitlin, M.D.
Hofstra Northshore-LIJ School of Medicine, New York, USA

R. Rabinowitz et al. (eds.), *Pediatric Urology for the Primary Care Physician*, Current Clinical Urology,
DOI 10.1007/978-1-60327-243-8_31, 

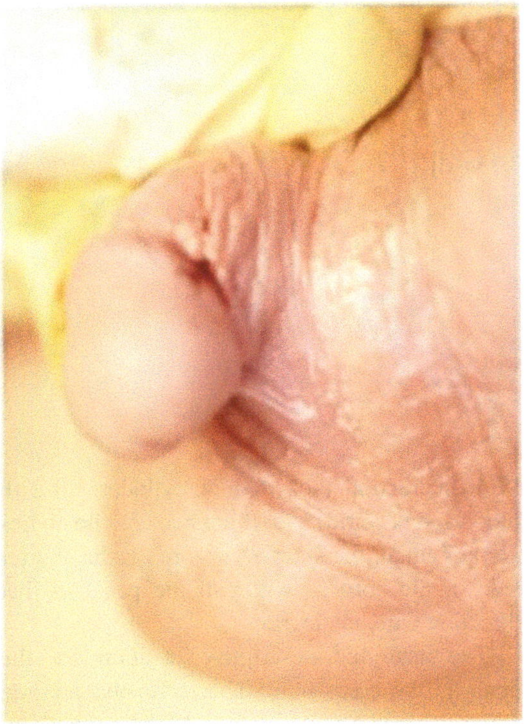

**Fig. 31.1** Penis with chordee

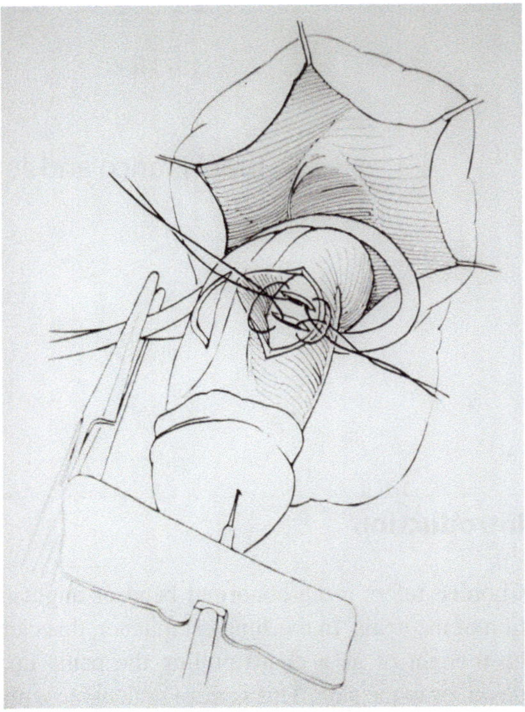

**Fig. 31.2** Nesbit plication technique (from Hinman's Atlas of Pediatric Urologic Surgery 2nd edition 2009 Ed. Frank Hinman, Jr and Laurence Baskin Saunders, Philadelphia, PA p. 676)

Early surgeons focused solely on hypospadias and ignored chordee. It wasn't until 1842 that Mattauer recognized skin tethering as a principal cause of chordee. In 1938 Byars described using preputial skin flaps to correct the skin tethering. Nesbit in 1941 described resecting part of the dorsal erectile body and placing sutures to correct the ventral bend and to make each side of the corporal bodies equal in length (Fig. 31.2). Lastly, in 2000, Baskin et al. [2] at UCSF reported on the anatomic position of the dorsal penile nerves, to help guide placement of sutures to correct chordee and avoid penile injury.

## Importance of Chordee

Aside from the cosmetic appearance of the penis from its curvature, the primary significance of chordee is the functional aspect. Specifically with intercourse, the bent penis can be an obstacle to successful penetration as well as painful for both partners.

The next significant aspect of chordee is its early and prompt recognition. There are several clues that chordee may exist. First, if the foreskin is not completely circumferential, then the lack of skin on one side may cause pulling/angulation and chordee. Next, in boys where the median raphae are off to the side, one should be suspicious about an underlying abnormality. Lastly, in boys with hypospadias, there is usually an associated chordee.

Recognition of chordee is imperative before proceeding with a newborn circumcision. In most forms of chordee there is a lack of ventral foreskin. It is imperative to save the dorsal skin to allow for reconstruction of the ventral penile skin at the time of chordee correction therefore obviating circumcision (Fig. 31.3).

All techniques for newborn circumcision rely on an intact, circumferential foreskin to be pulled up, and then clamped and finally, cut. Figure 31.4 demonstrates the normal foreskin. Figure 31.5

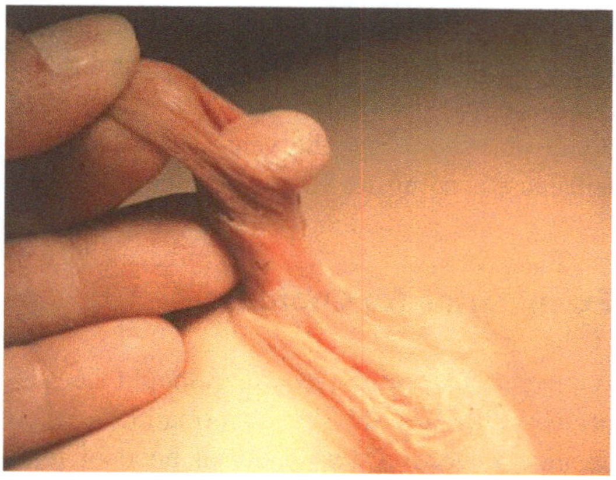

Fig. 31.3 Dorsal hood

demonstrates the Gomco clamp, and Fig. 31.6 demonstrates the Mogen clamp. Both techniques require that the foreskin be pulled up circumferentially, and then excised. If a circumcision is attempted in a patient with chordee and skin abnormalities where there is a lack of complete skin, it is possible that injury to the urethra can result. It is not uncommon to encounter large veins adjacent to the urethra in patients with chordee. These veins if transected can bleed profusely and may require suture ligature at the time of circumcision.

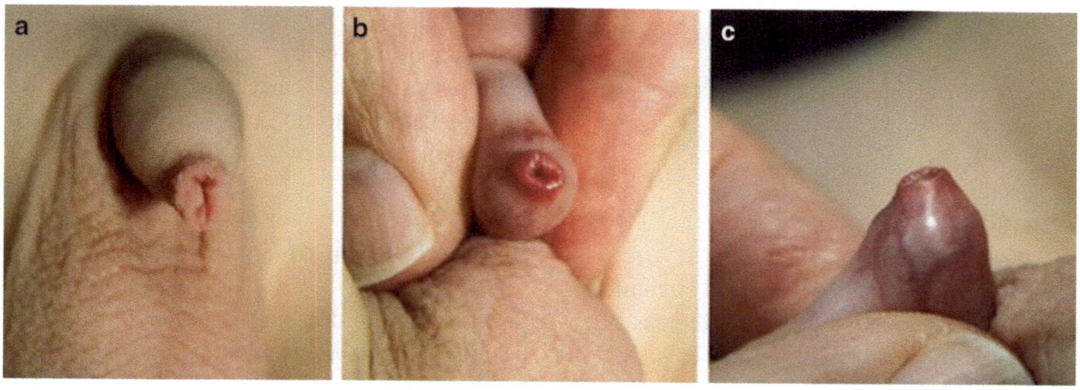


**Fig. 31.4** Variations on normal foreskin: (**a**) normal, (**b**) mild phimosis, and (**c**) moderate phimosis

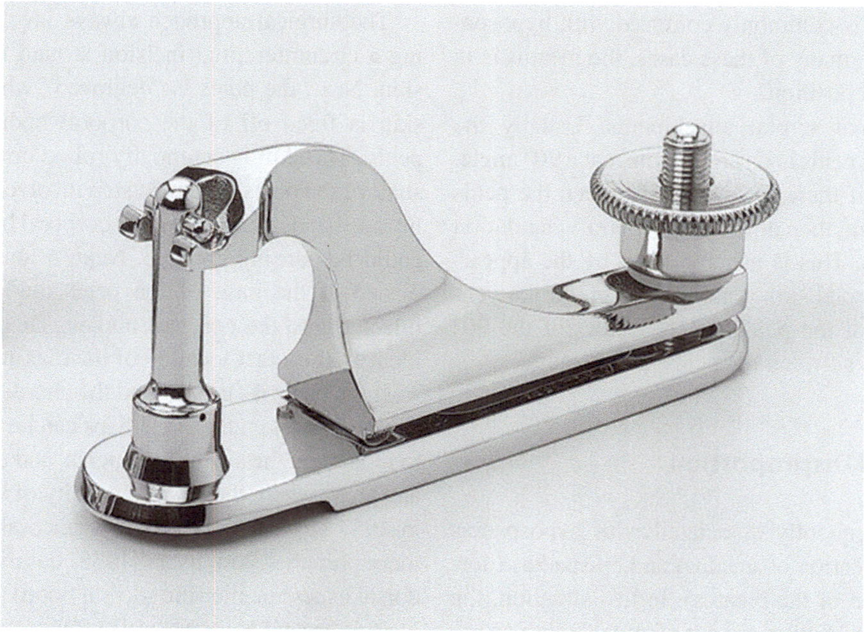

**Fig. 31.5** Gomco circumcision clamp

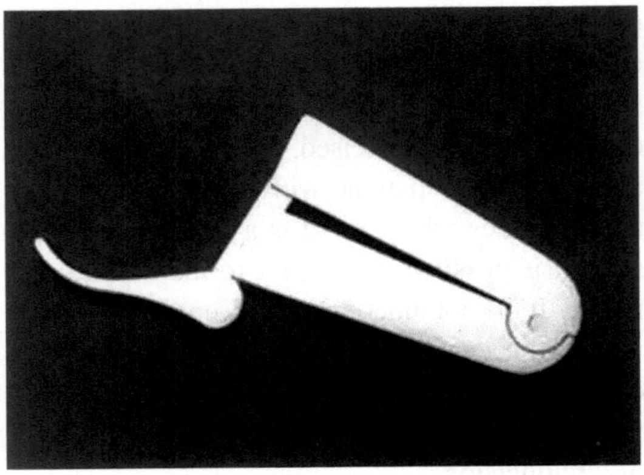

**Fig. 31.6** Mogen circumcision clamp

## Causes of Chordee

Chordee can be caused from a defect in one of the following:

### Skin

The penile skin is usually equal and circumferentially wrapped around the penis. If there is a deficiency in skin on either side of the penis, this will result in a bend towards that side. Frequently, this is seen in boys with a normal meatus, but lack of ventral foreskin. There is usually a hood of dorsal skin. This is commonly confused with hypospadias, but in many of these cases, the meatus is in the normal position.

Abnormal scrotal attachments: Usually the base of the penis and scrotum meet at a 90° angle. However, if there is webbing between the penis and scrotum, then downward (ventral) angulation may occur. This is usually noted by the appearance of scrotal skin coming up high on the ventral shaft of the penis. There is loss of the 90° angulation between the penis and scrotum.

### Corporal Disproportion

This is frequently associated with hypospadias (ventral location of meatus) and epispadias (dorsal location of the meatus). In this situation, the two corporal bodies are not of equal length on the ventral and dorsal aspects of the penis. This will lead to a bend to the side of the corpora (cylinder) that is shorter. In ventral chordee, the corporal bodies are shorter on the ventral side, and this will cause bending in a ventral manner (Fig. 31.1).

## Examination for Chordee

As mentioned earlier, chordee should be suspected if there are any skin abnormalities such as an incomplete foreskin, a dorsal hood of foreskin, or abnormal median raphae on the undersurface of the penis. Some parents may report seeing a bend when the baby has erections. This can be confirmed by the parents taking a digital photograph for review with the physician. If chordee is suspected, and repair is indicated, an intra-operative injection of saline into the penis will confirm its presence.

## Surgical Repair of Chordee

Surgery for chordee can be performed in most healthy children after 6 months of age. It is usually performed as an outpatient procedure, and recovery is rapid. Usually by the first postoperative day, there is no requirement for analgesia.

The surgical approach always involves making a circumferential incision around the penile skin. Next, the penis is "degloved" whereby the skin is freed off of the corporal bodies of the penis. The skin is essentially rolled down on the shaft of the penis. The next step involves excising fibrous bands of tissue on the corporal bodies that could be causing chordee. Next, a tourniquet is placed at the base of the penis, and saline is injected into the corporal bodies. This will help identify the exact location of the maximal bend.

If the penis is straight, and the chordee was due to abnormal skin, then skin flaps can be mobilized to re-surface the shaft of the penis, and correct for any areas where there was a paucity of skin. Firlit in 1987 [3] described using a mucosal collar of inner preputial skin. byars (1938) described using dorsal excess penile skin (dorsal hood) and bringing this around to the ventral surface of the penis.

If the chordee was due to scrotal webbing, then this can be corrected by degloving the penis and then the ventral penile skin is split along the midline into the scrotum. The scrotal fat and scrotal attachments are all removed from the penile shaft. The subepithelial tissue at the penoscrotal junction is tacked to the corporal bodies on each side. This fixes the penoscrotal angle in place. The excess foreskin then split and rotated to the front of the penis to cover the ventral skin defect that is usually associated with webbing. The ventral shaft skin is also closed in the midline, and the median raphe is reconstructed.

In cases where an artificial erection reveals a persistent bend, then the surgeon has two options. If the chordee is mild to moderate, a Nesbit plication may be performed. If there is ventral chordee due to ventral shortening of the corpora, then the plication will be performed on the opposite side (dorsal side) of the penis. Going in the midline (where there is an absence of nerves), sutures are placed to essentially shorten and "bunch up" the corporal body. This will help to correct the chordee by equalizing the size of the corporal body on each side. This technique can be applied to chordee of any direction. Basically, the surgeon goes to the side opposite of the chordee to place these plication sutures and straighten the bend (Fig. 31.2).

In cases of severe chordee, which is commonly associated with more severe forms of hypospadias, plication of the corpora may shorten the penis excessively and also leave a hump, which is unsightly. In such a case, a transverse incision can be made in the corporal body at the point of maximal bend. This will allow the penis to spring open and straighten out. However, there will then be an absence of tissue covering the corpora (tunica albuginea). Correction of this corporal defect will require some graft tissue to be used to make up the lack of tunica albuginea. The surgeon may then harvest a small piece of dermis from the groin [4, 5], SIS (subintestinal submucosa) [6], or tunica vaginalis from the scrotum to cover this defect [7] (Fig. 31.7). On some occasions the urethra is short and there may be no hypospadias and some of these urethras need to be transected and a graft inserted into the corpora. Six months are allowed to pass to allow for optimal wound healing and then the urethra is reconstructed.

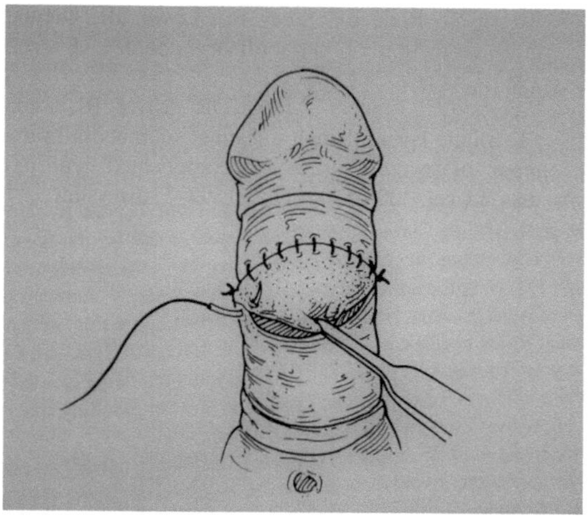

**Fig. 31.7** Dermal graft of the penile corpora technique (from Hinman's Atlas of Pediatric Urologic Surgery 2nd edition 2009 Ed. Frank Hinman, Jr and Laurence Baskin Saunders, Philadelphia, PA p 678)

Boys with severe chordee should be followed into adolescence, as there are reports of late recurrences of chordee [8]. In these children, the recurrence was due to fibrosis from the reconstructed urethra (32 %), corporal disproportion (36 %), and a combination of both in 32 % of boys.

In conclusion, chordee recognition is important in the newborn period to prevent improper circumcision and to plan for subsequent repair. The techniques used to correct chordee are very successful, with most boys having a normal-appearing and functioning penis.

## References


1. Smith ED. The history of hypospadias. Pediatr Surg Int. 1997;12(2–3):81–5.
2. Baskin LS, Erol A, Li YW, Liu WH. Anatomy of the neurovascular bundle: is safe mobilization possible? J Urol. 2000;164(3 Pt 2):977–80.
3. Firlit CF. The mucosal collar in hypospadias surgery. J Urol. 1987;137(1):80–2.
4. Lindgren BW, Reda EF, Levitt SB, Brock WA, Franco I. Single and multiple dermal grafts for the management of severe penile curvature. J Urol. 1998;160(3 Pt 2):1128–30.

5. Kogan SJ, Reda EF, Smey PL, Levitt SB. Dermal graft correction of extraordinary chordee. J Urol. 1983;130(5):952–4.
6. Weiser AC, Franco I, Herz DB, Silver RI, Reda EF. Single layered small intestinal submucosa in the repair of severe chordee and complicated hypospadias. J Urol. 2003;170(4 Pt 2):1593–5; disussion 5.
7. Hafez AT, Smith CR, McLorie GA, El-Ghoneimi A, Herz DB, Bagli DJ, et al. Tunica vaginalis for correcting penile chordee in a rabbit model: is there a difference in flap versus graft? J Urol. 2001;166(4):1429–32.
8. Vandersteen DR, Husmann DA. Late onset recurrent penile chordee after successful correction at hypospadias repair. J Urol. 1998;160(3 Pt 2):1131–3; discussion 7.

# 32 Epispadias

J. Todd Purves, Andrew A. Stec,
and John P. Gearhart

## Introduction

Epispadias consists of a dorsally located ectopic urethral meatus which is the result of a failure by the urethral plate to completely tubularize during embryologic development. It represents the least severe variant in the exstrophy-epispadias complex in that the abdominal wall and bladder are closed, and associated anomalies such as musculoskeletal defects, orthopedic abnormalities, vesicoureteral reflux, and hernias are less frequent or less pronounced.

Typically, epispadias is diagnosed at birth, although presentation is dependent on severity and gender of the patient. Unlike bladder exstrophy patients where the absence of a bladder can be easily seen on prenatal ultrasound, it is unlikely that the fetal abnormalities are significantly apparent to be found with screening during pregnancy. In males, the urethral meatus may be located on the dorsal aspect of the glans, penile shaft, or the penopubic junction and is usually obvious enough for immediate diagnosis. In all cases, there is some degree of upward curvature to the penis, commonly referred to as dorsal chordee. The penopubic variant is most commonly seen, affecting approximately 70 % of these patients. Called complete epispadias, this penopubic or complete form involves the entire urethral plate to the level of the bladder neck and includes a cleft striated sphincter (Fig. 32.1). As these patients lack a congenital continence mechanism, they are incontinent before surgical reconstruction and their lack of outlet resistance during infancy produces a thin-walled bladder with poor capacity. In contrast, the intermediate forms of epispadias at the penile shaft level, or the even more rare glandular variant, do not usually lead to incontinence because the bladder neck is intact. Their presentation is somewhat more subtle and in the glandular case, where the foreskin may be intact, a resulting delay of diagnosis may occur.

Being part of the exstrophy spectrum of birth defects, these patients have a similar array of associated anomalies. The bony pelvis will be outwardly and inferiorly rotated with a diastasis of the pubic symphysis that is bridged by an intrasymphyseal band. Compared to classic exstrophy pelves, however, the abnormalities are mild and usually do not require osteotomies at the time of surgical reconstruction. Vesicoureteral reflux has been reported to occur in between 30 and 85 % in some series, which is less than the 100 % in classic exstrophy cases. Obviously,

J.T. Purves, M.D., Ph.D.
Medical University of South Carolina,
96 Jonathan Lucas St., Suite 601, Charleston, SC
29425, USA
e-mail: purves@musc.edu

A.A. Stec, M.D. • J.P. Gearhart, M.D.,
F.A.A.P., F.A.C.S. (✉)
Division of Pediatric Urology, The Brady Urological
Institute, Johns Hopkins Hospital,
600 North Wolfe Street, Baltimore, MD 21287, USA
e-mail: jgearha2@jhmi.edu

R. Rabinowitz et al. (eds.), *Pediatric Urology for the Primary Care Physician*, Current Clinical Urology,
DOI 10.1007/978-1-60327-243-8_32, © Springer Science+Business Media New York 2015

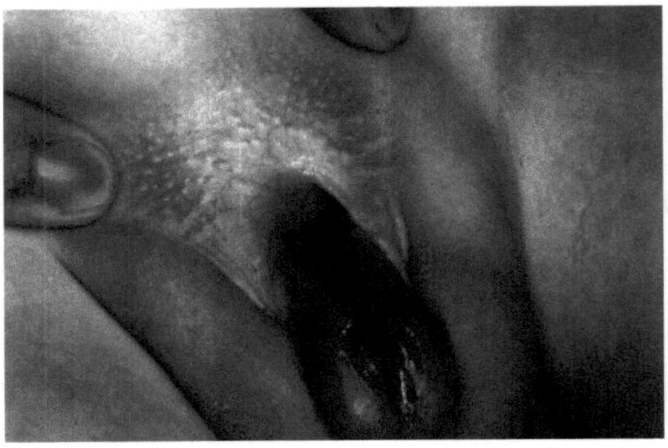

**Fig. 32.1** Complete male epispadias

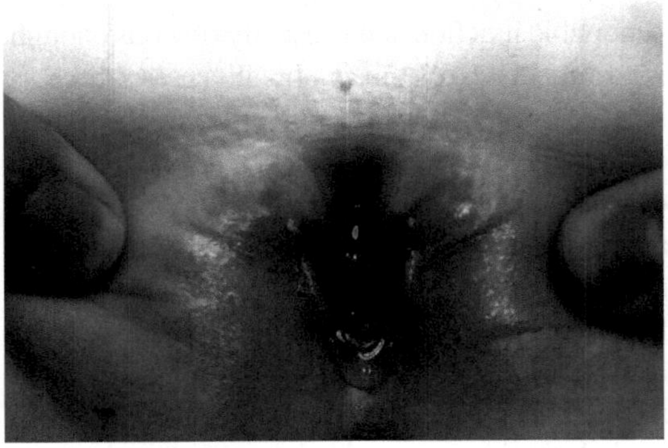

**Fig. 32.2** Complete female epispadias

screening for reflux must be done to assess the need for reimplantation. Finally, inguinal hernias have been found in 33 % of epispadias, again significantly lower than for classic exstrophy, but frequent enough to warrant careful examination.

Female patients present unique challenges as epispadias in girls is even more rare and the defects can be much less obvious than in males. In less severe forms, the urethral meatus may simply appear patulous or the entire urethra may be split along its entire length. It is not unusual for this to be missed at birth and rather present during toilet training as a constant wetness. In the most severe form, the entire urethra is affected and involves the bladder neck, thereby rendering the patient incontinent until bladder neck reconstruction is undertaken (Fig. 32.2). These children are often recognized at birth with a bifid clitoris and a depressed mons that is covered by smooth, glabrous skin which can be supported by moderate subcutaneous fat or can be closely applied to the anterior and inferior pubic symphysis. The labia minora are usually poorly developed and terminate anteriorly at the ipsilateral hemiclitoris, where there may be a rudiment of a preputial fold.

## Etiology

During the fifth week of gestation, the primordium of the genital tubercles migrates toward the midline, superior to the cloacal membrane, to form the genital tubercle. Aberrant migration results in the defect of the dorsal wall of the urethra known as epispadias [1].

Insights into the genetic and environmental factors that may contribute to epispadias have largely been gleaned from data on patients with classic bladder exstrophy which, at 1 in 35,000–50,000 live births, is significantly more common. Extrapolation of data seems reasonable as epispadias is an almost universal component to patients with the more severe forms of these pelvic midline defects. Perhaps the most credible evidence suggesting a genetic contributor is the fact that children born to women with exstrophy have a 1 in 100 chance of having exstrophy themselves. Family studies have found inheritance patterns between siblings, third degree cousins, and uncle/nephew pairings, all of which are indicative of complex inheritance phenomena involving multiple genes and possible environmental component. Indeed, the argument for environmental factors is supported by links between androgen disruptors, such as misoprostol, and increased incidence of exstrophy and other congenital anomalies. Geographical analysis of exstrophy in the United States shows that the incidence is higher in the South and Midwest with a significantly lower occurrence in the West, again supporting exogenous components. Other factors that appear to be associated with production of exstrophy-epispadias include decreased maternal age, Caucasian race, and conception through the use of in vitro fertilization.

## Surgical Management of the Male Epispadias Patient

Surgical management for patients with milder variants of epispadias consists of penile and urethral reconstruction while those with complete epispadias will require bladder neck reconstruction in addition to the penile procedures. In either case, penile surgery typically is performed when the child is between 6 months and 1 year of age in order to minimize anesthetic risks from operating on infants, while also decreasing the psychological trauma associated with genital surgery in older children. Most surgeons request that patients receive intramuscular injections of testosterone enanthate in order to increase penile size and, more importantly, increase the amount of penile skin which is often required for the creation of flaps or grafts during the repair. Often given by the patient's primary physician, the usual dose is 2 mg/kg and is injected at 5 and 2 weeks prior to the operation. In re-operative cases, 5 % testosterone cream applied to the urethral plate may enhance pliability and vascularity when prior scarring is an issue. Since many patients travel to specialized centers for their procedures, good communication between the operating surgeon and the primary care physician is essential for the proper timing and administration of the testosterone, which may decrease the complication rate from fistulae and strictures.

The goal of penile reconstruction is to create a cosmetically acceptable phallus that allows the patient to void through the tip of the penis and also to have normal sexual function. Regardless of the specific surgical strategy chosen, the issue of the dorsal chordee needs to be addressed and repaired during the first procedure. While many surgeons and the surgical literature report on means to achieve "penile lengthening," it is important to note that real gains in penile length rely on releasing the chordee and changing the angulation of the penis rather than actually achieving true increases in length. The reason for this, as gleaned from MRI studies of the exstrophy pelvis, is that these patients have an average corporal body length that is 50 % shorter, albeit 30 % greater in girth, than normal controls. It is possible to create a larger neo-phallus using plastic surgical techniques such as radial forearm flaps. However, the sacrifice in function and sensitivity when using non-erogenous tissues is so great that these methods are almost never employed in epispadias or exstrophy patients who typically are able to achieve satisfactory sexual performance with their natural phallus.

The two most commonly employed methods for penile reconstruction used today are the modified Cantwell-Ransley technique and the penile disassembly technique. With either strategy, the suspensory ligaments to the penis are divided and the corpora are dissected free from attachments to the inferior pubic rami. After release of the chordee, the urethral groove is lengthened, and medial rotation of the ventral corpora angulates the penis in a more downward direction. In unusual cases where more corporal length is required, a cavernostomy is performed with anastomosis or grafting. These are avoided, if possible, as there is no intrinsic deformity of the corporal bodies and the procedure requires mobilization of the neurovascular bundles which can be damaged with such a maneuver. With the penile disassembly, or Mitchell, repair, the three components of the penis, including the two corpora with their respective hemiglans, and the urethral wedge consisting of the urethral plate and underlying spongiosum, are dissected completely free from each other. In contrast, the modified Cantwell-Ransley repair leaves the distal 1 cm of the urethral plate attached to the glans penis. Supporters of the modified Cantwell-Ransley repair, including the authors, are discouraged by the fact that most patients undergoing complete disassembly are left with a hypospadias that will require a difficult second surgery to correct. They are also concerned by rare but devastating ischemic injuries that have resulted in loss of entire corporal bodies and glans tissue. Surgeons on either side of the debate, however, agree that the more important factor is the experience of the surgical team and that patients are best served when referred to large volume centers that have familiarity with this unusual anatomy.

After penile reconstruction, patients with complete epispadias will be totally incontinent owing to their lack of a continence mechanism. Bladder neck reconstruction is performed when the child is old enough and sufficiently motivated to participate in a voiding program, typically between 4 and 6 years of age. In the interim, the child will periodically undergo cystoscopy and gravity cystograms under general anesthesia which will permit the measurement of bladder capacity. Since ultimate continence is extremely dependent on bladder size, this information is critically important for surgical planning. Historically, bladder neck repair was performed before penile reconstruction until it was shown that primary urethroplasty and penile elongation in epispadias and exstrophy patients led to significant improvements in bladder capacity. This is believed to result from the increase outlet resistance that allows the bladder to experience a more normal cycle of filling and emptying. An important consequence of increased urethral resistance is that children with vesicoureteral reflux need to be identified and treated with prophylactic antibiotics during the period between penile surgery and the definitive procedure to protect the upper urinary tracts.

The continence procedure favored at our institution is the modified Young-Dees-Leadbetter bladder neck repair. Briefly, this consists of creating a tube of mucosa from the posterior bladder wall that is in continuity with the posterior urethra. A muscular funnel is created from bladder muscle flaps on each side of the tube to provide adequate resistance to outflow such that dryness is achieved during ordinary bladder volumes and pressures. A suprapubic tube is left indwelling for 3 weeks after surgery at which time voiding trials are initiated. These consist of clamping the suprapubic tube for progressively longer periods of time until the patient demonstrates the ability to completely empty the bladder. In cases of urinary retention, an 8 Fr Foley catheter is placed for 5 days and a subsequent trial is then initiated. As is universal in all patients who have had a bladder neck reconstruction, Foley catheters larger than 10 Fr should *never* be introduced per urethra as this will effectively destroy the repair.

Ureteral reimplantation to correct vesicoureteral reflux is undertaken at the time of bladder neck reconstruction. At our institution the Cohen repair is utilized, in which the ureters are brought through submucosal tunnels that extend transversely to the contralateral side of the bladder. Performing this procedure along with the bladder neck repair requires a significant amount of bladder tissue that would be extraordinarily difficult in an infant's small bladder. Ideally, a bladder capacity of 100 mL yields the best results in terms of continence rates and lower incidences of complications.

## Outcomes for Males

When parents are presented with the diagnosis of epispadias in their child, they will naturally inquire as to whether or not the child will ultimately have a normal appearing and functional penis and what potential for urinary continence exists. Outcomes data obtained from surgical series can be helpful in describing an accurate picture of what these patients can expect in the future. Since a child born with epispadias is structurally and clinically similar to a classic bladder exstrophy patient that has undergone a successful primary bladder closure, data from exstrophy studies is often extrapolated to the epispadias population.

Cosmetic results, in terms of a straight and downward angled penis, have been reported as quite good in series from North America and Europe. A study from the Mayo clinic found satisfactory cosmesis in 70 % of their patients when judged by the patient, parents, and experienced urologists. Within their population, 80 % of men reported satisfactory sexual intercourse and, of the 29 married patients, 19 had fathered children [2]. Since there is no associated testicular pathology with this condition, fertility is the rule. However, due to the fact that the reconstructed bladder neck does not respond to normal sympathetic input at the time of ejaculation, there remains a possibility that conception will be difficult or impossible via normal intercourse. With modern assisted reproductive technology, these men can expect to father children if desired.

Over half of boys born with epispadias will require bladder neck reconstruction to become continent, which is reflective of the proportion of patients with the complete epispadias variant of this condition. In a 1995 study from our institution, 82 % of patients were dry at night after continence surgery and were able to void spontaneously per urethra. Time to obtain initial continence after the operation was 90 days, significantly shorter than the 110 days seen for exstrophy patients [3]. This is likely due to the fact that the bladders of patients with epispadias are not exposed to the trauma of the external environment or surgical reconstruction and so remain more compliant, mobile, and more amenable to bladder neck reconstruction.

## Complications of Surgery

Urethrocutaneous fistula and urethral stricture are the most common complications incurred from penile reconstruction. Several series reporting on patients after the modified Cantwell-Ransley procedure estimate a fistula rate between 4 and 19 % and a stricture rate of 5–10 % [4]. Outcomes studies with the penile disassembly technique have reported a fistula rate from 2 to 20 % and one large study reported that 6 % of patients were rendered hypospadic and 1 % suffered from ischemic injury. One reason for a wide range of fistula formation is that many fistulae heal themselves over time without the need for surgical intervention. Therefore, groups who report follow-up at 3 months often have higher rates than those reporting out at 6 months or longer. Reoperation for fistula, stricture, or persistent chordee is uncommon but may occasionally be necessary.

With regard to persistent incontinence after bladder neck repair, many patients will be eligible for a second attempt which has shown relatively good salvage rates. Attempts have been made to improve continence by injecting the bladder neck with bulking agents such as collagen or deflux. Success rates are highly variable, with few groups reporting better than 25 % and the durability of this procedure is still questioned.

## Female Epispadias

Similar to males, the goals of epispadias repair are to create functional and cosmetically acceptable external genitalia and to achieve urinary continence while preserving renal function. At our institution, urethral and genitalia reconstruction are performed together as a single procedure, typically undertaken at 1 year of age. Bladder neck repair is then performed at 4–5 years of age when there has been adequate bladder development and the patient is mature enough to participate in a voiding program. Ureteral reimplantation is performed at the time of the bladder neck surgery. In a French series of 10 girls with epispadias, 9 of the patients had some degree of vesicoureteral reflux which suggests a relatively high frequency in this population [5]. We reimplant the ureters in all patients, even those without a prior history, because de novo reflux can arise as a result of increased bladder outlet resistance.

Several surgical series report urinary continence rates of better than 80 % with an infrequent need for intermittent catheterization, augmentation, or urinary diversion for failed repairs. When the urethra is reconstructed as a first-stage procedure, the bladder capacity can be expected to increase, significantly more than is seen in classic bladder exstrophy patients but it may not completely parallel the growth of normal children. Some surgeons advocate performing the genital, urethral, and bladder neck surgery all in one stage as it does appear to decrease the time interval over which complete dryness is obtained. However, we feel that the increased bladder growth obtained during the staged approach confers an important advantage when performing the bladder neck repair and ureteral reimplantation.

## Conclusion

Children born with epispadias have a generally good outlook in terms of having cosmetically acceptable and functional genitalia, urinary continence, and preservation of renal function. Management of this condition, however, is no small undertaking and requires experienced and dedicated medical, surgical, anesthesiology, and nursing staff. Although there is some variation with regard to the timing and performance of the procedures, it is universally agreed upon that patients have much better outcomes in dedicated exstrophy/epispadias center. Good communication between the consultants and referring physicians is paramount in terms of specific management steps and also for defining the reconstructive process in the context of the patient's overall health and well-being.

## References


1. Diamond DA, Ransley PG. Male epispadias. J Urol. 1995;154:2150–5.
2. Kramer SA, Mesrobian HG, Kelalis PP. Long-term followup of cosmetic appearance and genital function in male epispadias: review of 70 patients. J Urol. 1986;135:543–7.
3. Ben-Chaim J, Peppas DS, Jeffs RD, Gearhart JP. Complete male epispadias: genital reconstruction and achieving continence. J Urol. 1995;153:1665–7.
4. Baird AD, Gearhart JP, Mathews RI. Applications of the modified Cantwell-Ransley epispadias repair in the exstrophy-epispadias complex. J Pediatr Urol. 2005;1:331–6.
5. Mollard P, Basset T, Mure PY. Female epispadias. J Urol. 1997;158:1543–6.

# 33 Female External Genitalia

Marvalyn DeCambre

## Introduction

The first examination of a newborn infant allows clinicians to assess gender to correlate phenotype (external genitalia appearance) and genotype (e.g., 46XY, 46XX, 45X0, etc.). Variations in the appearance of the external genital anatomy in the female are normal. However, certain consistent landmarks in normal female anatomy exist. For example, in the normal girl, there are midline constant soft tissue structures such as the clitoris and the urethral and vaginal openings. There are also laterally located constant soft tissue structures: the paired labia majora and minora—together referred to as the vulva. The anus and palpable bony landmarks, which are the pubis and coccyx in the midline and the paired ischia laterally, are also normally located in fixed relationships to the above named midline soft tissue structures (Figs. 33.1 and 33.2). In 2001, one of our authors (MED, unpublished) performed surface measurements of the distance from the bony landmarks to the soft tissue landmarks. A reproducible ratio from the pubis to the midline soft tissue structures exists (Fig. 33.3). Using the distance from the pubis to coccyx as a denominator, the distance from the pubis to the clitoris as numerator is a fixed ratio of one third the distance, while the distance from pubis to the vaginal opening (os) is one half the distance. A normal female phenotype is illustrated here (Fig. 33.3). Normal anatomy as described above will be compared to abnormal anatomy to follow in this chapter.

M. DeCambre, M.D., M.P.H. (✉)
Poplar Bluff Regional Medical Center,
Poplar Bluff, MO, USA
e-mail: mer7sea@yahoo.com

## Labial Abnormalities

### Labial Adhesions

Estrogen deficiency in the neonate may promote an inflammatory reactivity of the external soft tissue of the genitalia. This results in denuded labial epithelial surfaces which adhere to one another, called labial adhesions [1] (Fig. 33.4a, b). Labial adhesion rarely occurs after the onset of puberty when estrogen is naturally prevalent. This supports the belief that hormonal deficiency has a significant role in the formation of labial adhesions. Substantiating the role of estrogen further is the beneficial effect of utilizing estrogen cream to facilitate the separation of the adherent labia [2]. Labial adhesions occur primarily between birth and 7 years at a rate of one to two in 100 female children [3]. Most girls are asymptomatic, and the majority will spontaneously resolve this problem and require no intervention. Because the hypoestrogenized labial epithelium is denuded, sometimes the passage of urine, which is naturally acidic, may produce symptoms such as burning, itchiness, and scratching activities among little girls with this condition.

R. Rabinowitz et al. (eds.), *Pediatric Urology for the Primary Care Physician*, Current Clinical Urology,
DOI 10.1007/978-1-60327-243-8_33, © Springer Science+Business Media New York 2015

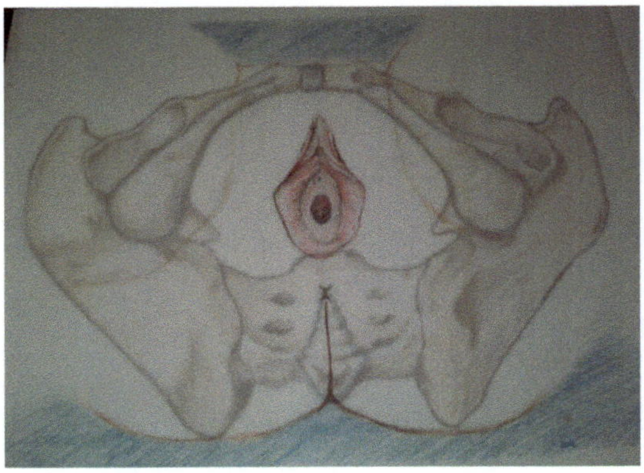

**Fig. 33.1** Structures of the perineum in relation to bony landmarks

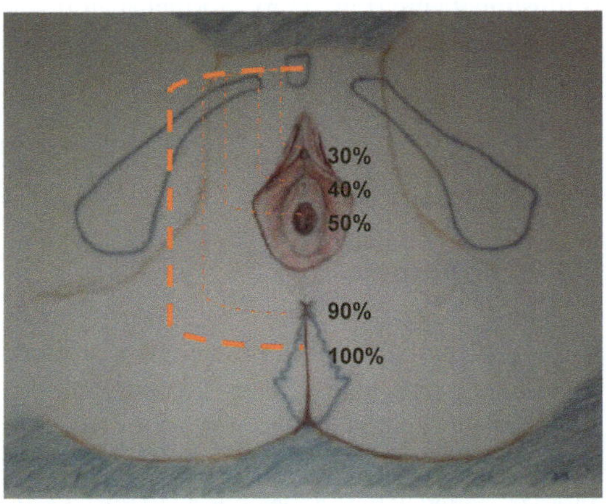


**Fig. 33.2** Depiction of the relationship of structures to the pubococcygeal distance. The clitoris is 1/3 the distance and the vaginal os is 1/2 the distance

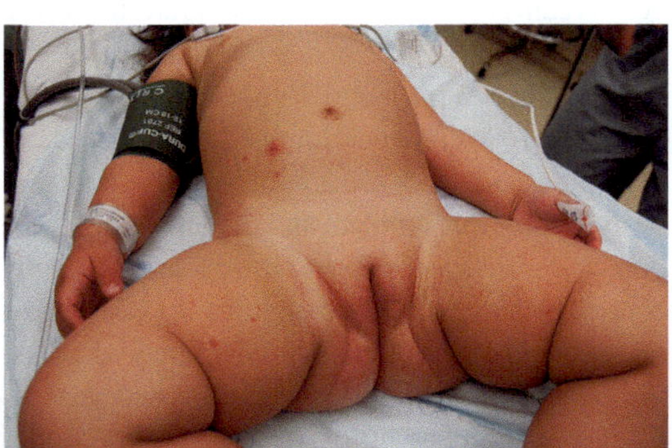

**Fig. 33.3** Normal female phenotypic appearance

These events can promote several bouts of vulvovaginitis (inflammation/irritation to the vulva and vaginal os), dysuria (burning with urination), and rare episodes of urinary tract infection, urinary pooling, and urinary retention. It is also likely the inflammatory process supports the persistent adhesions. Because this can be a frustrating problem for some families and traumatic for the child due to multiple genital inspections, consultation with a pediatric urologist may offer some solutions. Most often, labial adhesions require no intervention. The most common intervention for symptomatic labial adhesions is medical. A cotton tip application of topical estrogen cream/ointment to the line of fusion between the adhered labia minora once daily for 10–14 days followed by 6 weeks of three times daily application of a petroleum jelly-based product has worked well for some girls [4]. For dysuria and itching, utilization of warm water sitz baths may mitigate these symptoms. There are many recommendations for additives to warm sitz baths including: Epsom salt, sodium bicarbonate (baking soda), or vinegar with antiseptic such as iodine solution. It is the observation of our authors that recurrence strengthens adhesions, which creates a somewhat more fused line between the labia. Anecdotally, in-office separations under local analgesia without sedation, while efficient, may have an emotional, albeit temporary, impact on the child. Therefore, persistent symptomatic labial fusion may benefit from manual separation under anesthesia. One of our authors favors suturing over each denuded labia separately to help maintain the separation (Fig. 33.4b). Relative indications of surgical separation include recurrent infection and/or inflammation to the genital area and/or urinary tract. Referral to a pediatric urologist is appropriate at any point after labial adhesion has been uncovered by pediatrician or after a failed trial of topical estrogen.

## Labial Hypertrophy

The enlargement of one or both labia is known to as labial hypertrophy (Fig. 33.5). Labial hypertrophy primarily affects the labia minora. It may

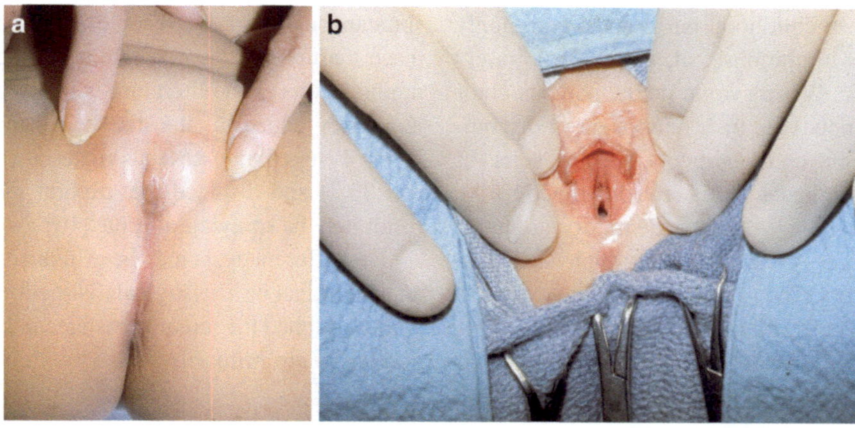


**Fig. 33.4** (**a**) Appearance of a typical child with labial adhesions. (**b**) Here is a demonstration of the surgical separation of the fused labia minora

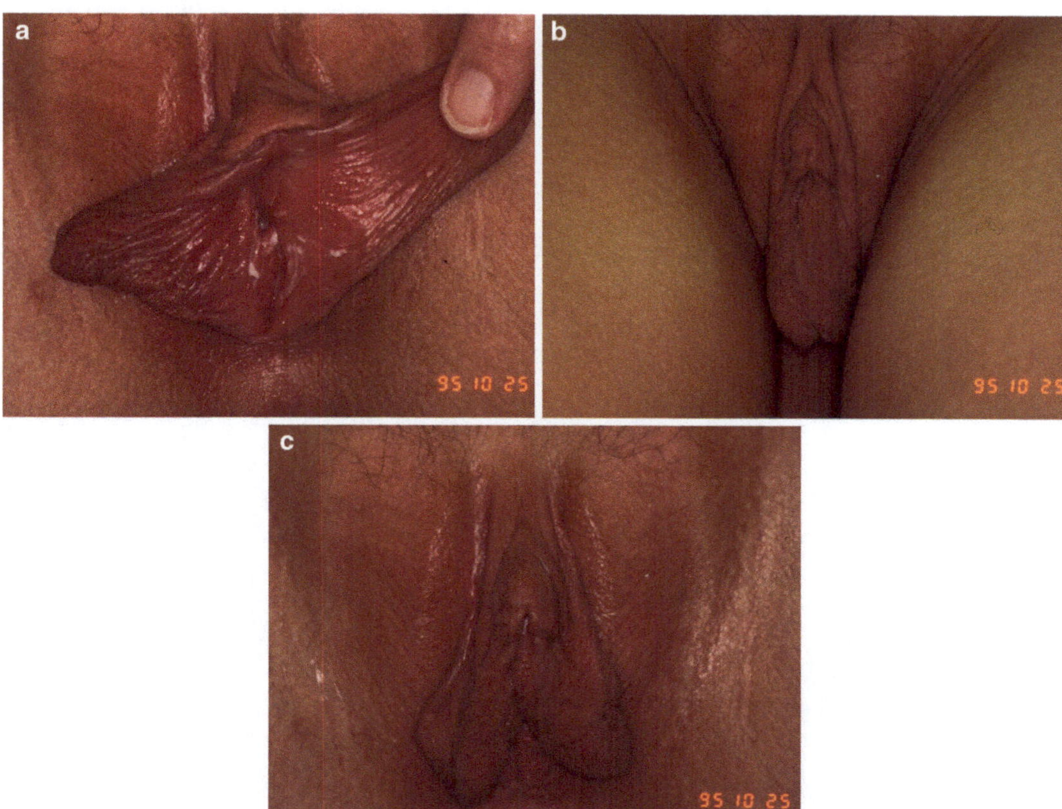


**Fig. 33.5** (**a–c**) Three different views of the same patient with significant labial hypertrophy

occur early in childhood but is most commonly uncovered with the onset of puberty. It is rarely symptomatic. When symptomatic, patients complain of dampness in their underwear or discomfort from tight undergarments, bathing suits, or pants if the elongated labia are constricted by the undergarments [5]. Some patients or parents of patients express concern for future physical sexual encounters. They may be reassured. Surgical reduction may be offered for management among symptomatic patients [6]. Referral to a pediatric urologist is necessary if patient or parent(s) request or express concern.

## Paraurethral Abnormalities

### Paraurethral Cysts

Paraurethral cysts represent several diagnoses including: Gartner's duct cysts, Bartholin glands, Skene's glands, and vaginal inclusion cysts [7] (Figs. 33.6 and 33.7). These cysts as a group occur primarily in the newborn period and are believed to form secondary to stimulation by maternal estrogens during development. They are relatively rare, occurring in 1 in 7,000–10,000 live births [8]. They are located around the urinary meatus (os or opening). As maternal estrogen levels subside, in the neonatal period, these introital cysts generally regress (Fig. 33.7b), or they may rupture spontaneously and as a result do not impinge/displace the urethra [9]. The rare reporting of paraurethral cysts in the literature is likely due to the temporary course of the disease, in most cases. When cysts contain caseous material (Figs. 33.6 and 33.7) and displace the urethral meatus, the result may be spraying of urine [10].

The different cysts may be evaluated for either an anatomical or histological distinction. Skene's glands, dubbed the female prostate, and Gartner's duct cysts are primarily located within the ante-

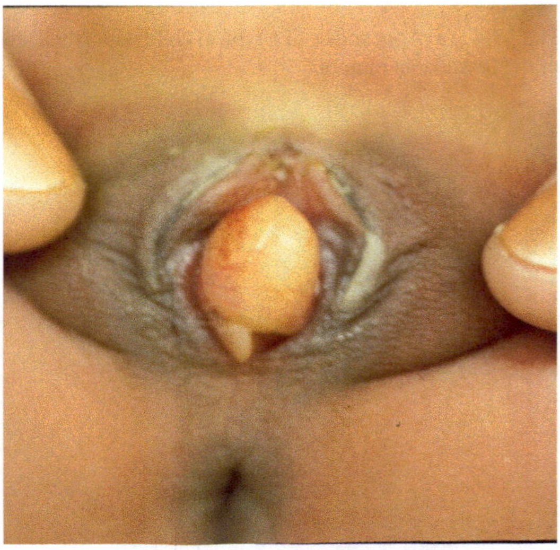

**Fig. 33.6** Paraurethral cyst projecting from the vaginal introitus. In this patient there is compression of the meatus which sprays the urine

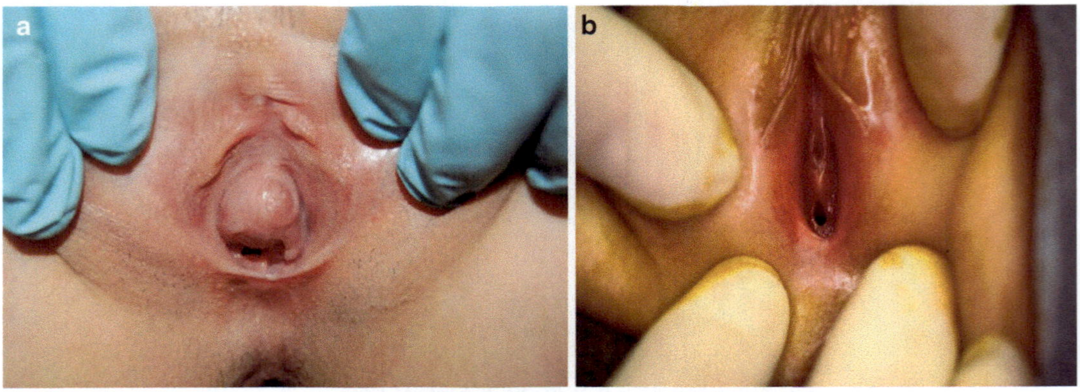

**Fig. 33.7** (**a**) Paraurethral cyst which contains obvious caseous material. (**b**) Small, regressing cyst just below the urethra in a teenage patient

rior and lateral vaginal wall (Fig. 33.7a). *Bartholin* gland cysts are located within the posterior lateral vagina and are within the labia majora [11]. They are most easily distinguished based on histologic appearance although Skene's glands, Gartner's ducts, and Bartholin gland cysts are of Wolffian duct origin. There are no reported tumor/cancers associated with paraurethral cysts. While most paraurethral cysts resolve spontaneously, a small group of paraurethral cysts (Fig. 33.7a, teenager) are refractory or persistent and require surgical manipulation including: incision and drainage, complete excision, or marsupialization.

MRI appears to be the best noninvasive imaging tool for determination of urethral pathology if a thorough physical exam is inconclusive or confirms the diagnosis [12]. MRI may also differentiate paraurethral cysts from urethral diverticula, ectopic ureteroceles, and imperforate hymen. Imaging does not replace the careful physical exam, however. So in evaluating these diagnoses, the physical examination should be completed first. If the physical exam threatens to traumatize the child, an exam under anesthesia (EUA) should be offered. While under anesthesia the urethra, bladder, and vagina may be inspected with the camera. Also under anesthesia, an evaluation with contrast may be placed in the ureteral orifice to evaluate the orientation of the ureter as the contrast travels up the ureter (retrograde pyelogram). Since imaging and physical examination may require specialist expertise to distinguish the aforementioned differential, a pediatric urologist is an appropriate first consultation.

## Ectopic Ureterocele and Ectopic Ureters

Ureteroceles are cystic dilation of the distal ureter likely secondary to congenital absence of opening of the distal ureter as it enters the bladder. Orthotopic ureteroceles are, by definition, found in the usual location for a ureter in the bladder. Ectopic ureteroceles (cecoureterocele) are found in an array of other locations and may prolapse into the urethra (Fig. 33.8). In doing so, ectopic ureteroceles may be an externally visible

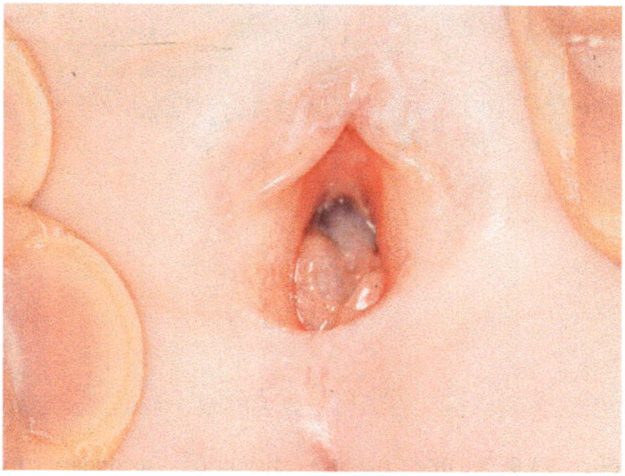

**Fig. 33.8** Ectopic ureteroceles can, in severe cases such as this, project from the urethral meatus

part of the genitourinary tract [13]. Ectopic ureteroceles may either obstruct the ureter or the urethra, which in either case promotes urinary stasis or retention [14]. Urinary retention requires urgent determination and management—this diagnosis may be aided by a simple physical examination (palpable bladder, see Fig. 33.9). If there is evidence of retention, the child's management should include immediate catheter drainage.

Ectopic ureters may be located distal to or outside to the urinary (external) sphincter and therefore promote continuous urinary leakage from an ectopic location (non-normal anatomic location, i.e., vagina). The patient or patient's parent(s) may express concern for continuous urinary leakage (i.e., "never dry"). Ectopic ureters may be associated with a nonfunctioning or poorly functioning upper pole of the kidney, when there is duplication.

Ultrasound is often diagnostic of ureteroceles. Voiding cystourethrogram (VCUG), renal scanning, and retrograde pyelogram provide additional useful information, such as associated urinary reflux and a poorly functioning portion of kidney, and can distinguish between a ureterocele and paraurethral cyst [15]. Magnetic resonance imaging of the urinary tract (MRU) is very helpful (if available in your local institution) for ruling out ectopic ureters when there are suspicious symptoms (i.e., persistent urinary incontinence). If the ureter is infected and obstructed, incision

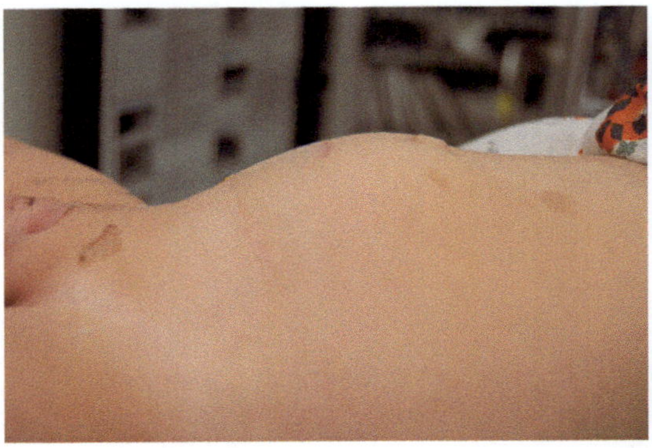

**Fig. 33.9** Visible bladder distention secondary to obstruction

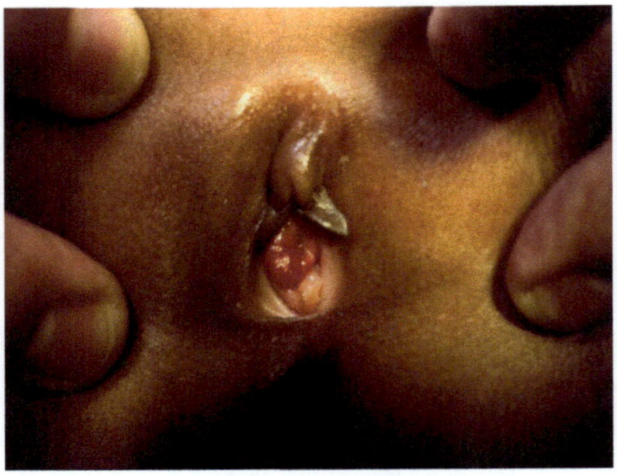

**Fig. 33.10** Circumferential prolapse of the urethral mucosa

and drainage may be necessary to avoid progression to urinary sepsis. Definitive repair would be undertaken later and may depend on results of VCUG, renal scan, retrograde pyelogram, and experience of the pediatric urologist. The management of ectopic ureteroceles is quite controversial, and the ranges of surgical options vary. If available, seek a pediatric urologist to help determine the best approach.

## Urethral Abnormalities

### Urethral Prolapse

Urethral prolapse is the circumferential eversion of the urethral mucosa out of the urethral meatus/orifice (Fig. 33.10). The everted mucosa may become edematous, friable, and necrotic. Symptoms include bleeding, dysuria (pain with urination), and frequency although some patients are asymptomatic. While urethral prolapse has been suggested to be more common in African-American girls, other populations of girls may also experience urethral prolapse as well. It is believed that estrogen deficiency is associated with this problem, and management has therefore included topical estrogen cream. For children having difficulty urinating or dysuria, Epsom salt sitz bath may offer some relief. If after conservative treatment the urethral prolapse persists, the next step is surgical management to reduce or excise the prolapsed area.

### Urethral Duplication

Urethral duplication is a rare entity and rarer in girls compared to boys [16] (Fig. 33.11). Only 35 cases of urethral duplication in females have been reported in the literature [17]. Epispadias, urinary incontinence, perineal discharge, and urinary tract infection may be associated with this problem. Imaging to evaluate for associated renal, spinal, and vaginal abnormalities is important. Urethral duplication may be associated with vaginal and anal duplication. Management often includes surgical reconstruction. Your local pediatric urology colleague is typically the most experienced in this management approach.

### Urogenital Sinus (Persistent Cloaca)

Urogenital (UG) sinus is the term used for a common opening that communicates with the urethra, vagina, and rectum during development (Figs. 33.12 and 33.13). A persistent urogenital sinus or cloaca is abnormal. It represents the failure of the cloacal membrane to dissolute and septum normally formed between the urinary and intestinal tract to be absent. The severity of persistent cloaca usually requires imaging: a genitogram, cystogram, and endoscopy of the urogenital sinus. A genitogram requires the placement of contrast dye into urogenital sinus (genitogram) to study its length

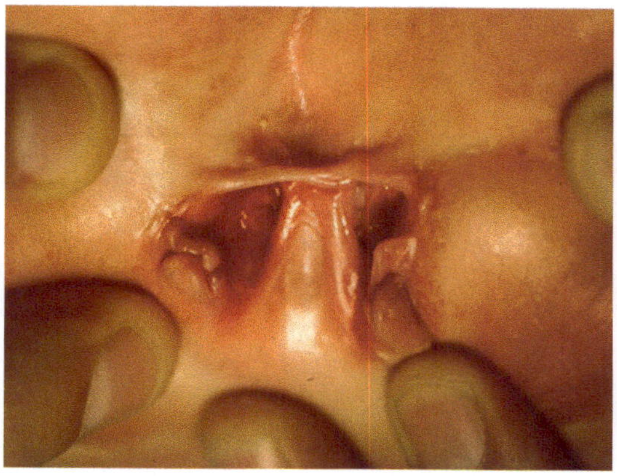

**Fig. 33.11** Urethral duplication is a rare condition with a complex treatment strategy

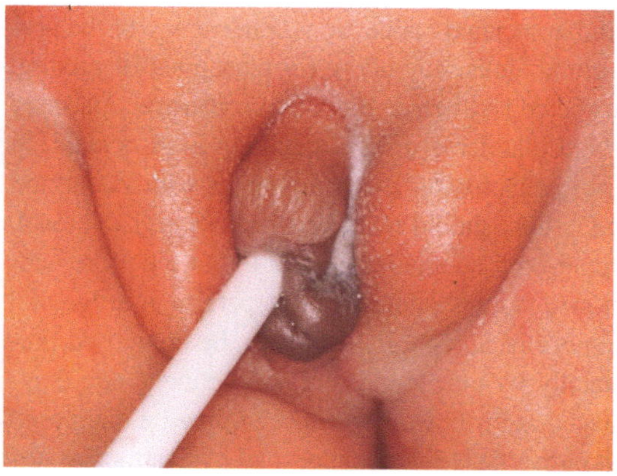

**Fig. 33.12** This catheter has been inserted into a common urogenital sinus which in this case drains both vagina and bladder (see Fig. 33.13)

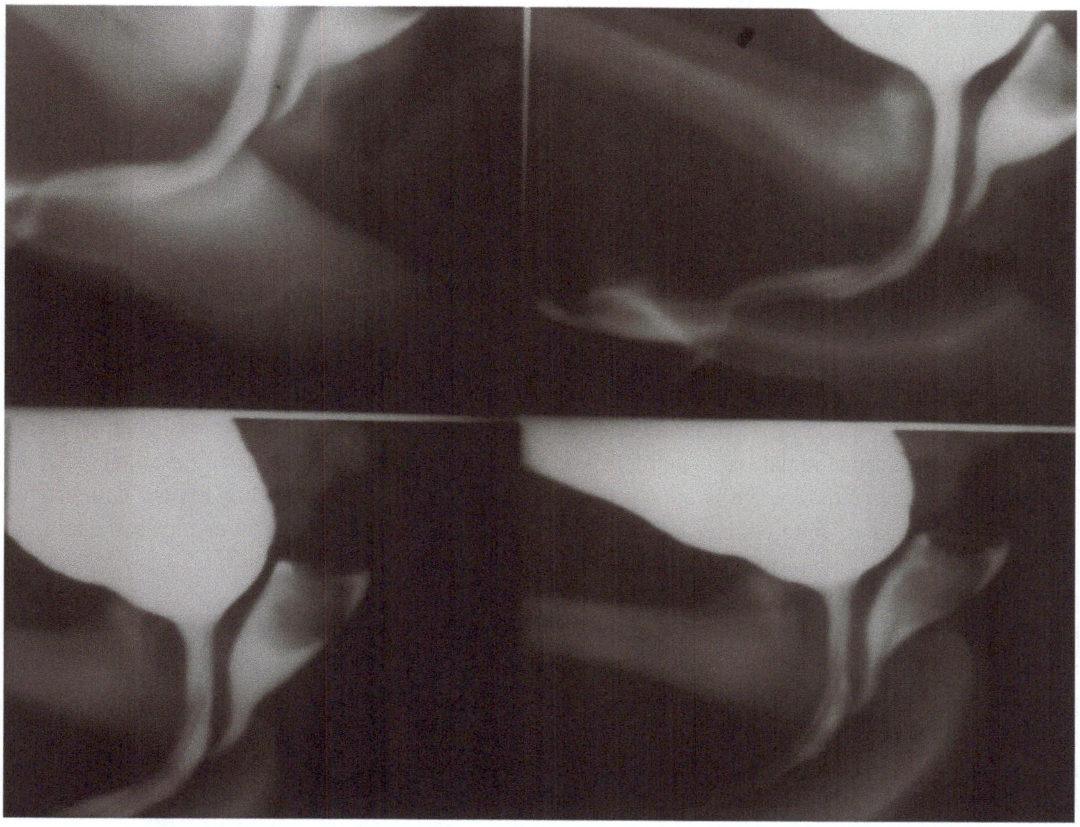

**Fig. 33.13** This genitogram demonstrates common urogenital sinus with the vagina and urethra converging distally (low, closer to the perineum)

and associated connections. Endoscopy of the urogenital sinus may allow for placement of urethral catheter just before definitive reconstruction or to drain bladder if urinary retention is associated. In the evaluation process, all patients with a common UG sinus should be evaluated for cardiac, spinal, renal limb anomalies in addition to the aforementioned studies to evaluate the persistent urogenital sinus/cloaca [18]. Patients may be diagnosed prenatally by ultrasound, but most patients are diagnosed at birth. Rarely, children may be diagnosed at pubarche [19]. Partial or total reconstructive surgery often occurs in infancy. With a longer urogenital sinus tract, the surgical repair to separate the single channel or externalize multiple channels within a single orifice is more complex than with shorter tracts [20]. Despite the strides in reconstructive techniques that have improved the continence rates over the years, fecal and urinary continence are common issues even after surgical reconstruction. A team approach including the expertise of pediatric urologist and pediatric general surgeons is important for the management of these patients.

## Hymenal Abnormalities

### Child Abuse

The normal hymen is a tissue that envelops the vaginal os, with multiple configurations around the opening, but in a normal female an opening exists. The shape and size of the hymen is not a reliable indicator of sexual intercourse, abuse, or molestation. Hymenal injury may occur secondary to digits, foreign objects, tampons, etc. Signs of blood, tears/fissures in the hymen, and purulent material emanating from the vaginal os should be pictorially documented proactively and investigated thoroughly. At times the suspicion for molestation is present and if so should be evaluated by the appropriate investigative organization in your medical system and appropriately managed or addressed for the benefit of ensuring a safe environment for the child. The primary clinician has an important role in evaluating female patients for such abnormalities in a routine physical exam, as well in cases of documented trauma/abuse.

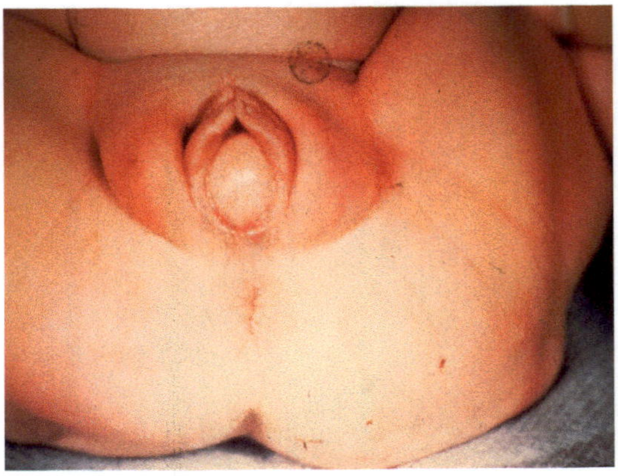

**Fig. 33.14** Imperforate hymen seen bulging between the labia in a newborn

### Imperforate Hymen

An imperforate hymen presents as a mass bulging from between the labia below the urethra [21] (Fig. 33.14). As the name suggests, an imperforate hymen is abnormally unopened vaginal os. In the neonate, the mass/bulge is from vaginal and uterine secretions due to maternal estrogen exposure. The treatment is often incision of the hymen and drainage of the vagina. In the case of a covered hymen (Fig. 33.14b) without a bulge, because secretions of vaginal glands are drained, there is typically an opening, usually toward the pubis. While an imperforate hymen requires intervention, a covered hymen does not. If there is confusion as to the diagnosis, consult your pediatric urologist. The primary care provider has an important role in evaluating female patients for such abnormalities in a routine physical exam.

### Hematometrocolpos

Hematometrocolpos may arise as a result of imperforate hymen, vaginal atresia, or status post vaginal reconstruction resulting in vaginal stenosis. It may be associated with uterine duplication [22] (Figs. 33.15, 33.16, and 33.17). Duplicated uteri when associated with patent duplicated vagina (Fig. 33.17), however, do not typically result in hematometrocolpos [23]. Hematometrocolpos constitutes painful monthly episodes because of monthly menstrual flow. Surgical management

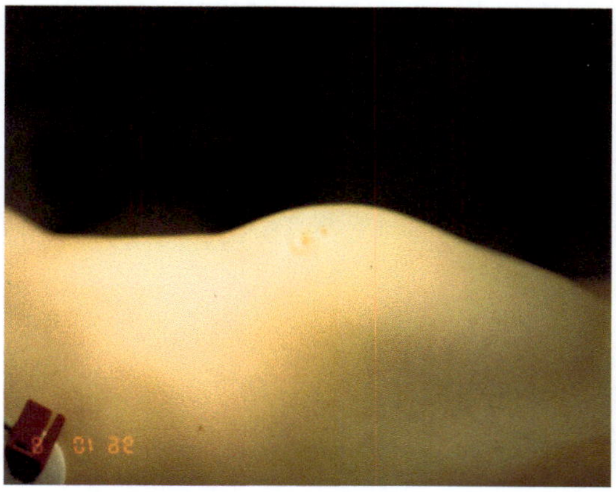

**Fig. 33.15** Distended abdomen in a patient with hematometrocolpos

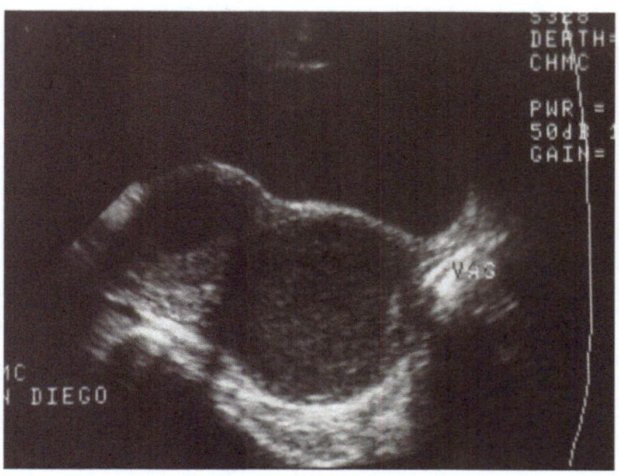


**Fig. 33.16** Pelvic ultrasound in a patient with hematometrocolpos demonstrating a dilated uterus

ranges from urgent percutaneous drainage to definitive hysterectomy due to painful symptomatology. Rarely, urinary retention occur secondary to the nearby obstructing mass compressing the urethra. Nonsurgical management may include hormonal therapy (Figs. 33.15 and 33.16) to suppress the cyclical menstrual flow. A urology/gynecology team approach may help with imaging determination and/or surgical reconstruction or ablation as is necessary.

## Hymenal Polyp

A hymenal polyp is a polypoid structure arising from the posterior aspect of the vagina. These patients are rarely symptomatic and intervention is rarely necessary (Fig. 33.18). Most hymenal polyps regress spontaneously. The lesion is believed to be a remnant of the urorectal septum [24]. If the polyp persists or symptoms occur, consult a pediatric urologist for further management.

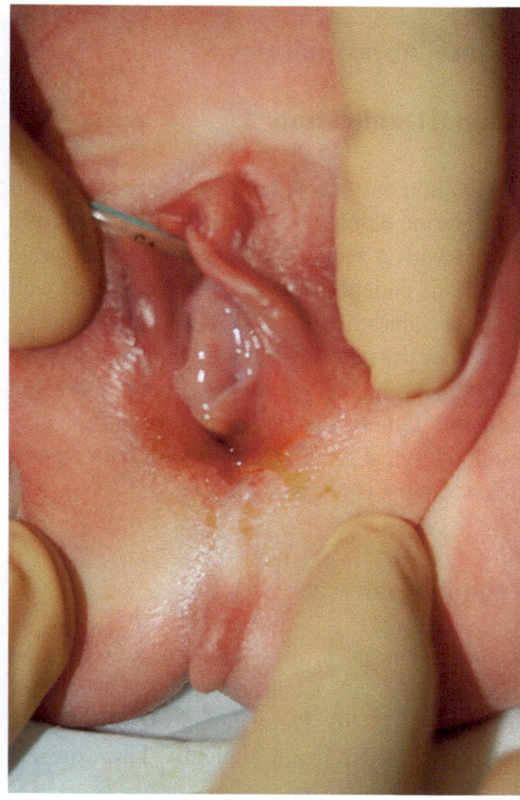

**Fig. 33.17** Duplication of the vagina

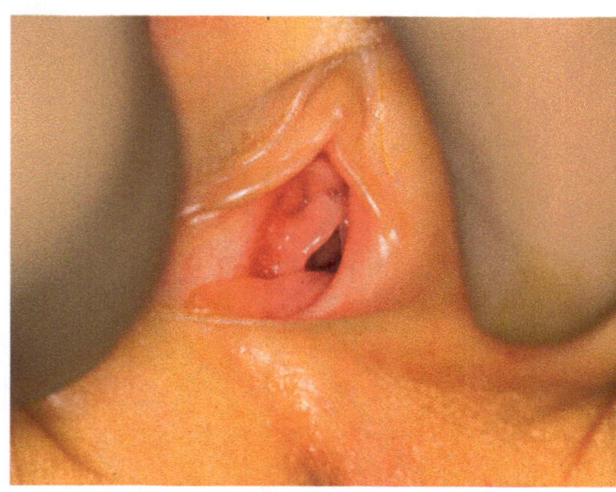

**Fig. 33.18** Hymenal polyp projecting from the posterior vaginal introitus

# Vaginal Abnormalities

## Vaginal Duplication

Duplication on the vagina is typically associated with uterine didelphys. Figure 33.19 illustrates a patient with a rectal fistula and an imperforate anus. This patient also has cardiac, renal, as well as spinal abnormalities. Vaginal duplication by itself does warrant surgical intervention but poses potential problems for menses, pregnancy, and delivery. Other associated abnormalities may require surgical repair. Consultation with a pediatric urologist is necessary.

## Vaginal Agenesis

Vaginal agenesis is most commonly associated with the Mayer-Rokitansky-Küster-Hauser syndrome (Fig. 33.20). These patients have a normal karyotype (46XX) and typically have present ovaries. Patients with vaginal agenesis have a normally placed urethral meatus with the clitoris at the 12 o'clock ventral position above it. Because of this relatively normal genital configuration, this problem may go undiagnosed until the age of menarche. These patients present with amenorrhea (absent onset of menses). On physical exam, a cotton tip may be use to assess the depth of the vagina. This condition may be related to renal anomalies, and a renal ultrasound should be considered. Treatment may range from serial dilation procedures to complete vaginal construction.

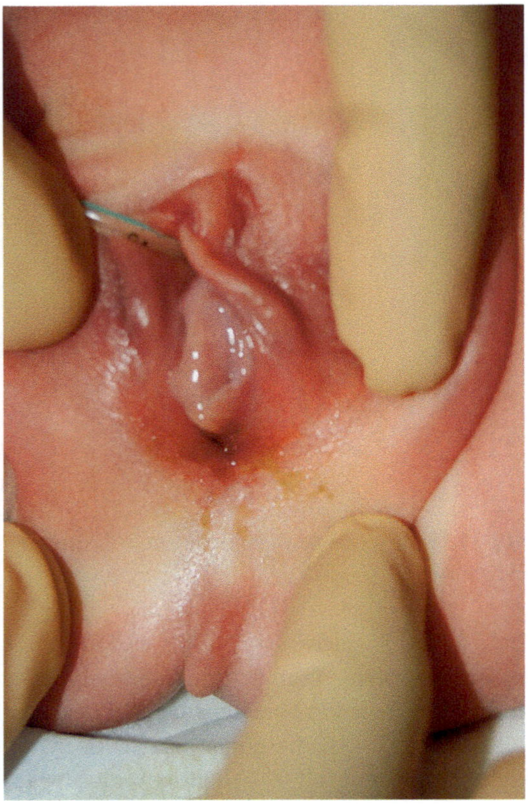

**Fig. 33.19** Duplication of the vagina

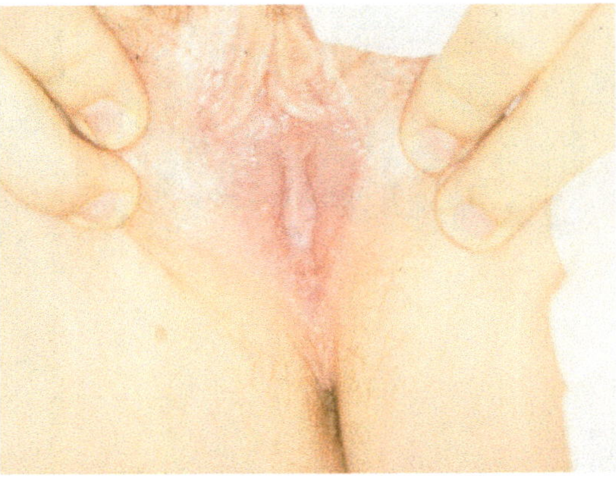

**Fig. 33.20** A patient with vaginal agenesis. Note the clitoral hood and normal urethral placement with an absent vaginal introitus

## Vulvovaginitis

Inflammation or infection of the vagina at the os or within the vault is called vulvovaginitis. The most common presentation is that of purulent vaginal drainage. The most common etiology of this presentation in a little girl is a foreign body. Although children explore themselves externally, very naturally, little girls often avoid placing foreign body into orifices unless they are witness to this behavior in others. This behavior when uncovered in a little girl should raise the suspicion of inappropriate sexual contact or behavior in front of the child. As in all cases of suspicion for molestation, additional questioning and evaluation is warranted, but the suspicious situations do in no way guarantee a misadventure toward the child prompted by inappropriate unsafe contact with child by parents or other contacts.

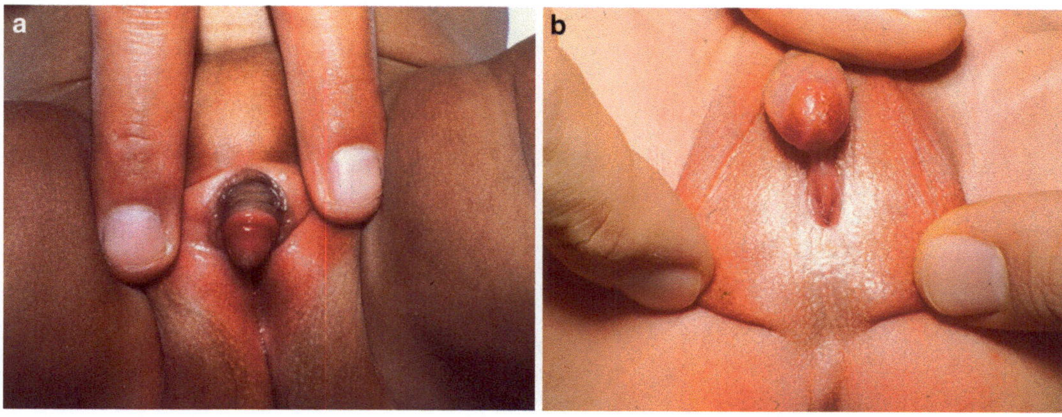


**Fig. 33.21** (**a, b**) These female patients with congenital adrenal hyperplasia have virilized genitalia and a common UG sinus which can easily be confused with a hypospadias penis

## Sarcoma Botryoides

Sarcoma botryoides is a soft tissue cancer (a subtype of embryonal rhabdomyosarcoma) that originates submucosally within gynecological structures (uterus, cervix, vulva, and vagina) and may present as a "bunch of grapes" at the perineum. The onset of presentation is often but not exclusively found in girls less than 5 years of age. The treatment includes radical surgery of pelvic organs, radiation therapy, and chemotherapy. Because the disease has a low survival rate, a sensitive discussion with patient and family members is critical from the onset of suspecting the diagnosis. A team approach to the management includes the expertise of pediatric oncologist, gynecologist, general surgeons, and urologist.

## Clitoral Abnormalities

### Congenital Adrenal Hyperplasia

Congenital adrenal hyperplasia is the most common intersex disorder (Fig. 33.21). It is a hereditary disorder that primarily affects the female fetus. When it affects genotypic females in utero, external female genitalia become virilized, and the clitoris has the appearance of a hypospadias penis. Genetic females do not have palpable external gonads [25]. The most common genetic mutation associated with congenital adrenal hyperplasia is 21-hydroxylase deficiency [26]. 11-Beta-hydroxylase and 3-beta-hydroxylase deficiencies are less common forms of congenital adrenal hyperplasia. The phenotype of an affected patient is not the only issue. Affected patients can have electrolyte abnormalities and may be hemodynamically unstable secondary to salt wasting. Electrolytes are a critical part of the evaluation and may require urgent management to correct the abnormalities. This is especially important in the immediate neonatal period for males in which diagnosis is not as obvious since the additional virilizing hormones would make no difference phenotypically. Children affected by CAH may benefit from endocrine hormone replacements [27]. A pediatric endocrinologist would likely be helpful in confirming the diagnosis of CAH and managing the dosing of hormonal replacements. Lab evaluation generally consists of plasma cortisol, 17-hydroxyprogesterone, androstenedione, renin, aldosterone, and urinary ketosteroids. The mother of children with CAH may take dexamethasone to prevent virilization of the phallus in the female fetus. Dexamethasone is implemented in the first trimester of pregnancy and continued at least until the XX karyotype may be determined. A female fetus would need continued maternal administration of dexamethasone, and male fetus would not. A pediatric urologist is particularly helpful with reconstructing a female phallus and creating a neovagina. Surgical reconstruction early may be useful for parents, but the reconstruction may be delayed. Controversy exists about the timing of surgery for these children.

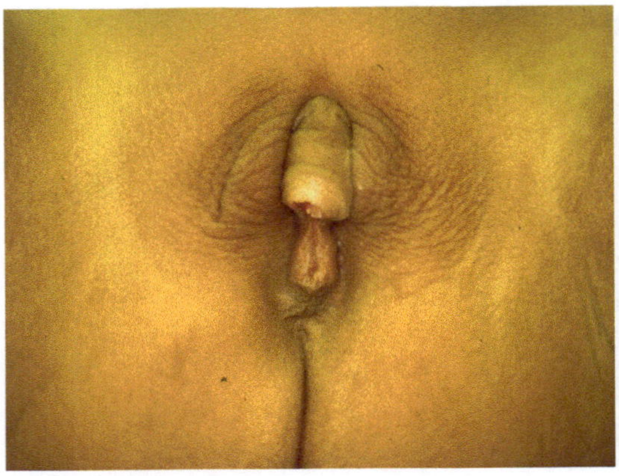

**Fig. 33.22** Androgen exposure in utero can lead to a wide variety of phenotypes depending on the degree of exposure. In this case, the labia are more darkly pigmented and have ruggated skin; the clitoris is also enlarged

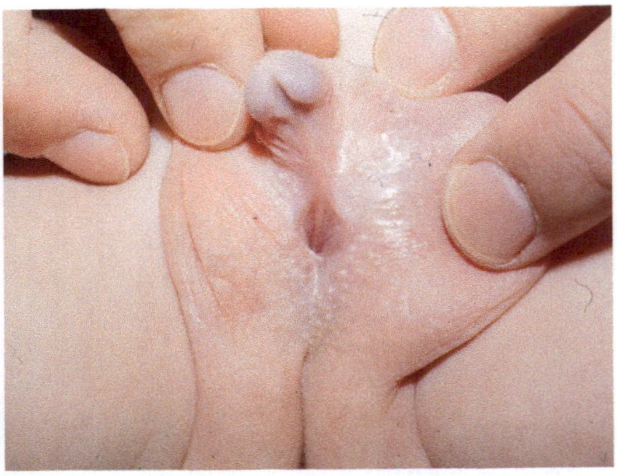

**Fig. 33.23** In mixed gonadal dysgenesis, the presence of asymmetrical labia—in this case secondary to a descended testis—can point toward the diagnosis

## Prenatal Androgen Exposure

Prenatal androgen exposure can virilize a female fetus (Fig. 33.22). Because there is no ongoing genetic perturbation, electrolytes and endocrine hormones are normal. Surgical reconstruction is likely all that is necessary for management. Consult your pediatric urologist.

## Mixed Gonadal Dysgenesis

Mixed gonadal dysgenesis is the second most common intersex disorder [28] (Fig. 33.23). The most common genotypes associated with this disorder are 45X0 and 46XY. The phenotype may be a hypospadias phallus, asymmetric labioscrotal folds, or unilateral palpable gonad. A palpable gonad typically has testicular tissue, and the other gonad is usually a streak [29]. This neonate deserves a pelvic ultrasound to confirm the absence of female internal genital structures. Gender assignment is less controversial in these populations, and a male gender assignment is more common [30]. Consult a pediatric urologist.

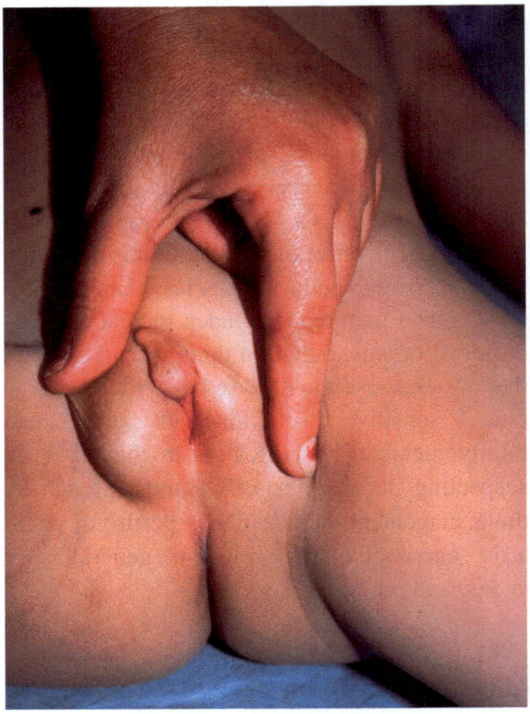

**Fig. 33.24** Patients with 5-alpha-reductase deficiencies are genotypic males who have undervirilized genitalia. Here, one can see a common UG sinus and small phallus

## 5-Alpha Reductase Deficiency

5-Alpha reductase deficiency is a form of male pseudohermaphroditism where the genotype is 46XY and the gonads are testes but testosterone cannot be converted to dihydrotestosterone (DHT) (Fig. 33.24). Since DHT is responsible for virilization of the external genitalia of the male fetus, the external genitalia may look ambiguous [31]. Diagnosis of the 5-alpha reductase deficiency may be difficult and requires a high index of suspicion. The phenotype is a wide spectrum

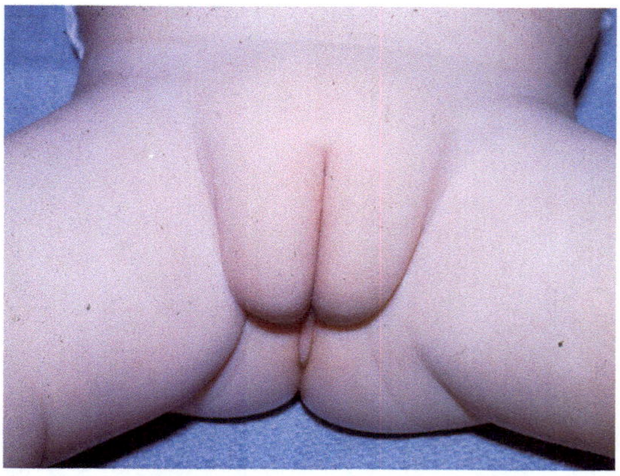

**Fig. 33.25** This patient with complete androgen insensitivity, while appearing phenotypically female, is a genotypic male

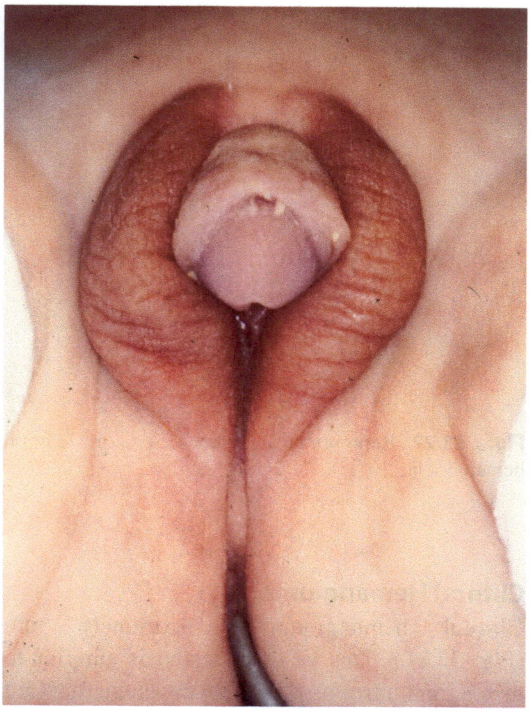

**Fig. 33.26** True hermaphroditism is defined as the presence of both ovarian and testicular tissue. The phenotypic presentation is variable

of ambiguity, and most have a female phenotype and appear to have an enlarged clitoris and single urogenital sinus opening. By this ambiguous genital appearance, electrolytes, a karyotype, and endocrine hormones are appropriate next steps to distinguish this entity from other intersex states. When there is high index of suspicion, testosterone/dihydrotestosterone ratio and HCG stimulation test levels should be obtained. Imaging studies should include pelvic ultrasound and genitogram. Although there is not much of a phallus in these children and reconstruction may be difficult, there is androgen imprinting in utero that impacts on sexual identity later in life. The sex of rearing is controversial, and so gender reassignment early in life is premature [32].

## Testicular Feminization

Testicular feminization or complete androgen insensitivity syndrome occurs as a result of a defect in the androgen receptor (Fig. 33.25). These children therefore lack virilization of the genitalia in a male child. The child appears phenotypically female but is genetically male. This child may present with groin bulge representing a hernia in a phenotypic female [33]. A hernia in a female always warrants a karyotype and evaluation by pediatric urologist to manage hernia and confirm the diagnosis [34]. A blood karyotype and pelvic ultrasound are appropriate to aid diagnosis. Typically these phenotypically female children are expected to have menses in puberty, and a diagnosis is made when they are amenorrheic [35].

## True Hermaphrodite

True hermaphroditism is an intersex state in which both an ovary and a testis exist in the same patient (Fig. 33.26). The gonads have variable presentation: 1/3 have ovotestes bilaterally, another 1/3 have ovotestis/ovary combination, and the remaining third have either ovotestis/testis or ovary/testis [36]. Associated with this wide spectrum of gonads are their ipsilateral internal structure phenotypes which favor the female default when an ovotestis is present [37]. The diagnosis is aided by obtaining the karyotype, gonadal tissue biopsy, and pelvic ultrasound. Sex assignment may be difficult and is controversial. Sex of rearing will determine the gonad removed [38].

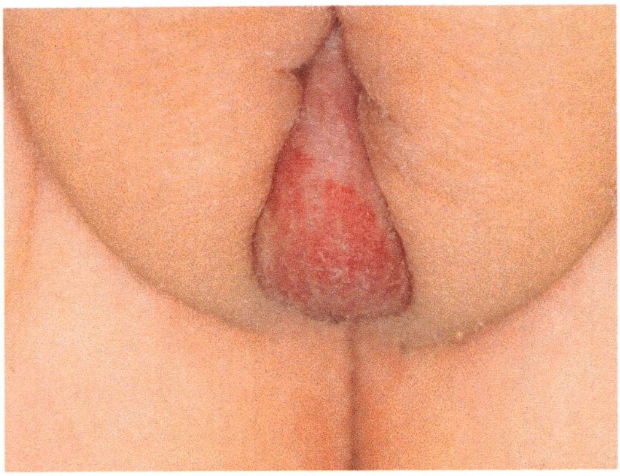

**Fig. 33.27** Representative photo of a clitoral hemangiomas

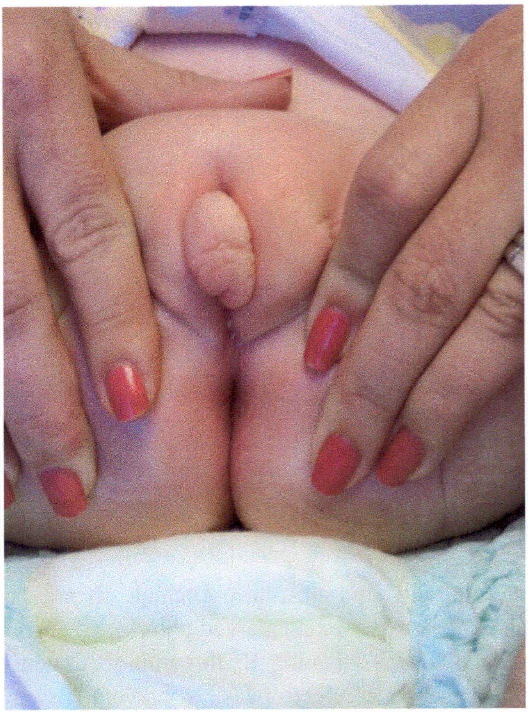

**Fig. 33.28** Representative photo of a patient with clitoral lymphedema. Etiology of the edema is often never found

### Clitoral Hemangioma

Clitoral hemangioma is extremely rare (Fig. 33.27). This vascular lesion is anterior to the vaginal introitus [39]. Few cases are reported in the literature. Management trends toward surgical excision [40]. No laboratory or imaging studies are necessary. The natural history of these lesions is unknown.

### Clitoral Lymphedema

Clitoral lymphedema is rare and may be self-limited (Fig. 33.28). The etiology is often unknown, and treatment is supportive although an effort to uncover an etiology is often pursued. Consult pediatric urology, gynecology, and oncology for infectious disease.

### Clitoral Agenesis

Clitoral agenesis is a rare condition and may be accompanied by other abnormalities including other genital hypoplasia. A urologic evaluation is appropriate.

### Epispadias

It is a forme fruste of exstrophy. There is an associated pubic diathesis. Urinary incontinence may be a feature of this anomaly. Urologic reconstruction may help with both cosmesis and functional abnormality.

### Female Circumcision

Clinicians in the United States of America are increasingly exposed to unfamiliar cultural customs. One of which is the operation of the female external genitalia. Since the practice is not commonly accepted or encouraged in non-Islamic cultures, it is especially important to be respectful and not subject the patient to undue stress because of this performed procedure. The practice includes a variation of manipulation of clitoral, vulval, and hymenal tissues that involves both cutting and suturing typically performed by a local village practitioner in some countries outside of the USA. There may be complications from genital manipulation process called "female circumcision." Urologic or gynecologic evaluation is not necessary unless the patient, family, or primary care physician requests further evaluation.

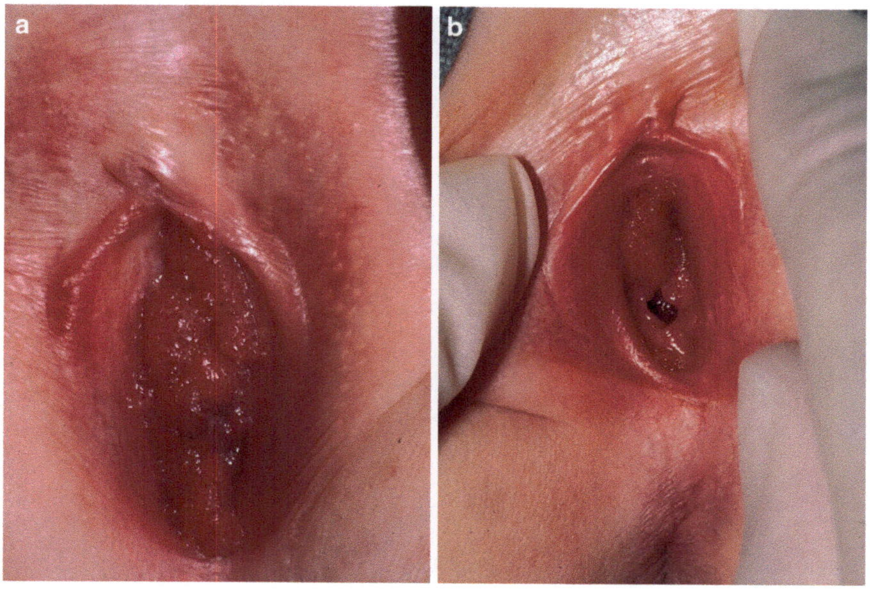

**Fig. 33.29** Condyloma may present on any genital surface or around the anus and raises suspicion for sexual abuse

## Infection/Inflammation

### Condyloma

Condyloma is due to human papilloma virus, and location is typically a site of microtraumas (Fig. 33.29). These lesions may be associated with sexual intercourse, sexual abuse, passage through the birth canal, etc. Symptoms are usually itching and vulvar pain. These lesions may occur on any location on the genitals. Acetic acid (vinegar) whitens these lesions and may be diagnostic. Topical agents such as Aldara 5 % of Podophyllin are therapeutic. Dermatologists or urologists are appropriate tertiary care consultants. Urologic evaluation of internal structures may be appropriate to evaluate the extent of the lesions as lesions may be found within the vagina. Biopsies of the lesions are rarely indicated given the characteristic appearance of the lesions [41].

### Molluscum Contagiosum

A characteristic umbilicated lesion that may be seen on any body part is molluscum contagiosum. As the name suggests, it is contagious. Concern for sexual molestation is not unwarranted but not guaranteed. Therefore care providers ought to critically question or evaluate for additional evidence that may substantiate a sexual molestation evaluation [42]. The questioning of care providers around the topic of molestation is challenging and should be handled with care. Molluscum contagiosum may be managed with a number of different methods ranging from topical medications to surgical excision.

## Bony Abnormalities

### Spinal Dysraphism

A spinal column congenital abnormality associated with spinal cord and meningeal abnormality is called spinal dysraphism (Fig. 33.30). Spinal dysraphism encompasses a broad spectrum of these abnormalities at varying thoracic levels, including caudal agenesis and spina bifida. The external genitalia of these patients are typically normal. On occasion, the bony abnormalities of the lower extremities make it difficult to expose the child for evaluation of external genitalia. A pediatric urologist is one of many in a team of

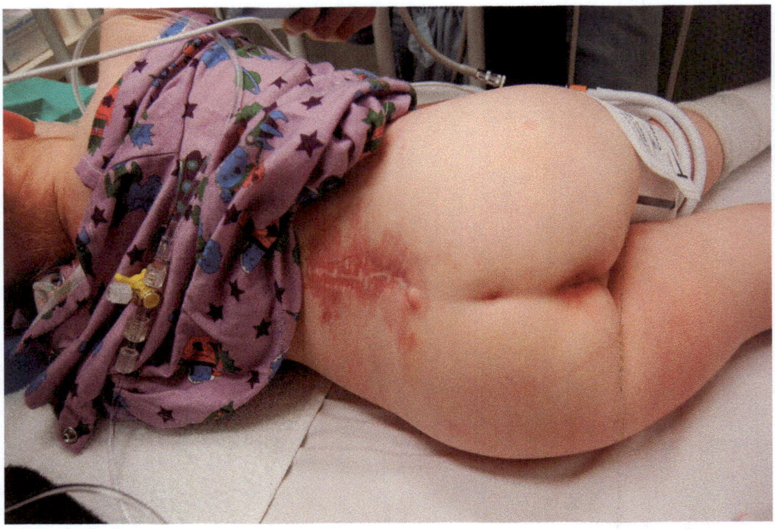

**Fig. 33.30** A child after closure of a lumbar-sacral spinal defect

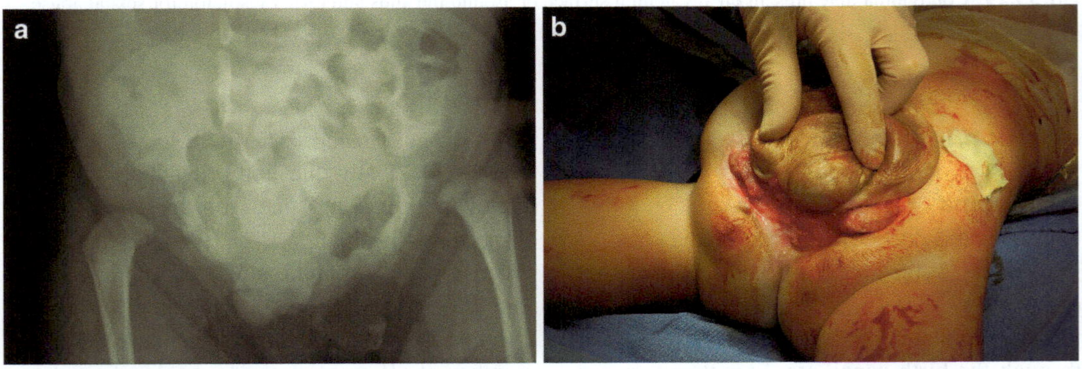


**Fig. 33.31** (**a**) Abdominal X-ray in a newborn with classic exstrophy. Note the external rotation of the hips secondary to the pubic diathesis. (**b**) Representative photo of a child with an omphalocele, exstrophy of the bladder, imperforate anus, and spinal dysraphism (OEIS complex)

doctors that are typically involved in the care of these patients because of their complex constellation of symptoms which includes urinary and bowel retention or incontinence.

## Exstrophy

The bladder is a spherical structure that is normally internal to the abdominal wall in an extraperitoneal location just superior and dorsal to the pubic bone within the pelvis (Fig. 33.31). When the bladder is plate flush with the abdominal wall and the pubic bone is separated (pubic diathesis), this is called exstrophy. There are two categories of exstrophy: classic isolated bladder exstrophy and cloacal exstrophy. Classic bladder exstrophy is about 10× less common than cloacal exstrophy (1 in 400,000). Cloacal exstrophy requires the expertise of a pediatric general surgeon, pediatric orthopedic surgeon, and pediatric urologist to manage the bowel, bone, and bladder abnormalities, respectively. Classic bladder exstrophy usually requires a pediatric urologist and pediatric orthopedic surgeon who have experience in the management of the bladder and bony abnormalities as well as the timing of repair.

## References


1. Starr NB. Labial adhesions in childhood. J Pediatr Health Care. 1996;10:26–7.
2. Myers JB, Sorensen CM, Wisner BP, Furness PD, Passamaneck M, Koyle MA. Betamethasone cream for the treatment of pre-pubertal labial adhesions. J Pediatr Adolesc Gynecol. 2006;19:407–11.
3. Leung AK, Robson WL, Tay-Uyboco J. The incidence of labial fusion in children. J Paediatr Child Health. 1993;29:235–6.
4. Clair DL, Caldamone AA. Pediatric office procedures. Urol Clin North Am. 1988;15:715.
5. Lynch A, Marulaiah M, Samarakkody U. Reduction labioplasty in adolescents. J Pediatr Adolesc Gynecol. 2008;21(3):147–9.
6. Rouzier R, Louis-Sylvestre C, Paniel BJ, Haddad B. Hypertrophy of labia minora: experience with 163 reductions. Am J Obstet Gynecol. 2000;182 (1 Pt 1):35–40.
7. Deppisch LM. Cysts of the vagina: classification and clinical correlations. Obstet Gynecol. 1975;45(6):632–7.
8. Herek O, Ergin H, Karaduman D, Cetin O, Akşit MA. Paraurethral cysts in newborn: a case report and review of literature. Eur J Pediatr Surg. 2000; 10(1):65–7.
9. Ceylan H, Ozokutan BH, Karakök M, Buyukbese S. Paraurethral cyst: is conservative management always appropriate? Eur J Pediatr Surg. 2002; 12(3):212–4.
10. Fujimoto T, Suwa T, Ishii N, Kabe K. Paraurethral cyst in female newborn: is surgery always advocated? J Pediatr Surg. 2007;42(2):400–3.
11. Kondi-Pafiti A, Grapsa D, Papakonstantinou K, Kairi-Vassilatou E, Xasiakos D. Vaginal cysts: a common pathologic entity revisited. Clin Exp Obstet Gynecol. 2008;35(1):41–4.
12. Holmes M, Upadhyay V, Pease P. Gartner's duct cyst with unilateral renal dysplasia presenting as an introital mass in a new born. Pediatr Surg Int. 1999; 15(3–4):277–9.
13. Ilica AT, Kocaoğlu M, Bulakbaşi N, Sürer I, Tayfun C. Prolapsing ectopic ureterocele presenting as a vulval mass in a newborn girl. Diagn Interv Radiol. 2008;14(1):33–4.
14. Merlini E, Lelli Chiesa P. Obstructive ureterocele-an ongoing challenge. World J Urol. 2004;22((2)):107–14. Epub 2004 Jun 15.
15. Berrocal T, López-Pereira P, Arjonilla A, Gutiérrez J. Anomalies of the distal ureter, bladder, and urethra in children: embryologic, radiologic, and pathologic features. Radiographics. 2002;22(5):1139–64.
16. Stephens F. Abnormal embryology-cloacal dysgenesis: congenital malformations of the urinary tract. New York: Praeger Publishing Scientific; 1983. p. 15–52.
17. Cost NG, Lucas SM, Baker LA, Wilcox DT. Two girls with urethral duplication. Urology. 2008;72(4): 800–2.
18. Diamond DA. Sexual differentiation: normal and abnormal. In: Walsh PC, Retik AB, Darracott Vaughan E, Wein AJ, editors. Campbell's urology. 8th ed. Philadelphia: WB Saunders; 2002. p. 2395–427.
19. Maclellan DL, Diamond DA. Recent advances in external genitalia. Pediatr Clin North Am. 2006; 53(3):449–64.
20. Kryger JV, Gonzalez R. Urinary continence is well preserved after total urogenital mobilization. J Urol. 2004;172(6 Pt 1):2384–6.
21. Winderl LM, Silverman RK. Prenatal diagnosis of congenital imperforate hymen. Obstet Gynecol. 1995;85(5 Pt 2):857–60.
22. Tseng JJ, Ho JY, Chen WH, Chou MM. Prenatal diagnosis of isolated fetal hydrocolpos secondary to congenital imperforate hymen. J Chin Med Assoc. 2008;71(6):325–8.
23. Dhombres F, Jouannic JM, Brodaty G, Bessiere B, Daffos F, Bénifla JL. Contribution of prenatal imaging to the anatomical assessment of fetal hydrocolpos. Ultrasound Obstet Gynecol. 2007;30(1):101–4.
24. Borglin NE, Selander P. Hymenal polyps in newborn infants. Acta Paediatr. 1962;51(S135):28–31.
25. Hughes IA. Early management and gender assignment in disorders of sexual differentiation. Endocr Dev. 2007;11:47–57. Review.
26. Ghizzoni L, Cesari S, Cremonini G, Melandri L. Prenatal and early postnatal treatment of congenital adrenal hyperplasia. Endocr Dev. 2007;11:58–69. Review.
27. Brown J, Warne G. Practical management of the intersex infant. J Pediatr Endocrinol Metab. 2005; 18(1):3–23.
28. Federman DD, Donahoe PK. Ambiguous genitalia–etiology, diagnosis, and therapy. Adv Endocrinol Metab. 1995;6:91–116.
29. Hsu LY. Prenatal diagnosis of 45, X/46, XY mosaicism–a review and update. Prenat Diagn. 1989; 9(1):31–48.
30. Bidarkar SS, Hutson JM. Evaluation and management of the abnormal gonad. Semin Pediatr Surg. 2005;14(2):118–23.
31. Imperato-McGinley J, Zhu YS. Androgens and male physiology the syndrome of 5alpha-reductase-2 deficiency. Mol Cell Endocrinol. 2002;198(1–2):51–9.
32. Byne W. Developmental endocrine influences on gender identity: implications for management of disorders of sex development. Mt Sinai J Med. 2006; 73(7):950–9.
33. Galani A, Kitsiou-Tzeli S, Sofokleous C, Kanavakis E, Kalpini-Mavrou A. Androgen insensitivity syndrome: clinical features and molecular defects. Hormones (Athens). 2008;7(3):217–29.
34. Gottlieb B, Pinsky L, Beitel LK, Trifiro M. Androgen insensitivity. Am J Med Genet. 1999;89(4):210–7.

35. Balducci R, Ghirri P, Brown TR, Bradford S, Boldrini B, Sciarra F, Toscano V. A clinician looks at androgen resistance. Steroids. 1996;61(4):205–11.
36. Walker AM, Walker JL, Adams S, Shi E, McGlynn M, Verge CF. True hermaphroditism. J Paediatr Child Health. 2000;36(1):69–73. Review.
37. Yordam N, Alikasifoglu A, Kandemir N, Caglar M, Balci S. True hermaphroditism: clinical features, genetic variants and gonadal histology. J Pediatr Endocrinol Metab. 2001;14(4):421–7.
38. Luks FI, Hansbrough F, Klotz Jr DH, Kottmeier PK, Tolete-Velcek F. Early gender assignment in true hermaphroditism. J Pediatr Surg. 1988;23(12):1122–6.
39. Strayer SA, Yum MN, Sutton GP. Epithelioid hemangioendothelioma of the clitoris: a case report with immunohistochemical and ultrastructural findings. Int J Gynecol Pathol. 1992;11(3):234–9.
40. Ishizu K, Nakamura K, Baba Y, Takihara H, Sakatoku J, Tanaka K. Clitoral enlargement caused by prepucial hemangioma: a case report. Hinyokika Kiyo. 1991;37(11):1563–5.
41. Khachemoune A, Guldbakke KK, Ehrsam E. Infantile perineal protrusion. J Am Acad Dermatol. 2006;54(6):1046–9.
42. Pandhi D, Kumar S, Reddy BS. Sexually transmitted diseases in children. J Dermatol. 2003;30(4):314–20.

# Ambiguous Genitalia

# 34

Luis Henrique Perocco Braga
and Joao Luiz Pippi Salle

## Definition

Ambiguous genitalia is a rare condition in which a newborn's external genitalia is not clearly male or female (Fig. 34.1).

It is caused by congenital conditions in which chromosomal, gonadal, or anatomical sex is atypical. There are four main categories of disorders of sex differentiation (DSD): 46XX DSD, 46XY DSD, ovotesticular DSD, and gonadal dysgenesis, either pure or mixed.

## Causes of Disorders of Sex Differentiation

1. Chromosomal abnormalities—Abnormalities in the number or structure of the sex chromosomes can cause abnormal gonadal differentiation resulting in deficient hormone production.
2. Partial or total androgen insensitivity can result in incomplete masculinization of the male fetus.
3. Primary endocrine disorders can alter androgen levels and cause undervirilization of a male or virilization of a female fetus.

L.H.P. Braga, M.D.
McMaster Children's Hospital, McMaster University, Hamilton, ON, Canada

J.L.P. Salle, M.D., Ph.D., F.R.C.S.C., F.A.A.P. (✉)
University of Toronto, Toronto, ON, Canada

The Hospital for Sick Children, Toronto, ON, Canada
e-mail: pippi.salle@sickkids.ca

## Who Should Be Investigated?

Evaluation to rule out DSD should be undertaken whenever two out of the three genital structures (penis and two testes) are abnormal. As shown in Fig. 34.2, the following possibilities may arise warranting investigation:

- Bilateral impalpable testes
- Hypospadias + unilateral undescended testis (Fig. 34.3)
- Micropenis + unilateral undescended testis
- Clitoral enlargement

Other situations that also call for investigation of DSD include:

1. Patients with ambiguous genitalia at birth. Although not typically classified as ambiguous, this includes males with a very small penis or girls with an enlarged clitoris or posterior labial fusion.
2. Adolescent girls with amenorrhea, inappropriate breast development, virilization, or onset of cyclical "hematuria."

## Evaluation of Patients with Ambiguous Genitalia

The goals of evaluating a child with ambiguous genitalia are (1) to establish genetic sex, (2) to determine the hormonal milieu, (3) to evaluate the anatomy of internal and external genitalia and gonads, and (4) in older children, to assess the phenotypic and psychological sex.

R. Rabinowitz et al. (eds.), *Pediatric Urology for the Primary Care Physician*, Current Clinical Urology,
DOI 10.1007/978-1-60327-243-8_34, © Springer Science+Business Media New York 2015

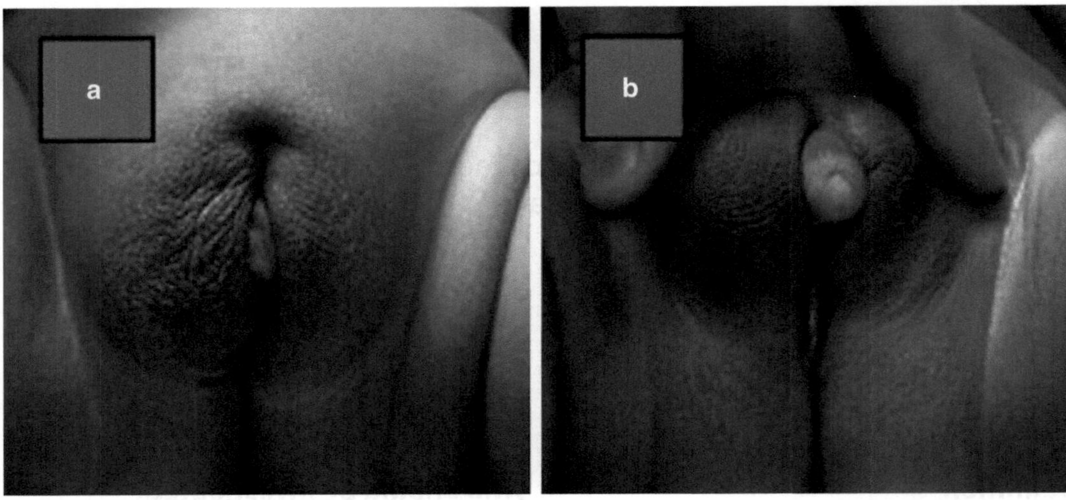


**Fig. 34.1** (**a**) Ambiguous genitalia in an infant who was thought to be a girl. (**b**) After investigation, clitoral enlargement and labia majora turned out to be a small phallus with perineal hypospadias and bifid scrotum

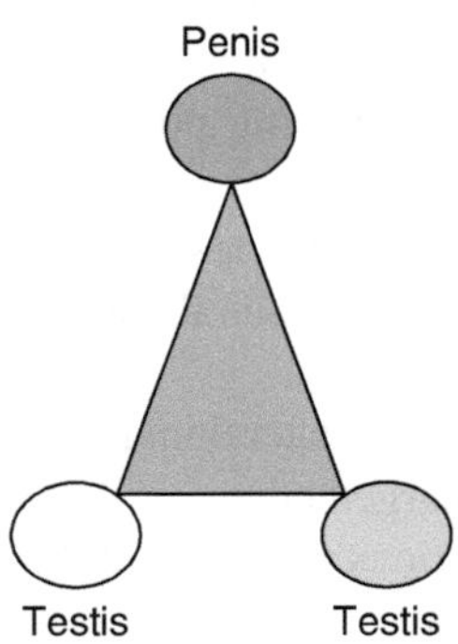


**Fig. 34.2** Rule of thumb for deciding when investigating for DSD

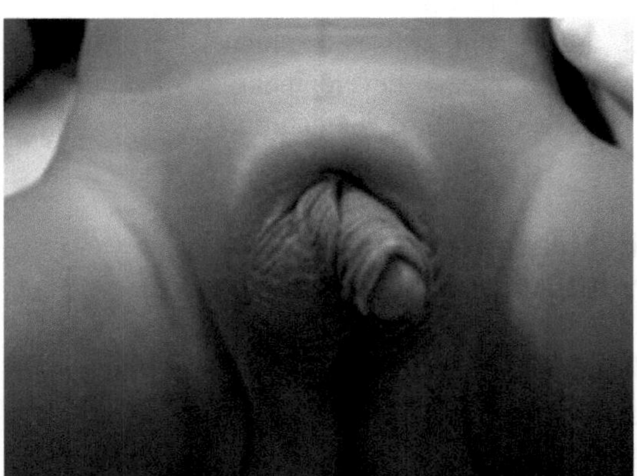

**Fig. 34.3** Unilateral undescended testis (empty left hemiscrotum) and hypospadias in a 2-year-old child with mixed gonadal dysgenesis raised as a boy

A newborn with ambiguous genitalia should have rapid assessment and, if possible, early gender assignment to minimize emotional trauma to the family. However, ethical implications should be considered and careful evaluation and discussion undertaken, as about one quarter of these patients as adults are now known to be dissatisfied with the sex of rearing that was allocated by the family and physicians. A multidisciplinary approach involving endocrinologist, pediatric urologist, neonatologist, geneticist and genetic counselor, pediatric gynecologist, psychologist, and social worker is required, and the decisions should always include the family. It should be based on the anatomo-physiological findings as well as the likely prognosis for behavior and gender orientation.

The four types of DSD mentioned above can present with sexual ambiguity at birth. The algorithm in Fig. 34.4 shows a simplified approach to establish the diagnosis in the first days of life. This method alone is enough to classify the ambiguous genitalia into one of the four main categories of DSD in more than 80 % of the cases. This approach involves physical examination to check for symmetry or asymmetry of the external genitalia, palpability of gonads, presence of vaginal and urethral openings, and determination of sex chromosome markers such as SRY or sexual chromatin (inactivated X chromosome).

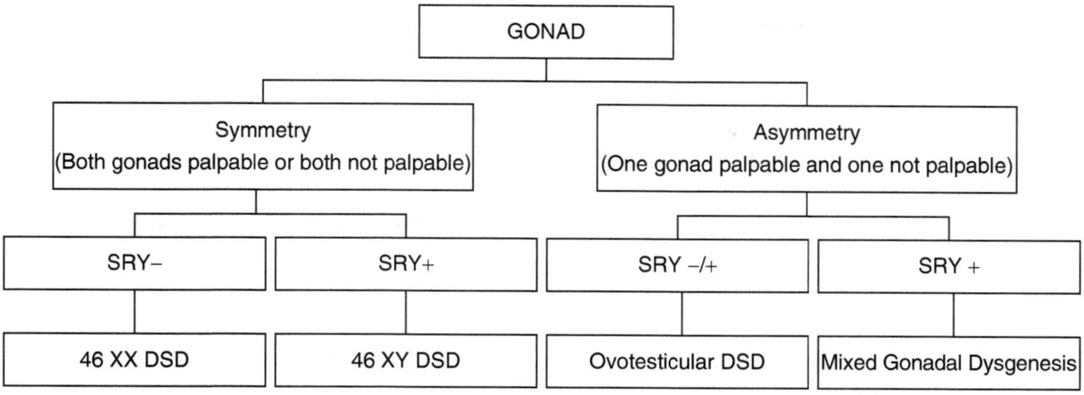


**Fig. 34.4** Rapid diagnostic algorithm for newborns with ambiguous genitalia

The sexual chromatin can be detected on examination of a buccal smear, but due to lack of accuracy with this diagnostic method, most centers have replaced it by the detection of the distal arm of the Y chromosome using fluorescent markers.

Several aspects are important in the investigation of ambiguous genitalia:

1. *History and physical examination*: Special emphasis should be placed on identifying other family members with DSD conditions [recessive inheritance—congenital adrenal hyperplasia (CAH)] or early postnatal deaths. Maternal medications taken during pregnancy should receive careful attention. Physical examination should include retraction of the labia in order to adequately visualize the urethral and vaginal orifices in females. A careful assessment should be made for scrotal asymmetry and the presence of palpable gonads. Hyperpigmentation secondary to adrenocorticotropic hormone secretion may be present in the genital region and areola. Signs of dehydration and hypertension are suggestive of CAH.
2. *Ultrasound*: It is important to check for the presence of Müllerian remnants and uterus. It is also helpful to investigate the presence of intra-abdominal gonads (occasionally) as well as hydrocolpos/hydronephrosis.
3. *Karyotype*: To confirm an XX or XY chromosomal background. Mosaicism and structural abnormalities can also be identified.
4. *Metabolic studies*: Serum electrolytes, 17-hydroxyprogesterone, 17-ketosteroids, and pregnanetriol testosterone (maternal and infant). In specific cases a βHCG stimulation test or an assessment of response to the administration of exogenous testosterone may be necessary.
5. *Genitogram*: Retrograde contrast injection into the urogenital sinus can delineate the confluence between the urethra and the vagina which has importance for surgical strategy. In boys with severe hypospadias, the presence of an enlarged utricle can be determined.
6. *Gonadal histology*: In most cases of DSD, with the exception of the adrenogenital syndrome and some cases of androgen insensitivity, gonadal histology is essential to establish the correct diagnosis. The biopsy should involve the deep portion of the gonad since the ovotestes may have the testicular and ovarian tissue overlying each other. Internal gonads can be biopsied using a traditional open laparotomy or, more recently, using laparoscopic techniques.

## Classification of Disorders of Sex Differentiation

The classification is based on gonadal histology and is divided in four main groups.

1. 46XX DSD—Only histologically normal ovarian tissue is found in an XX individual. It is the most common cause of DSD, and CAH is the usual diagnosis in virilized girls.

2. Ovotesticular DSD—Both ovarian and testicular tissues are present in the same child, variable karyotype, but 70 % of the cases have 46XX karyotype. This group used to be referred as true hermaphrodites in the past.
3. Gonadal Dysgenesis
   (a) Mixed gonadal dysgenesis—Dysgenetic testis in one side and a streak gonad in the other. Karyotype 45XO/46XY (mosaic) is seen in 70 % of the cases.
   (b) XY gonadal dysgenesis (Swyer syndrome)—Bilateral streak gonads in an XY individual.
4. 46XY DSD—Testicular tissue is present in an XY patient. This group includes patients with undervirilized genitalia that can be classified into eight basic etiologic categories: (1) Leydig cell failure, (2) testosterone biosynthesis defects, (3) androgen insensitivity syndrome, (4) 5α-reductase deficiency, (5) persistent Müllerian duct syndrome, (6) testicular dysgenesis, (7) primary testicular failure, and (8) exogenous insults. For the purpose of this chapter, we will focus on the most common conditions: partial or total androgen insensitivity, 5α-reductase deficiency, and Leydig cell failure.

## 46XX DSD

Virilization of the female fetus occurs as a result of endogenous exposure or exogenous administration of androgens. The main etiologies are:

- CAH—Deficiencies of 21-hydroxylase and 11β-hydroxylase are the most common types (95 %).
- Maternal ingestion of compounds with androgenic activity (e.g., progesterone) during pregnancy.
- Maternal androgen-secreting tumors.

## Congenital Adrenal Hyperplasia

This is the most common etiology of 46XX DSD. Deficiencies of 21-hydroxylase or 11β-hydroxylase represent the two most common defects. The loss of enzymatic activity results in the accumulation of 17-hydroxyprogesterone. Accumulation of 17-hydroxyprogesterone leads to the overproduction of androgens including dehydroepiandrosterone (DHEA), androstenedione, and testosterone. Virilization of the female fetus as well as the salt-loosing defect occurs in varying degrees, depending on the penetrance of the genetic defect. The severity of virilization exhibits a wide spectrum and has been classified into five types according to Prader (Fig. 34.5).

There may be only mild clitoral hypertrophy, the absence of labioscrotal fusion, and genital pigmentation (Fig. 34.6).

In more severe cases, the urethra and vagina may enter a common urogenital sinus, or there may be a phallic urethra (Figs. 34.7 and 34.8).

For technical reasons it is important to determine the length of the urogenital sinus. A high confluence between the urethra and vagina may present a significant technical challenge when an attempt is made to bring both orifices down to the perineum. The internal reproductive organs including the uterus and fallopian tubes are normal. Rarely an ovary may be found inside the

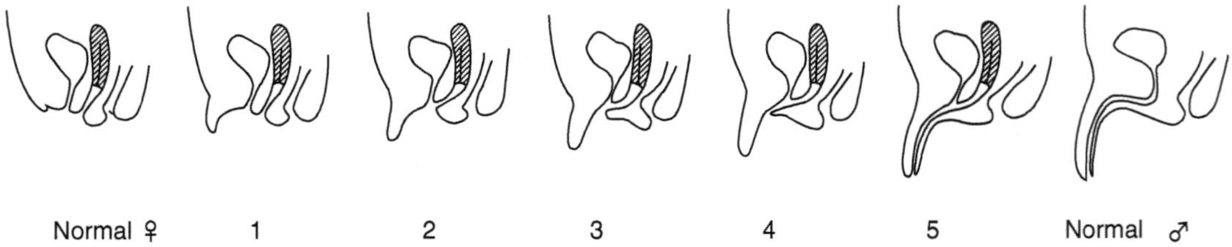


**Fig. 34.5** Prader classification for the severity of virilization of the external genitalia in patients with CAH

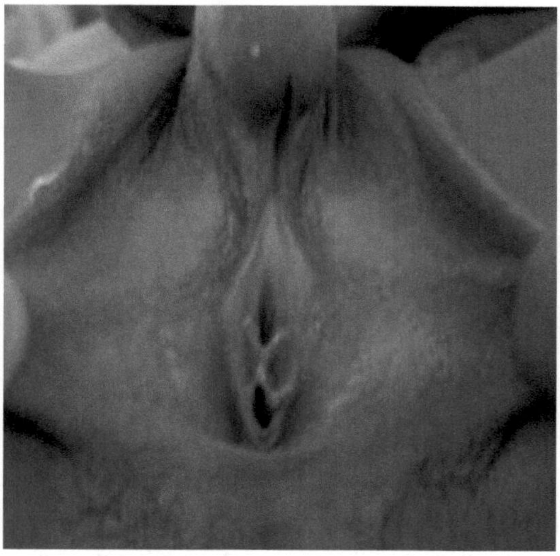

**Fig. 34.6** Prader II—External genitalia of a child with CAH showing mild clitoral hypertrophy, separate urethral and vaginal openings, and the absence of labioscrotal fusion

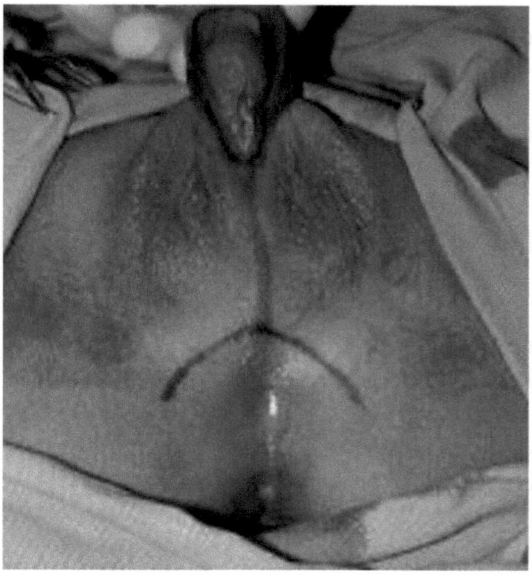

**Fig. 34.7** Prader IV—More pronounced clitoral enlargement, labioscrotal fusion, and urethra and vagina joining a common channel that opens at the base of the phallus

inguinal hernia sac. Therefore, in the great majority there are NO PALPABLE GONADS on physical examination.

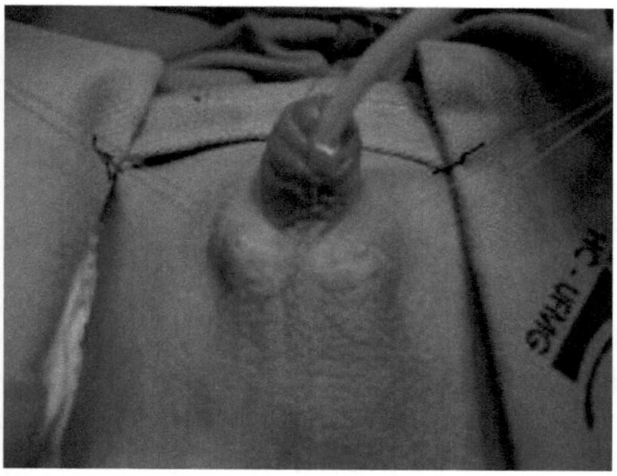

**Fig. 34.8** Prader V—Severe clitoral hypertrophy, complete labioscrotal fusion, phallic urethra, and bilateral impalpable gonads

## 21-Hydroxylase Deficiency

Approximately 90 % of cases of CAH are secondary to a 21-hydroxylase deficiency. The disorder is recessively inherited and can affect both sexes but the male fetus does not present genital ambiguity. The degree of female virilization may vary however, in the classic form of the disease, the genitalia is usually ambiguous.

Investigation:

1. Serum electrolytes: 21-hydroxylase deficiency causes a lack of cortisol and aldosterone production. Salt wasting occurs in approximately 75 % of cases. Since maternal cortisol and deoxycortisol are present at birth, most babies do not manifest clinical symptoms during the first 2 weeks of life. Subsequently, the undiagnosed infant may present with adrenal shock (dehydration, vomiting, hyponatremia, hyperkalemia), which is unresponsive to hydration alone, and the urgent administration of steroids is imperative. Hyperkalemia and hyponatremia are typical of adrenal shock and the key to establish the diagnosis. The low serum aldosterone levels lead to an elevation in plasma renin activity.
2. 17-Hydroxyprogesterone levels may be elevated 50- to 100-fold.

3. Ultrasound—presence of uterus.
4. Genitogram—to assess the length of the urogenital sinus.

## Management

The child with CAH should be raised as female because of potential normal reproductive female life if glucocorticoid and mineralocorticoid replacement therapy is provided and appropriate reconstructive surgery is performed. Patients are started on glucocorticoid supplementation such as hydrocortisone (Cortef, 10–20 mg/m$^2$/day) and mineralocorticoid supplementation such as fludrocortisone (Florinef, 0.1 mg daily) in case of high plasma renin. Long-term follow-up with an endocrinologist is necessary, since lifelong treatment and adjustment of medication dosage will be required. Prenatal treatment can be offered to a mother who had a previous child with CAH since it is the only DSD condition where sex ambiguity can be prevented. Suppression of the overproduction of androgen by the fetal adrenal gland can be achieved by giving the mother an appropriate dose of glucocorticoid (a daily dose of 20 μg of dexamethasone/kg of maternal weight, split in two or three doses).

# Ovotesticular DSD

Ovotesticular DSD varies widely in the appearance of their external genitalia. The majority however tend to have a male external genitalia and present with severe hypospadias, chordee, and asymmetric labioscrotal folds (Fig. 34.9).

The karyotype is variable, but most cases reported have been 46XX (70 %) and from African American origin. Mosaicism or a 46XY karyotype has been documented in the remaining cases.

As for the other classes of ovotesticular DSD, the external appearance of the genitalia is not diagnostic of the type of disorder. Gonadal biopsies are essential for diagnosis. By definition, both ovarian and testicular tissue must be present. These can be found in varying combinations but the most common type of gonad found is the ovotestis. The ovarian or testicular tissue can have a polar distribution within the gonad or tissue of one type may be localized deep within the hilar region of the gonad. For this reason an adequate biopsy should incorporate both gonadal poles as well as the hilar region. The hormonal function of the gonad parallels the histological findings, although there is a tendency to require supplemental testosterone administration in ovotesticular DSDs raised as males. Genitogram can demonstrate the presence of a vagina and ultrasound may reveal uterus and fallopian tubes.

Patients with a reasonable-sized phallus are usually raised as males. In cases where ovarian tissue predominates, the phallus may be quite rudimentary and the patient is usually raised as a female, requiring vaginoplasty and clitoroplasty with removal of discordant gonadal tissues. Supplemental testosterone administration is often required at puberty in patients raised as males.

# Gonadal Dysgenesis

These conditions are characterized by a failure or interruption in gonadal development.

## Mixed Gonadal Dysgenesis

This disorder is relatively common and is characterized by the presence of a dysgenetic or histologically normal testis on one side and a streak gonad on the other. In the great majority of cases the karyotype is 46XX/45XO. Patients have been diagnosed antenatally following discovery of a 46XX/45XO karyotype at amniocentesis. Urological evaluation for antenatal counseling has become increasingly more common in recent years. When counseling such cases it is important to take several points into consideration:

1. The majority of fetuses diagnosed antenatally with a 45XO/46XY karyotype will have a normal male genitalia.
2. The majority will need hormonal supplementation at puberty even if a fully descended and histologically normal testicle is present.
3. Many patients will develop an important learning disability.

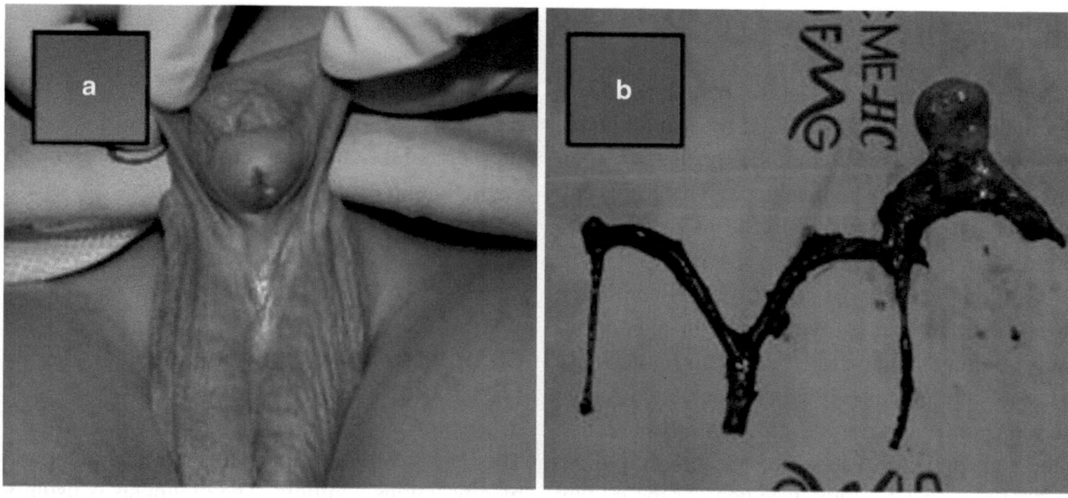


**Fig. 34.9** (**a**) Male external genitalia with right testis in the scrotum. (**b**) Internal genitalia showing rudimentary uterus, fallopian tubes, and left ovotestis

4. The risk of malignancy in the dysgenetic or normal testicle can be as high as 30 % if it is located in the abdominal cavity. Descended testes have a lower rate of malignancy. Streak gonads also have up to a 15 % risk of malignancy. The current recommendation is to leave the dysgenetic gonads untouched until puberty to allow for full pubertal development and, only after the maturation process is over, remove the gonads.
5. The internal structures usually parallel the gonadal findings. A well-developed fallopian tube and a rudimentary hemiuterus are usually found on the side of the streak gonad (no production of MIS). An epididymis is typically associated with the dysgenetic or normal testis. The decision to raise the child as a male or female is dependent on the degree of virilization and the size of the phallus. Müllerian structures and the streak gonad are removed and the penis is reconstructed utilizing some of the available techniques for hypospadias repair in patients reared as males. Females will require a vaginoplasty and clitoroplasty.

## Pure Gonadal Dysgenesis

These patients have a 46XY karyotype, low or absent virilization, Müllerian structures, and bilateral streak gonads. Diagnosis is usually made during evaluation for delayed puberty or primary amenorrhea.

Although Turner syndrome is included in the pure gonadal dysgenesis group due to the presence of bilateral streak gonads, it will not be discussed here because it is not associated with ambiguous genitalia.

## 46XY DSD

This is the most difficult group to diagnose and manage. Male XY DSD present with histologically normal testes. Undervirilization is the result of either an insensitivity of the target tissues to testosterone or a deficiency in the production of the androgens testosterone or dihydrotestosterone (DHT). Testosterone is converted by 5α-reductase to DHT. Virilization of the male external genitalia is dependent on the action of DHT.

## Leydig Cell Agenesis

This is a rare disorder characterized by the absence of Leydig cells. Genital ambiguity may be present. The internal ductal structures are of Wolffian derivatives.

## 5α-Reductase Deficiency

The deficiency of 5α-reductase, type 2, results in genital ambiguity characterized by a small penis, perineal hypospadias, and the presence of an enlarged utricle (pseudovagina). The testes are undescended and can usually be palpated in the inguinal or labial regions (Fig. 34.10).

Familial variants of the disorder have been described. Unfortunately, because of phenotypically female characteristics many of these patients are mistakenly raised as females and undergo an inappropriate clitoroplasty. Later in life, high pubertal testosterone levels may drive either the type 1 5α-reductase gene or the mutant gene to produce enough DHT to induce virilization. Patient may then start to develop male sexual characteristics such as deepening of the voice, hair growth in the body distribution of a male, and some descent of the testes. More importantly the great majority of patients demonstrate a male gender identity. For these reasons, it is important to make the diagnosis early and it is recommended that these patients be raised as males.

The diagnosis is established by demonstrating an increased ratio of testosterone to DHT in the blood. Testosterone levels may be low in infants and children and as a result measurement of the testosterone/DHT ratio must be performed following gonadotropin stimulation. The diagnosis in children may also be made using cultured genital fibroblasts and measuring their in vitro ability to transform testosterone to DHT.

The recommendation is to raise children with type 2 5α-reductase deficiency as males. Despite supplemental androgen treatment the mean penile length achieved has been reportedly small. In patients raised as female, gonadectomy and a genitoplasty should be performed.

## Complete Androgen Insensitivity (Testicular Feminization)

This is a hereditary condition, not characterized by ambiguous genitalia. The diagnosis is usually made during an inguinal hernia repair for phenotypic females when the surgeon is faced with the presence of a normal-looking testicle inside the hernia sac. The need of bilateral orchiectomy has been debated because risk of malignant degeneration is low and females undergoing gonadectomy tend to lose their libido. Therefore timing of testicular removal remains controversial. Some advocate early orchiectomy and induction of puberty by exogenous estrogen administration. Others, including ourselves, prefer to leave the testicles in place until puberty is entered spontaneously. These patients produce high levels of testosterone at puberty. Aromatase can convert testosterone to estrogen and bring about the development of spontaneous and satisfactory

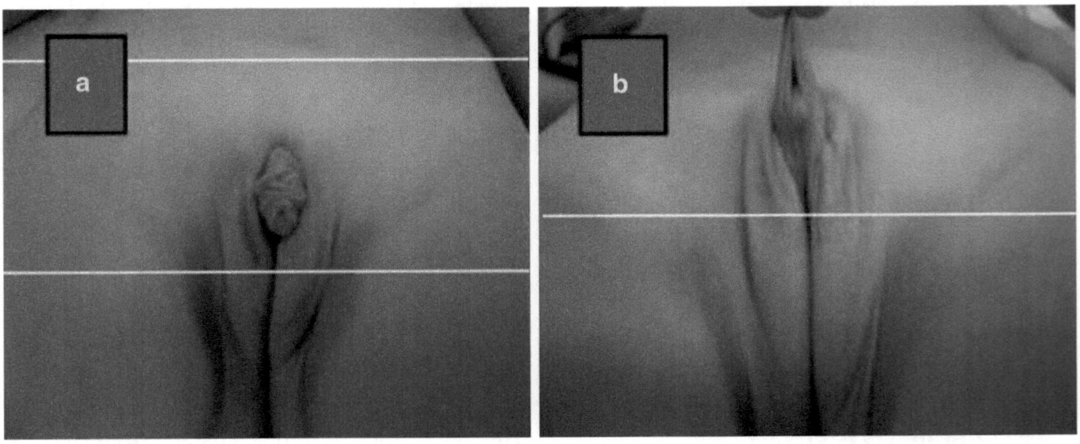


**Fig. 34.10** (**a**) Empty scrotum due to bilateral undescended testes. (**b**) Perineal hypospadias associated with bifid scrotum

secondary female sexual characteristics. We prefer this approach since we believe that spontaneous puberty is more desirable from a psychological perspective and the incidence of prepubertal testicular tumors is exceedingly rare. Vaginoplasty may be required in cases where the vagina is very short and unresponsive to dilatations.

## Partial Androgen Insensitivity

These patients present the most difficult management problems among the disorders of sexual differentiation. When raised as males the degree of virilization at puberty may be inadequate. The adequacy of the penile growth in response to the administration of exogenous testosterone has been used to help in gender assignment. Management however should be based on multidisciplinary decision-making. Ablative surgery should be avoided in early childhood, regardless of the decision to raise as female. As well, clitoroplasty and vaginoplasty may be deferred until later in life if clitoral enlargement is not so prominent. If male gender is assigned, genitoplasty incorporates the principles of hypospadias repair.

## Gender Assignment

Factors that influence gender assignment include diagnosis, genital appearance, surgical options, need for lifelong replacement therapy, potential for fertility, views of the family, and, sometimes, circumstances relating to cultural practices.

More than 90 % of patients with 46XX CAH and all patients with 46XY CAIS assigned female in infancy identify themselves as females. Therefore evidence supports the current recommendation to raise markedly virilized 46XX infants with CAH as female.

Approximately 60 % of 5α-reductase-deficient patients assigned female at infancy choose to be reassigned as males at puberty. Among those with partial androgen insensitivity syndrome (PAIS), androgen biosynthetic defects, and incomplete gonadal dysgenesis, there is dissatisfaction with the sex of rearing in approximately 25 % of individuals whether raised male or female. The decision to rear an undervirilized neonate as male or female depends on several factors as mentioned above. The main arguments that should be taken into account to make a decision are listed in Table 34.1. A full discussion should be made by the multidisciplinary team and must include the parents. It is important to keep in mind that there is no perfect choice of sex of rearing and the most reasonable outcome should be considered.

**Table 34.1** The main arguments for the choice of sex of rearing (according to Nicolino N et al. BJU Intern suppl 3, 93:20–5, 2003)

| In favor of | |
|---|---|
| Female gender | Male gender |
| Small size of clitoris (1–2 cm) | Size of the phallus (>2 cm) |
| Presence of uterus | Normal scrotum containing testis |
| Bilateral undescended testes | No vagina or small prostatic utricle |
| Gonads to be removed | Good/normal response to hCG |
| Vaginal pouch >2 cm | Androgen insensitivity |
| Low testosterone response to hCG | Prediction of normal stature |
| Prediction of small stature | Parental adherence |
| Parental adherence | |

When making a decision on the sex of rearing for children with ovotesticular DSD, one should think about the potential for fertility on the basis of gonadal differentiation and genital development and assuming that the genitalia can be consistent with the chosen sex. In the case of MGD, factors to consider include prenatal androgen exposure, testicular function at or after puberty, phallic development, and gonadal location.

## Feminizing Genitoplasty

Female genitoplasty is indicated in severely virilized cases of CAH (46XX DSD) and other selected DSD conditions. According to the 2006 consensus statement on management of DSD, CAH patients with mild clitoris hypertrophy (Prader I or II) should be managed expectantly and not undergo clitoroplasty until at least after puberty, when the children would be able to participate in the decision-making process. Furthermore, timing of vaginoplasty still remains controversial, but there has been an agreement that patients with a very high urethrovaginal confluence and hypoplastic vaginas should have their vaginoplasty performed after puberty as most substitution vaginoplasty techniques need frequent postoperative dilatations and often require revisions later. The classic feminizing genitoplasty consists of clitoroplasty, labiaplasty, and vaginoplasty. Based on the 2002 consensus for management of patients with CAH, feminizing genitoplasty, when indicated, should be performed within the first 6 months of life.

## Clitoroplasty

Many techniques have been described. The fundamental surgical principles involve preservation of the neurovascular bundle supplying the glans clitoris as well as the mucosa of the clitoris to create a mucosal-lined vestibule. All efforts should be made to avoid resection of the glans clitoris tissue even in cases of severely enlarged clitoral head, to reduce the risk of diminishing clitoral sensitivity. Currently, the trend towards a more conservative approach for the management of DSD has prompted development of surgical techniques that might be reversible such as the recently reported corporal sparing dismembered clitoroplasty, which does not excise the corporal bodies. Instead, this procedure separates each hemi-corpora of the clitoris and buries them free into the labioscrotal pouches (5).

## Vulvoplasty

Vulvar reconstruction attempts to restore the normal anatomic appearance of the vulva. The labia minora are constructed with the prepuce of the clitoris and should end at the lateral aspect of the vaginal introitus. Unfortunately several described techniques fail to appreciate this anatomic configuration and, as a result, do not achieve optimal surgical outcomes that should be representative of the normal female anatomy.

## Vaginoplasty

Several surgical techniques have been reported. Most recently Pena described the principle of total urogenital sinus mobilization, thereby avoiding the technically difficult process of separating the vagina from the urethra that leads to formation of urethrovaginal fistulas. Mobilization of the entire urogenital sinus can be accomplished in cases where the length of the sinus is no longer than 3 cm, from the level of the perineum. It is important to create a large opening in the posterior vaginal wall in order to minimize the postoperative incidence of vaginal stenosis.

## Suggested Reading

Bidakar SS, Hutson JM. Evaluation and management of the abnormal gonad. Semin Pediatr Surg. 2005;14:118–23.

Husmann DA. Intersex. In: Gillenwater JY, Grayhack JT, Howards SS, Mitchell ME, editors. Adult and pediatric urology, chap. 52C, vol. 3. 4th ed. Philadelphia: Lippincott Williams & Wilkins; 2002. p. 2533–64.

Lee PA, Houlk CP, Ahmed F, Hughes IA. Consensus statement on management of intersex disorders. Pediatrics. 2006;118:488–99.

Mouriquand PDE. The management of ambiguous genitalia. Proceedings of a symposium, Lyon, France, April 2003. BJU Intern. 2003;93(Suppl. 3):1–65.

Pippi Salle JL, Braga LP, Macedo N, Rosito N, Bagli DJ. Corporeal sparing dismembered clitoroplasty: an alternative technique for feminizing genitoplasty. J Urol. 2007;178:1796–81.

# Myelodysplasia: From Birth to Adulthood

35

Stuart B. Bauer

## Introduction

The assessment and management of children with myelodysplasia is an ever-changing condition. The expansion of its understanding and treatment over the last 50 years has been just remarkable. In the mid-1950s, there were few insights and minimal alternatives to being in diapers or wearing an appliance over an abdominal wall stoma. As a result many individuals who survived infancy were ostracized from secondary schooling and/or sequestered away at home with few opportunities to actively engage with peers or become socially involved in society. Starting with the development of adequate X-ray assessment and reliable urodynamic investigation, the advent of clean intermittent catheterization (CIC), artificial urinary sphincter implantation, continent urinary conduit creation, and a plethora of bladder-specific drugs that modulate lower urinary tract function, a great deal of information has been learned about the pathophysiology, pathogenesis, and efficient treatment of the urologic manifestations of this disorder. With the promise of tissue engineering, nerve refunctionalization, and stem cell therapy, new vistas for treatment seem to be on the horizon.

S.B. Bauer, M.D., F.A.A.P., F.A.C.S. (✉)
Department Of Urology, Children's Hospital Boston, Harvard Medical School, 300 Longwood Avenue, Boston, MA 02115, USA
e-mail: stuart.bauer@childrens.harvard.edu

The terminology used throughout this manuscript will conform to the standardization document recently published in the *Journal of Urology* [1].

## Myelomeningocele

Myelodysplasia is a descriptive term applied to several types of anatomic abnormalities of the developing spinal column that include spina bifida occulta, myelocele, myelomeningocele, lipomyelomeningocele, and anterior meningocele (Fig. 35.1). *Spina bifida occulta* is a lesion occurring predominantly at the L5 vertebrae in which there is failure of fusion of the posterior spinal arch. Usually the cord and nerve roots are unaffected by this defect and the abnormality is typically found incidentally on a KUB or CT scan. No cutaneous manifestation is seen in the skin overlying the defect and no neurologic deficit is apparent on neurologic examination assessment or urodynamic testing. A *myelocele* is a posterior protrusion of the dura due to a defect in the formation of the posterior arches of the vertebral bodies, but this outpouching contains no neural elements. Thus, except for the meningocele sac with or without a skin covering, no neurologic deficit is present. *Myelomeningocele* refers to a condition that is similar to a myelocele but into which neural elements have evaginated. Consequently, there is a variable neurologic deficit picture that involves the lower extremities and/or the bladder and urethral and anal sphincter

R. Rabinowitz et al. (eds.), *Pediatric Urology for the Primary Care Physician*, Current Clinical Urology, DOI 10.1007/978-1-60327-243-8_35, © Springer Science+Business Media New York 2015

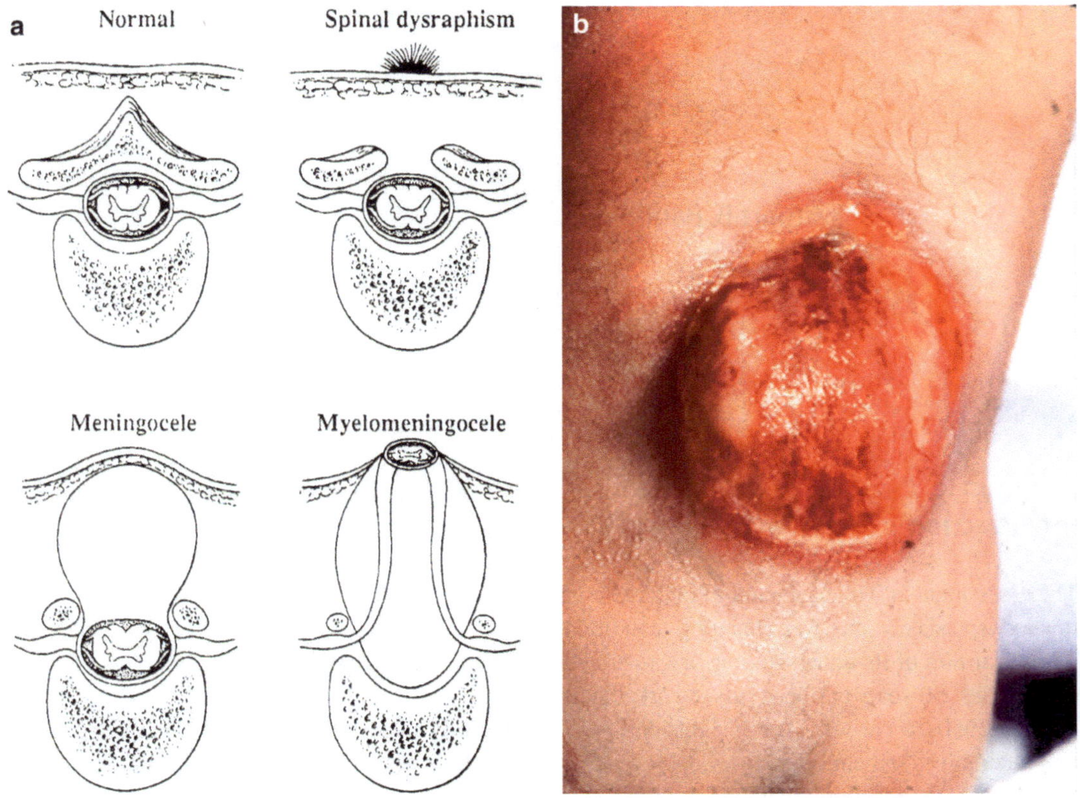


**Fig. 35.1** Schematic of the cross-sectional pathology of the various lesions involved in myelodysplasia (**a**). An open skin lesion involving the spine in a newborn with myelodysplasia before closure of the defect (**b**). (**a**) Reprinted from McLellan DL, Bauer SB: Bladder dysfunction. In: Avner EA, Harmon WE, Niaudet F, eds Pediatric Nephrology 5th Ed. Philadelphia: Lippincott, Williams & Wilkins, 2004; 1077-90

muscle mechanisms. A *lipomyelomeningocele* is present when fatty tissue has infiltrated into the meningocele sac. Again, the neurologic picture is very individualized and one that cannot be predicted from the location or size of the lesion. Myelomeningocele accounts for more than 90 % of all open spinal dysraphic states [2].

## Etiology and Embryology

The exact cause of these lesions is not known, but folate vitamin deficiency, teratogenic agents, and antibodies during pregnancy have been implicated in its formation [3, 4]. The developing spinal canal begins its formation on the 18th day of gestation and is completed by day 35, with neural tubularization occurring late in a caudad direction starting from the cephalic end of the fetus. Failure of the canal to close completely and for mesodermal in-growth over the developing spinal cord results in an open spinal lesion, most commonly in the lumbosacral area, with a decreasing incidence taking place in the thoracic and cervical areas, respectively (Table 35.1). The exposed spinal cord and its nerve roots, some of which may protrude into the meningocele sac, and tension on the spinal cord as the cord "rises up" the canal with elongation of the fetus (from L2–L3 in mid to late fetal life to L1 at birth)

**Table 35.1** Spinal bony level of myelomeningocele (uppermost vertebral abnormality)

| Location | Incidence (%) |
|---|---|
| Cervical—high thoracic | 2 |
| Low thoracic | 5 |
| Lumbar | 26 |
| Lumbosacral | 47 |
| Sacral | 20 |

contribute to a variable picture of neural tissue injury to the lower urinary tract, rectal sphincter mechanism, and lower extremities [5]. Coupled with obstruction of the aqueduct to the fourth ventricle (Chiari malformation) resulting in possible herniation of the brain stem and compression injury to the center for micturition coordination (the pontine mesencephalic center), additional layers of dysfunction are added to those peripheral nerve pathways already affected.

## Prenatal Assessment and Intervention

Prenatal ultrasound examination of the spinal column in the last trimester of pregnancy has excellent correlation with the level of affected vertebrae but not in predicting the type of neurologic function of the lower urinary tract that is noted on postnatal assessment [6]. There have been several reports regarding the beneficial effects of prenatal repair of the meningocele defect at 21–23 weeks of fetal life that include a much lower need for ventriculoperitoneal shunting and the findings of stable lower extremity function after birth [7, 8]. No careful analysis of lower urinary tract function has been included in these reports. The only study that does exist is one that evaluated six prenatally treated children 1 year after birth with urodynamic assessment. All these babies had complete denervation of the urethral sphincter and an overactive bladder; this resulted in four children having hydronephrosis and all requiring intervention to achieve continence beyond CIC and drug therapy [9]. A long-term efficacy study regarding prenatal intervention for children with meylodysplasia has been published that showed improved cognitive function and reduced need for ventriculoperitoneal shunting but no significant improvement in lower urinary tract function [10].

## Newborn Assessment and Initial Management

The major overriding issue at birth is whether or not the infant can empty his/her bladder completely at low pressure and does the child have detrusor external urethral sphincter dyssynergy or incoordination. Thus, it is recommended that as soon as feasible after birth, the child's residual urine should be measured following a spontaneous void, and if high, a repeat measurement recorded after a Credé maneuver. Then, when appropriate, a renal and bladder ultrasound is performed to assess kidney size and appearance, parenchymal echogenicity, degree of collecting system dilation, presence of ureteral dilation (especially distally), and bladder size and wall thickness [11], and a calculation of residual volume is done if the child voids during the study. A serum creatinine level should be measured after about 7 days of age to eliminate the influence of maternal renal function. Within the first 3 weeks to 1 month of life, urodynamic studies are undertaken to evaluate detrusor function (compliance, overactivity, and contractility). It is imperative to know the level of detrusor pressure both at capacity and when the child voids or leaks. In addition, knowledge of external urethral sphincter function is important (baseline electrical activity, response to various sacral reflexes, and reaction of the sphincter to bladder filling and emptying). This study thus provides a clear picture of the neuro-urologic status of the lower urinary tract in the newborn [12]. Consequently, it can be used to determine if subsequent studies represent a change that warrants either urologic or neurosurgical intervention. In addition, these newborn findings can dictate whether or not the child needs to be treated prophylactically with intermittent catheterization (CIC) and/or drug therapy to prevent upper and/or lower urinary tract deterioration from taking place, rather than having the child managed expectantly. Lastly, it allows the treating physician to counsel the child's family about future bladder, bowel, and sexual function.

Interestingly, it has been noted in our series that all infants with radiologic abnormalities in the newborn period (5–10 % with hydronephrosis or reflux) had active bladder outlet obstruction in the form of bladder sphincter dyssynergia on their initial neonatal study. Undoubtedly, the high voiding or leaking pressures (above 40 cm $H_2O$) during fetal life caused these changes to occur in utero [13].

**Table 35.2** Indications for and type of proactive intervention based on assessment

| | |
|---|---|
| *Urodynamic findings* | |
| Bladder changes | |
| Overactivity | Anticholinergics |
| Poor compliance | Anticholinergics |
| Urethral sphincter | |
| Bladder sphincter dyssynergy or non-relaxation during a bladder contraction or at expected capacity | CIC |
| Leak point pressure ≥40 cm $H_2O$ from denervation fibrosis | CIC |
| *Radiologic findings* | |
| Ultrasound | |
| Hydroureteronephrosis | CIC + anticholinergics |
| Thick-walled bladder | Anticholinergics |
| Voiding or radionuclide cystogram | |
| Reflux ≥3 (scale of 5) | CIC ± anticholinergics |
| Incomplete emptying (↑ pvr) | CIC |

Anticholinergics anticholinergic medication, i.e., oxybutynin, tolterodine, trospium
*CIC* clean intermittent catheterization

Furthermore, the presence of elevated detrusor filling pressure, bladder sphincter dyssynergy, or high bladder outlet pressure (from fibrosis of the denervated striated muscle component of the external urethral sphincter) can result in upper urinary tract deterioration in as many as 63 % of affected children if they are treated expectantly and not proactively (Table 35.2) [14]. When proactive treatment in the form of CIC and anticholinergic medication is initiated in newborns at risk, the incidence of urinary tract deterioration is greatly diminished [15–18]. Thus, many centers treating large numbers of these newborns advocate a renal and bladder ultrasound and a catheterized measure of residual urine after the infant either voids or leaks urine, within the first 2–3 days of life, a serum creatinine after 7 days, and a urodynamic study that incorporates both detrusor pressure measurements, as well as external urethral sphincter electromyography within the first month. Voiding cystography is undertaken when hydronephrosis is present on the newborn examination and/or the urodynamic study indicates bladder outlet obstruction with either increased leak point pressure at capacity or bladder sphincter dyssynergy. The risk for reflux when there is functional bladder outlet obstruction can range as high as 50 % [19].

Although some clinicians still preach watchful waiting if the renal and bladder ultrasound is normal and the residual urine is minimal and do not recommend urodynamic studies in the newborn period, opting instead for instituting CIC and drug therapy only with the first sign of ureteral or renal pelvic dilation [20, 21], most centers within the USA now advocate for full investigation of the lower urinary tract and initiate prophylactic treatment if there are signs of bladder outlet obstruction and/or elevated bladder filling or voiding pressure [22, 23]. The incidence of urinary tract deterioration can be greater than 50 % [11] when children with the potential for deterioration are followed with expectant and not preemptive therapy. Even though these "watchful waiters" have demonstrated they can reduce the presence of hydronephrosis and possibly reflux, the changes in detrusor dynamics are not as easily reversed, and the need for subsequent aggressive management of the bladder to control incontinence and a poorly compliant bladder are commonplace as well as challenging (Table 35.2). Therefore, CIC is promoted when either detrusor sphincter dyssynergy, elevated leak point pressures greater than 40 cm $H_2O$ from denervation fibrosis, or reflux grade III or higher (on a scale of I to V) are present. Instituting CIC and anticholinergic therapy in infancy have produced many advantages over time [24, 25]: both the parents and the child adapt to the routine of CIC much more easily than they would have if it were to be begun when the child is older; the bladder often remains very compliant, expanding as the child grows and maintaining appropriate wall thickness as noted on bladder echography; hydronephrosis and vesicoureteral reflux develop in less than 10 % of children treated with proactive therapy; continence is readily achieved in greater than 50 % with no additional maneuvers needed because the detrusor muscle maintains good compliance; and the need for augmentation cystoplasty to maintain a reasonable organ for storage is markedly reduced from almost 60 to 16 % when compared to children followed with expectant therapy [15].

The disadvantages are few, including a higher rate of bacteriuria (60–70 % versus 30 %) but a lower rate of symptomatic urinary tract infection (20 % versus 40 %) during childhood as compared to children followed expectantly [26]. Because the subsequent risk of vesicoureteral reflux is lower, the effect on renal function and the development of scarring are reduced when these prophylactically treated children are compared to those monitored with watchful observation [27].

## Vesicoureteral Reflux

When vesicoureteral reflux is present, CIC can effectively lower intravesical emptying pressure by bypassing the high bladder outlet resistance from either detrusor external sphincter dyssynergy or denervation fibrosis. In addition, the adjunctive use of anticholinergic medication not only works to lower detrusor filling pressure but also abolishes detrusor overactivity, which is often a response to the functional bladder outlet obstruction from the dyssynergy. Lowering detrusor filling and emptying pressures have proven to be very beneficial in the management of vesicoureteral reflux; 30–50 % of children resolve their reflux within 2–3 years of its discovery and initiation of this therapy [28].

Credé voiding is not an efficacious maneuver for emptying the bladder in children with myelodysplasia, especially if the urethral sphincter is partially or fully innervated [29]. Because most children have intact motor function above the L1 level, any increase in abdominal pressure from a Credé maneuver can lead to a reflexive increase in urethral sphincter activity, thus producing an increase in bladder outlet resistance resulting in "high voiding pressure" (Fig. 35.2). Potentially, this can be a particularly noxious reaction in children with moderate to severe grades of reflux [29]. As a result, Credé voiding should only be employed when it is definitely known that the urethral sphincter is unresponsive to increases in abdominal pressure, as noted on urodynamic testing that includes an assessment of urethral sphincter function. In these instances, there will be no corresponding increase in urethral sphincter activity and thus, no increase in bladder outlet resistance. The bladder may be emptied without a substantial rise in pressure beyond the measured leak point pressure. Another disadvantage to Credé voiding occurs as the child grows, because the bladder comes to reside more in the true pelvis and is less intra-abdominal. This change in position further reduces the effectiveness of the Credé maneuver.

The indications for antireflux surgery in children with myelodysplasia are not substantially different from that advocated for children with normal bladder function [30]. These indications include: recurrent urinary tract infection despite appropriate antibiotic therapy, anatomic abnormalities at the ureterovesical junction that preclude its disappearance (i.e., ectopic position, large diverticula into which the ureter drains), failure of at least improvement if not complete resolution of higher grades of reflux during an acceptable period of observation in a child with good bladder compliance, failure of renal growth over a 2–3 year time period (Table 35.3), progressive decrease in uptake or the development of scarring on DMSA renal scanning, and the need for surgery to increase bladder outlet resistance to achieve continence because this may lead to a worsening in the grade of reflux as the bladder retains urine for longer periods of time following surgery.

Recently, several clinicians have not advocated antireflux surgery in children with mild to moderate grades of reflux when these children are about to undergo augmentation cystoplasty [31–33]. In these studies it was noted that low and moderate grades of reflux (grades I to III) will resolve concomitant with a decrease in intravesical pressure achieved by the augment. However, there is still no consensus regarding this and there is no data regarding higher grades of reflux.

With the evolution of an effective endoscopic bulking agent over the last 20 years, this alternative surgical approach is now a viable option for treating vesicoureteral reflux [34].

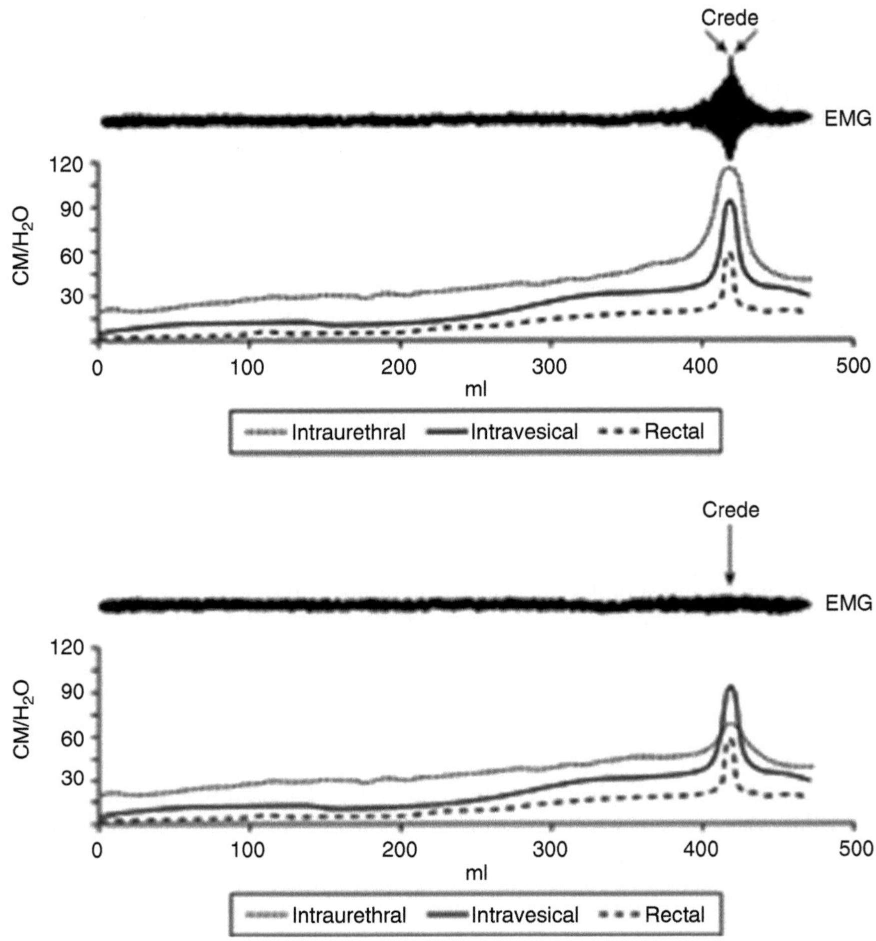


**Fig. 35.2** When the external urethral sphincter EMG is reactive (*top*), a Credé maneuver leads to an increase in urethral sphincter activity, a rise in intraurethral resistance, and "high" voiding pressure from the Credé. When the sphincter EMG is nonreactive (*bottom*), there is no corresponding rise in intraurethral resistance and voiding pressures are lower

**Table 35.3** Indications for antireflux surgery in neurogenic bladder dysfunction

| |
|---|
| Recurrent UTI despite appropriate antibiotics |
| Anatomic abnormality at the ureterovesical junction |
| Failure of resolution (or improvement) after 3–4 years |
| Failure of renal growth over 2–3 years |
| Progressive loss of function on DMSA scan |
| Anticipated bladder outlet surgery in the presence of reflux |

DMSA = $T^{99}$-labeled dimercaptosuccinic acid radionuclide renal scan

Prior to the use of Deflux, a hyaluronic acid polymer encased in microspheres, all bulking agents injected submucosally at the ureterovesical junction seemed to migrate and/or resorb and not be a good long-term effective treatment [35]. Deflux appears to have much greater staying power and, thus, may be a more permanent solution (Fig. 35.3). Deflux has been reported to be effective in approximately 80 % of children with grades I to III and 65 % in children with grade IV reflux [36, 37]. For this technique to be effective, however, it is imperative that detrusor compliance and overactivity must be managed with sufficient anticholinergic medication and CIC employed to insure complete emptying of the bladder at low pressure. Even when these prerequisites are met, it remains to be seen if Deflux will remain such an effective agent on a long-term basis.

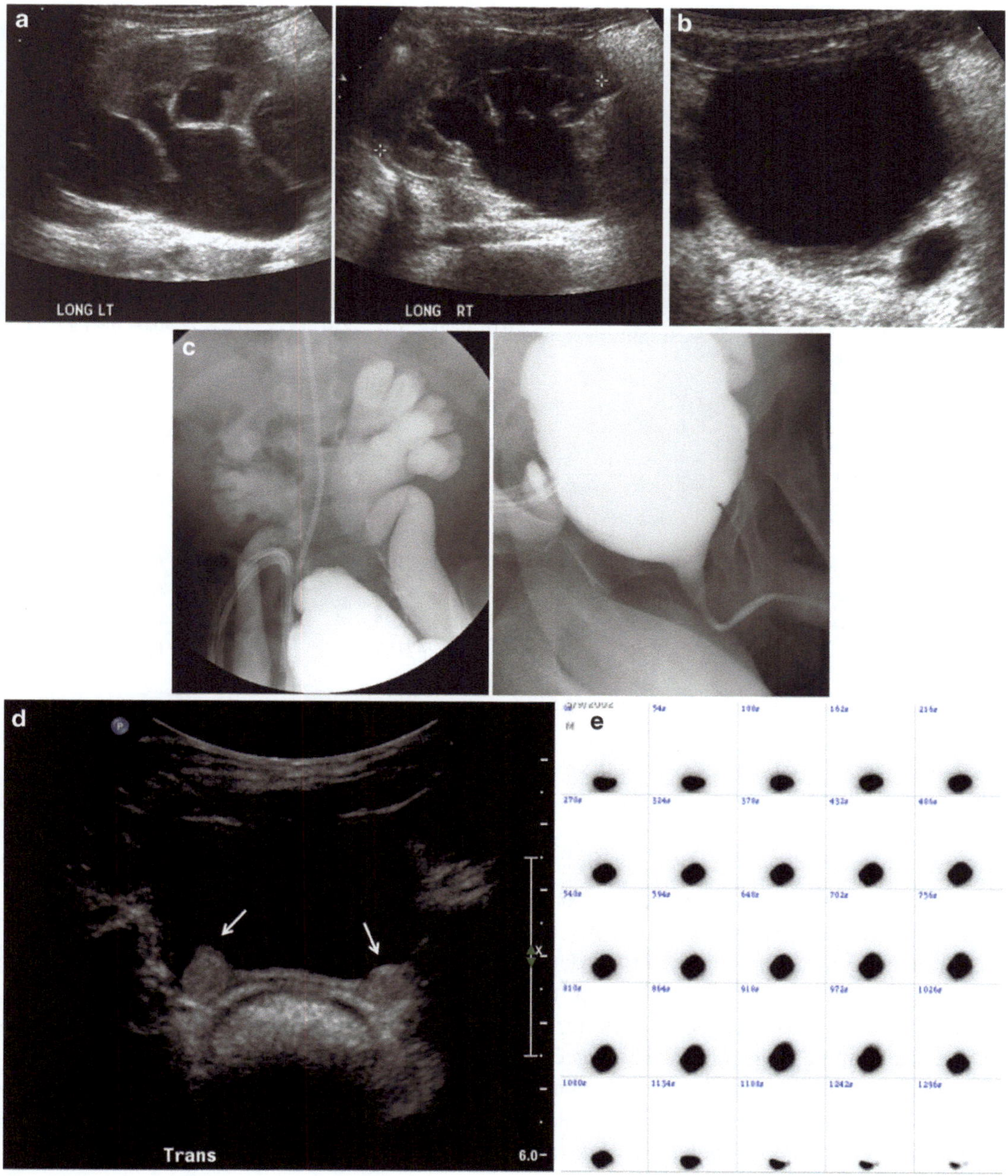


**Fig. 35.3** A 3-year-old boy with myelodysplasia who had severe bilateral hydroureteronephrosis (**a**, **b**, ECHO) secondary to bilateral grade 5/5 reflux (**c**, VCUG). Following Deflux injections bilaterally the mounds can be seen (**d**, ECHO) and the reflux has resolved (**e**, nuclear cystogram)

## Medical Management of the Bladder During Childhood

The key to a stable bladder and, consequently, renal function is the maintenance of a good capacity highly compliant detrusor muscle combined with periodic and complete emptying of the bladder at low pressure, as has been advocated throughout this manuscript. Anticholinergic medication (primarily oxybutynin, tolterodine, glycopyrrolate, hyoscyamine, or trospium) (Table 35.4) and CIC achieve that in a majority of children and provide an added benefit of continence

**Table 35.4** Drugs that affect lower urinary tract function

| Type | Dosage | |
|---|---|---|
| | Minimum | Maximum |
| Cholinergic | | |
| Bethanechol (Urecholine) | 0.7 mg/kg TID | 0.8 mg/kg QID |
| Anticholinergic (T = tertiary or Q = quaternary amines) | | |
| Propantheline (Pro-Banthine) (Q) | 0.5 mg/kg BID | 0.5 mg/kg QID |
| Oxybutynin (Ditropan) (T) | 0.2 mg/kg BID | 0.2 mg/kg QID |
| Glycopyrrolate (Robinul) (Q) | 0.01 mg/kg BID | 0.03 mg/kg TID |
| Hyoscyamine (Levsin) (Q) | 0.03 mg/kg BID | 0.1 mg/kg TID |
| Tolterodine (Detrol) (T) | 0.01 mg/kg BID | 0.04 mg/kg BID |
| Trospium chloride (Sanctura) (Q) | 0.3 mg/kg BID | 0.5 mg/kg BID |
| Darifenacin (Enablex) (T) | 0.0625 mg/kg BID | 0.125 mg/kg BID |
| Sympathomimetic | | |
| Phenylpropanolamine (alpha) | 2.5 mg/kg TID | 2.5 mg/kg QID |
| Ephedrine (alpha) | 0.5 mg/kg TID | 1.0 mg/kg TID |
| Pseudoephedrine (alpha) | 0.4 mg/kg BID | 0.9 mg/kg TID |
| Sympatholytic | | |
| Prazosin (alpha) (Minipress) | 0.05 mg/kg BID | 0.1 mg/kg TID |
| Phenoxybenzamine (alpha) | 0.3 mg/kg BID | 0.5 mg/kg TID |
| Propranolol (beta) | 0.25 mg/kg BID | 0.5 mg/kg BID |
| Alfuzosin (alpha) | 0.05 mg/kg BID | 0.1 mg/kg BID |
| Smooth muscle relaxant | | |
| Flavoxate (Urispas) | 3.0 mg/kg BID | 3.0 mg/kg TID |
| Dicyclomine (Bentyl) | 0.1 mg/kg TID | 0.3 mg/kg TID |
| Others | | |
| Imipramine (Tofranil) | 0.7 mg/kg BID | 1.2 mg/kg TID |

if the child has reasonable bladder outlet resistance [15]. When these agents combine with M2 and M3 antimuscarinic receptor sites in the detrusor, they block the uptake of acetylcholine that stimulates the detrusor muscle to contract. Unfortunately, these drugs do not have specific M-receptor site selectivity, so side effects abound, such as dry mouth, facial flushing, tiredness, overheating, constipation, mood changes, and dilated pupils, when these M-receptor sites in these other organ locations are stimulated as well. There are several newer drugs (darifenacin, solifenacin, and propiverine) that supposedly have better and more selective affinity for the bladder muscle M receptors. In addition, these drugs do not cross the blood–brain barrier, thus reducing debilitating CNS effects, but their full efficacy and tolerability in children still need to be tested.

Alpha 1α sympathomimetic agents (Table 35.4) (ephedrine, pseudoephedrine, and phenyl propanolamine) are known to increase bladder outlet resistance, but unfortunately, the degree of predictability regarding their efficacy is poor. It has been shown that there is a concentration of alpha 1α receptors in the trigone and posterior urethra in males and females that should be responsive to medical stimulation, but this is not always the case in clinical practice. Currently, these medications may be prescribed in children with a low leak point pressure who have incontinence despite maximal anticholinergic therapy and frequent emptying with CIC.

## Surgical Options for Achieving Continence

When drug therapy fails to achieve continence or improve poor detrusor compliance, especially if the latter is the cause of any hydroureteronephrosis, several surgical options are available to counteract these conditions. Botulinum toxin A can be injected directly into the detrusor muscle endoscopically (100–200 *IU* [international units] are injected into 20–30 sites within the detrusor, but not the trigone), with a very effective short-term (6 months) response. A repeat series of injections has resulted in a more prolonged paralysis of the detrusor muscle, but a sustained response (years) has yet to be achieved [37, 38].

Alternatively, augmentation cystoplasty using a segment of detubularized intestine or stomach has been a mainstay for enlarging the bladder and lowering intravesical pressure for the past 25 years. However, a plethora of complications has been seen the longer the bowel segment remains in place within the bladder: problematic mucus, stone formation, electrolyte imbalance, and recurrent urinary infection have been reported in multiple series with long-term follow-up [39]. In children with a gastric augment, a hematuria-dysuria-type syndrome is not an uncommon occurrence [40], and hyponatremic hypochloremic metabolic acidosis may develop following a bout of viral gastroenteritis. Therefore, it is critical that children with this type of augment be followed very carefully and have adequate fluid and electrolyte replacement with any gastrointestinal disturbance [41]. Recent reports have described the late occurrence of cancer either in the augmented segment or at its anastomotic site with the bladder [42–44]. These concerns have spearheaded a call for close surveillance of these patients 10 or more years after their augment; some clinicians have even raised the specter of a moratorium on the use of bowel segments for bladder augmentation.

Management of the incompetent bladder outlet is controversial as well. When a child does not respond to alpha 1α stimulation, then a fascial sling using either a strip of autologous rectus muscle fascia or small intestine submucosa (SIS) has been effective in elevating and compressing the bladder neck against the undersurface of the pubic symphysis to achieve dryness [45–47]. Alternatively, the placement of an artificial urinary sphincter with the cuff positioned around the bladder neck (or bulbar urethra in older teenage boys) has been more than 80 % effective with 10 years of follow-up [48, 49]. The attractiveness of this latter procedure is that if the individual can strain to empty before surgery, complete emptying is still possible in more than 60 % of the patients postoperatively. As a result, it is not mandatory to start CIC following sphincter implantation as is needed for other surgeries that increase bladder outlet resistance. One disconcerting long-term effect of increasing bladder outlet resistance is the development of reduced detrusor compliance over time [49–51]. This phenomenon is often silent because the increased outlet resistance prevents urinary leakage at the expense of diminished upper urinary tract drainage, resulting in hydroureteronephrosis and possibly diminished kidney function. Therefore, all children undergoing a bladder outlet procedure to increase resistance, especially those having an artificial urinary sphincter implanted, need periodic surveillance of their bladder dynamics and upper urinary tract imaging even though they may be perfectly continent.

The creation of a continent catheterizable urinary stoma has become fashionable in children with difficulty catheterizing their native urethra, either due to body habitus limitations for easy CIC access (obesity, poor eye-hand coordination, inability to balance hands-free on the toilet), intractable incontinence, or difficulty with urethral catheterization following bladder outlet surgery [52, 53]. The appendix, distal ureter (with a transureteroureterostomy of the proximal ureter to the contralateral ureter), or a very short segment of reconfigured small intestine has been used successfully as a continent catheterizable conduit to bridge the gap from the bladder to an anterior abdominal wall stoma either at the umbilicus or right lower quadrant [54, 55]. The ease of subsequent bladder catheterization with no leakage from the stoma has been an attractive option for older patients as they attempt to become independent of caregivers [56, 57]. Stomal stenosis, however, is a not insignificant long-term complication [57].

Within the last 10 years, a novel approach to improving bladder storage capabilities has been developed that involves obtaining a biopsy specimen from the diseased bladder wall, growing its cells in tissue culture, seeding them onto a polyglycolic acid polymer, and finally transferring the entire construct to the bladder 6–8 weeks later [58]. Phase 1 trials of the advanced technique in 5 children have proven to be effective over a 2–3-year period. Phase 2 studies are currently underway to determine the efficacy and safety of this process.

## Bowel Function

Bowel function in children with myelodysplasia is often similarly and extensively affected. The lower rectum and internal and external sphincter mechanisms are innervated exactly as the lower urinary tract is, from the thoracolumbar and S2 and S3 areas in the spinal cord and along the same peripheral nerve pathways involving the hypogastric, pelvic, and pudendal nerves. The brain stem region coordinates lower GI function, but it is under cortical control, just as it is for the lower urinary tract. Bowel incontinence is frequently unpredictable and not associated with the attainment of urinary control. It is often related to the consistency of fecal material and how rapidly the upper rectum refills after each evacuation. However, fecal incontinence is more devastating socially than urinary incontinence, especially in older children and adolescents [59]. Most bowel regimens begin in early infancy and are modulated throughout childhood to achieve the most normal level of function possible. Children are placed on diets intended to create a formed but not constipated stool. Fiber is an integral part of the child's intake. Suppositories to help evacuate the rectum are used regularly in order to train the lower bowel to fill and empty. Enemas are encouraged by some clinicians, but it is difficult for some children to retain the fluid that stimulates a bowel movement due to the laxity of the external anal sphincter. Biofeedback training has been used on occasion, but it may not be effective due to sphincter muscle denervation [60].

When diet, medications, and manual evacuation fail to achieve predictable bowel emptying without soiling, a continent cutaneous pathway from the lower abdominal wall to the cecum may be created using the vermiform appendix; this is called the ACE procedure, for Antegrade Continence Enema [61]. When the appendix is unavailable, a small segment of the bowel may be reconfigured to act as a catheterizable conduit [55]. Enemas consisting of either GoLYTELY, saline, or tap water sometimes in combination with bisacodyl are instilled daily or every other day to evacuate the colon. Cleansing the colon in this manner has resulted in complete continence in 89 % of children in whom it has been tried [62–64]. Older children readily become independent in managing their bowel function leading to improved self-esteem and sociability [65, 66].

## Sexuality and Quality of Life

Sexuality has become an increasingly important issue as these individuals mainstream into society and live longer more productive and satisfying lives. Increasingly more studies exist looking at quality of life assessments and sexual function [67, 68]. Females have no hormonal disturbances other than the onset of early puberty (possibly due to central nervous system effects on pituitary function) [69]. Thus, the ability to get pregnant is not impaired. Carrying a fetus to term and vaginal delivery may be difficult in some women with complete denervation of the pelvic floor [67, 70]. High-risk obstetrical centers often advocate for a planned Cesarean section to minimize complications at delivery. The ability of women to have an orgasm and to feel satisfied sexually is very variable, partly dependent on the degree of sensory nerve impairment. From quality of life assessment, sexual satisfaction is related to the presence of hydrocephalus, increased ambulation, and the degree of continence [71].

Males have varying degrees of sexual impairment as well, with impotency and ejaculatory dysfunction related to brain stem, spinal cord, and/or peripheral nerve root injury [72]. Sensory as well as motor function loss is the cause. The degree of physical impairment in males cannot be predicted based on the level of CNS dysfunction, as noted on neurologic assessment or urodynamic evaluation. Recent quality of life studies reveal that a substantial number of men can achieve an erection but maintaining it is harder to accomplish [73]. Sildenafil has been effective in counteracting

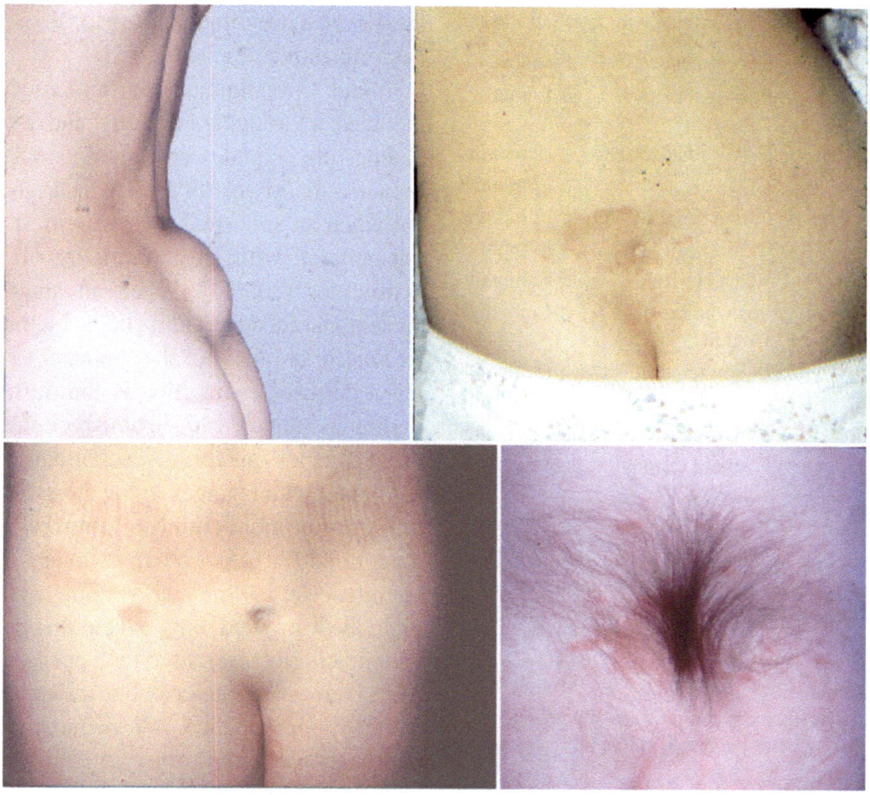

**Fig. 35.4** Typical skin manifestations on the lower back that suggest the presence of an underlying occult spinal dysraphism

this shortcoming [60]. A not insignificant number of men have claimed fatherhood in questionnaire studies to date, but no specific meaningful percentage of this capability is known [67, 74].

## Occult Spinal Dysraphism

Occult spinal dysraphism is being diagnosed with increasing frequency since the advent of spinal ultrasound and MR imaging [75]. An intraspinal lipoma or lipomeningocele, a diastematomyelia, a fatty filum with tethering of the cord, or a dermal sinus tract preventing the cephalad migration of the cord make up the extent of these disorders. More than 90 % of affected individuals have a cutaneous lesion on the lower back [76]. These lesions include a subcutaneous mass, dermal vascular malformation, hypertrichosis (hair patch), a midline dimple or sinus tract, a skin tag, or an asymmetric gluteal cleft (Fig. 35.4). These lesions often signify an underlying bony and/or spinal cord malformation. Ultrasound within the first 3 months of life can easily visualize the intraspinal space. Thus, most pediatricians should now image the back with a spinal ultrasound in any newborn whenever there is a suspicion of an occult dysraphism, based on finding one of these skin manifestations or an abnormality in the lower extremities. After this window in the newborn period has lapsed, MR imaging is needed to diagnose and/or confirm the presence of a spinal dysraphic state.

Most infants have no other manifestations of this disease (other than the cutaneous lesion) because lower extremity neurologic function is normal. In the past, before intraspinal imaging was feasible, these lesions often went undetected until urinary and/or fecal incontinence became problematic or lower limb difficulties became evident [76–79]. This change frequently occurs around the time of a pubertal growth

**Table 35.5** Surveillance in infants with myelodysplasia[a]

| Sphincter activity | Recommended tests | Frequency |
|---|---|---|
| Intact—synergic | Postvoid residual volume | q 4 months |
| | IVP or renal ECHO | q 12 months |
| | UDS | q 12 months |
| Intact—dyssynergic[b] | IVP or renal ECHO | q 12 months |
| | UDS | q 12 months |
| | VCUG or RNC[c] | q 12 months |
| Partial denervation | Postvoid residual volume | q 4 months |
| | IVP or renal ECHO | q 12 months |
| | UDS[d] | q 12 months |
| | VCUG or RNC[c] | q 12 months |
| Complete denervation | Postvoid residual volume | q 6 months |
| | Renal ECHO | q 12 months |

*IVP* intravenous pyelogram, *ECHO* sonogram, *UDS* urodynamic study, *VCUG* voiding cystourethrogram, *RNC* radionuclide cystogram
[a]Until age 5 years
[b]Patients receiving intermittent catheterization and anticholinergic agents
[c]If detrusor hypertonicity or reflux is already present
[d]Depending on degree of denervation (the more severe the less often)

spurt when increased traction on the spinal cord takes place [80]. As imaging techniques have evolved and urodynamic studies in children are being performed at an early age to assess sacral cord function, it has become clear that most babies have minimal neurologic impairment at first but that the neurologic lesion is likely to progress with advancing age [81] (Table 35.5).

The pathophysiology involves the apparent tension on the lower end of the spinal cord as the child grows. Normally, the conus medullaris ends at L1 and L2 at birth but "rises" cephalad to T12 and L1 at puberty. The differential growth rate between the spinal cord and the vertebral bodies stretches the lower cord and cauda equina due to fixation of the filum terminale to the bottom of the vertebral canal. Alternatively, the nerve roots emanating from the spinal cord become compressed by an expanding intraspinal lipoma. With time, this stretching and/or compression affect the oxidative process of the neural tissue, and this leads to impaired function of the lower extremities and/or lower urinary and gastrointestinal tracts [82, 83].

Initial investigation of an affected child includes a urodynamic study and a renal and bladder ultrasound. Urodynamic studies in children less than 1 year of age are invariably normal, but when an abnormality is present, it is usually not coupled with an abnormality of the lower extremities [80, 84]. When an abnormality is present, partial denervation in the urethral sphincter muscle or failure of the sphincter to relax during a detrusor contraction is the most common finding in infancy, while extensive denervation of the sphincter and/or an acontractile detrusor combined with changes in lower extremity function are the most common abnormalities in an older child [85]. As noted previously for myelomeningocele children, a voiding cystourethrogram is warranted only when the urodynamic parameters suggest risk to the upper urinary tract from increased bladder outlet resistance or poor detrusor compliance. Vesicoureteral reflux, hydronephrosis, and urinary incontinence are all managed in the same fashion one would treat children with similar neurologic impairment due to an open spinal abnormality.

The abnormal condition tends to improve following spinal cord de-tethering in the infant, but this normalization is unlikely when an older child is operated on [80, 85–87]. Therefore, specific urologic therapy is not instituted following delineation of an abnormality in infants until urodynamic studies are repeated 3 months or so after the condition has been repaired. If the findings have not changed or the child is older (when the chance that the neurologic abnormality will not improve), treatment based on the principles outlined in the section on open spinal lesions is instituted.

Thirty per cent of children operated on early in infancy will have secondary spinal cord tethering over time, some as late as puberty or just beyond it, when the last major growth spurt occurs [76, 85, 87]. Therefore, careful surveillance and repeat assessment are warranted at the first sign of urinary and/or fecal incontinence or a change in lower extremity function. No child is considered risk-free until he/she has reached their full adult height.

## Sacral Agenesis

The partial or complete absence of the most caudad vertebral bodies has been labeled sacral agenesis. The condition can range from missing part or all of just the last two or three sacral bodies to the absence of all sacral and several lumbar bones (sirenomelia). The condition is seen in the offspring of insulin-dependent diabetic mothers (1 %) [88], but it may be part of a genetic disorder due to a deletion of part of chromosome 7 (7q36) leading to the absence of an important transcription factor that plays a role in the development of the caudal end of the spinal cord and vertebral column [89]. In familial cases of sacral agenesis associated with the Currarino triad syndrome (presacral mass, sacral agenesis, and anorectal malformation), deletions in chromosome 7 (7q) resulting in HLXB9 genetic mutations have been found [90]. A mutation in HLXB9, a homeodomain gene of a 403 amino acid protein, which appears to be responsible for neural plate infolding, has been identified in 20 of 21 patients with familial and in 2 of 7 sporadic cases of Currarino triad syndrome [91, 92]. Heterozygote carriers within these families have also been identified [93]. Thus, sacral agenesis may represent one point on a spectrum of abnormalities that encompass both a sacral meningocele and anorectal malformations [94].

In the newborn period (and even afterwards), these affected infants appear normal with no lower extremity abnormality. Unless thought of when evaluating a newborn of a diabetic mother, these babies often go undiagnosed. With time, as the child has difficulty with toilet training or has urinary infection, it becomes evident that there is a problem [88, 95]. On physical examination, a subtle but pathognomonic sign is absence of the upper end of the gluteal cleft with flattened buttocks (Fig. 35.5). Lower extremity motor and sensory function usually remain normal, but there may be minor changes with weakness of the toes and/or diminished sensation in the S1 dermatome if the lesion affects these higher nerve roots. When considering this diagnosis, a lateral spine film (or a spinal ultrasound in infants under 3 months of age) will confirm the abnormality (Fig. 35.6). A spinal MR reveals a sharp cutoff to the cord at about T12 with nerve roots streaming from it. About 90 % of the children develop neurogenic bladder dysfunction [96].

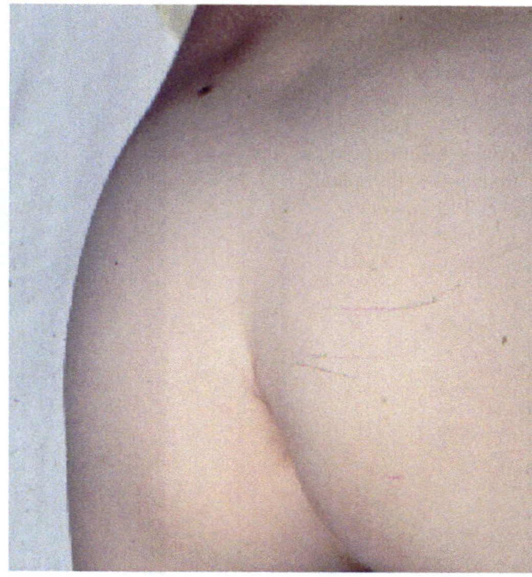

**Fig. 35.5** The typical appearance of the lower back in a child with sacral agenesis (note the flattened buttocks and absence of the gluteal crease extending very cephalad

Of the children with a neurologic deficit, an almost equal number have either an overactive detrusor with sphincter dyssynergy (46 %) or an acontractile detrusor with complete denervation in the urethral sphincter (41 %) [95, 97]. The former is often associated with recurrent urinary infection and vesicoureteral reflux, whereas the latter produces continuous incontinence, urinary as well as fecal [96]. The type of neurologic impairment affecting the lower urinary tract cannot be predicted from the level of absent or abnormal vertebral bones [95]. Obviously, management depends on the type of dysfunction present. CIC, anticholinergic medication, and antibiotics are instituted in those children with an upper motor neuron-type lesion, while surgical measures that increase bladder outlet resistance, as outlined in the section for myelomeningocele, coupled with CIC are needed in those with an incompetent urethral sphincter mechanism.

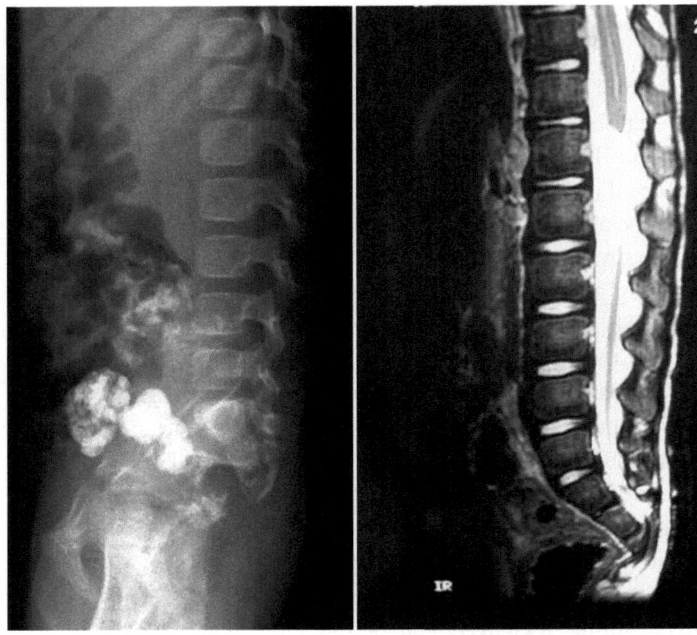

**Fig. 35.6** A lateral spine film (*left*) confirms the absence of the lowermost vertebrae (*arrow*), and a spinal MRI (*right*) reveals no conus medullaris and a sharp cutoff to the spinal cord at T12 (*arrow*)

## References


1. Austin PF, Bauer SB, Bower W, Chase J, Franco I, Hoebeke P, Rittig S, Vande Walle J, von Gontard A, Wright A, Yang SS, Neveus T. Standardization of terminology of lower urinary tract function in children and adolescents: update report from the standardization committee of International Children's Continence Society. J Urol. 2014;191:1863–66.
2. Stark GD. Spina bifida: problems and management. Oxford: Blackwell Scientific; 1977.
3. Centers for Disease Control and Prevention. Spina bifida and anencephaly before and after folic acid mandate—United States, 1995-1996 and 1999-2000. MMWR Morb Mortal Wkly Rep. 2004;53:362–5.
4. Williams LJ, Rasmussen SA, Flores A, Kirby RS, Edmonds LD. Decline in the prevalence of spina bifida and anencephaly by race/ethnicity: 1995–2002. Pediatrics. 2005;116:580–6.
5. Bauer SB, Labib KB, Dieppa RA, Retik AB. Urodynamic evaluation in a boy with myelodysplasia and incontinence. Urology. 1977;10:354–62.
6. Assessment of neural tube defects in fetuses: accuracy of imaging and correlation of findings with neurourologic outcomes. In: The annual meeting of the European Society of Pediatric Urology, Brugge, Belgium; 27 April 2007.
7. Bruner JP, Tulipan N, Paschall RL, et al. Fetal surgery for myelomeningocele and the incidence of shunt dependent hydrocephalus. JAMA. 1999;282:1819–25.
8. Holzbeierlein J, Pope JC, Adams MC, et al. The urodynamic profile of myelodysplasia in childhood with spinal canal closure during gestation. J Urol. 2000; 164:1336.
9. Koh C, DeFilippo R, Bauer SB, Borer JG, Khoshbin S. Lower urinary tract function after fetal closure of myelomeningocele. J Urol. 2006;176:2232–6.
10. Adzick NS, Thom EA, Spong CY, Brock JW 3rd, Burrows PK, Johnson MP, Howell LJ, Farrell JA, Dabrowiak ME, Sutton LN, Gupta N, Tulipan NB, D'Alton ME, Farmer DL. MOMS Investigators. N Engl J Med. 2011;364(11):993–1004.
11. Yeung CK, Sreedhar B, Leung VT, Metreweli C. Ultrasound bladder measurements in patients with primary nocturnal enuresis: a urodynamic and treatment outcome correlation. J Urol. 2004;171:2589–94.
12. Bauer SB. Myelodysplasia, newborn evaluation and management. In: McLaurin RL, editor. Spina bifida: a multidisciplinary approach. New York: Praeger; 1984. p. 262–7.
13. Bauer SB, Hallet M, Khoshbin S, Lebowitz RL, Winston KR, Gibson S, Colodny AH, Retik AB. The predictive value of urodynamic evaluation in the newborn with myelodysplasia. JAMA. 1984;152:650–2.
14. Edelstein RA, Bauer SB, Kelly MD, Darbey MM, Peters CA, Atala A, Mandell J, Colodny AH, Retik AB. The long-term urologic response of neonates with myelodysplasia treated proactively with intermittent catheterization and anticholinergic therapy. J Urol. 1995;154:1500–4.
15. Kaefer M, Pabby A, Kelly M, Darbey M, Bauer SB. Improved bladder function after prophylactic treatment of the high risk neurogenic bladder in newborns with myelomeningocele. J Urol. 1999;162:1068–71.
16. Dik P, van Gool JD, de Jong-de V, van Steenwijk CC, de Jong TP. Early start therapy preserves kidney function in spina bifida. Eur Urol. 2006;49:908–13.
17. Geranoitis E, Koff SA, Enrile B. Prophylactic use of clean intermittent catheterization in treatment of infants

and young children with myelomeningocele and neurogenic bladder dysfunction. J Urol. 1988;139:85–6.
18. Wu H-Y, Baskin LS, Kogan BA. Neurogenic bladder dysfunction due to myelomeningocele: neonatal versus childhood treatment. J Urol. 1997;157:2295–7.
19. Bauer SB. The management of spina bifida from birth onwards. In: Whitaker RH, Woodard JR, editors. Paediatric urology. London: Butterworths; 1985. p. 87–112.
20. Hopps CV, Kropp KA. Preservation of renal function in children with myelomeningocele managed with basic newborn evaluation and close followup. J Urol. 2003;169:305–8.
21. Teichman JMH, Scherz HC, Kim KD, Cho DH, Packer MG, Kaplan GW. An alternative approach to myelodysplasia management: aggressive observation and prompt intervention. J Urol. 1994;152:807–11.
22. Perez LM, Khoury J, Webster GD. The value of urodynamic studies in infants less than one year old with congenital spinal dysraphism. J Urol. 1992;148: 584–7.
23. Seki N, Akazawa K, Senoh K, Kubo S, Tsunoda T, Kimoto Y, Naito S. An analysis of risk factors for upper urinary tract deterioration in patients with myelodysplasia. Br J Urol. 1999;84:679–82.
24. Joseph DB, Bauer SB, Colodny AH, Mandell J, Retik AB. Clean intermittent catheterization in infants with neurogenic bladder. Pediatrics. 1989;84:78–82.
25. Bauer SB. Neuropathic dysfunction of the lower urinary tract. In: Wein AJ, Kavoussi LR, Novick AC, Partin AW, Peters CA, editors. Campbell—Walsh urology. 9th ed. Philadelphia: Saunders Elsevier; 2006. p. 3625–55.
26. Schlager TA, Clark M, Anderson S. Effect of a single-use sterile catheter for each void on the frequency of bacteriuria in children with neurogenic bladder on intermittent catheterization for bladder emptying. Pediatrics. 2001;108:E71.
27. Cohen RA, Rushton HG, Belman AB, Kass EJ, Majd M, Shaer C. Renal scarring and vesicoureteral reflux in children with myelodysplasia. J Urol. 1990;144:541–4.
28. Agarwal SK, McLorie GA, Grewal D, Joyner BD, Bägli DJ, Khoury AE. Urodynamic correlates of resolution of reflux meningomyelocele patients. J Urol. 1997;158:580–2.
29. Barbalais GA, Klauber GT, Blaivas JG. Critical evaluation of the Credé maneuver: a urodynamic study of 207 patients. J Urol. 1983;130:720.
30. Bauer SB. Vesico-ureteral reflux in children with neurogenic bladder dysfunction. In: Johnston JH, editor. International perspectives in urology, vol. 10. Baltimore: Williams & Wilkins; 1984. p. 159–77.
31. Nasrallah PF, Aliabadi HA. Bladder augmentation in patients with neurogenic bladder and vesicoureteral reflux. J Urol. 1991;146:1991.
32. Simforoosh N, Tabibi A, Basiri A, Noorbala MH, Danesh AD, Ijadi A. Is ureteral reimplantation necessary during augmentation cystoplasty in patients with neurogenic bladder and vesicoureteral reflux? J Urol. 2002;168:1439–41.
33. Juhasz Z, Somogyi R, Vajda P, Oberritter Z, Fathi K, Pinter AB. Does the type of bladder augmentation influence the resolution of pre-existing vesicoureteral reflux? Urodynamic studies. Neurourol Urodyn. 2008;27:412–6.
34. Elder JS. Therapy for vesicoureteral reflux: antibiotic prophylaxis, urotherapy, open surgery, endoscopic injection, or observation? Curr Urol Rep. 2008;9: 143–50.
35. Elder JS, Diaz M, Caldamone AA, Cendron M, Greenfield S, Hurwitz R, Kirsch A, Koyle MA, Pope J, Shapiro E. Endoscopic therapy for vesicoureteral reflux: a meta-analysis. I. Reflux resolution and urinary tract infection. J Urol. 2006;175:716–22.
36. Kirsch AJ, Perez-Brayfield M, Smith EA, Scherz HC. The modified sting procedure to correct vesicoureteral reflux: improved results with submucosal implantation within the intramural ureter. J Urol. 2004;171: 2413–6.
37. Schulte-Baukloh H, Knispel HH, Stolze T, Weiss C, Michael T, Miller K. Repeated botulinum-A toxin injections in treatment of children with neurogenic detrusor overactivity. Urology. 2005;66:865–70.
38. Akbar M, Abel R, Seyler TM, Bedke J, Haferkamp A, Gerner HJ, Möhring K. Repeated botulinum-A toxin injections in the treatment of myelodysplastic children and patients with spinal cord injuries with neurogenic bladder dysfunction. BJU Int. 2007;100: 639–45.
39. Metcalfe PD, Rink RC. Bladder augmentation: complications in the pediatric population. Curr Urol Rep. 2007;8:152–6.
40. Nguyen DH, Bain MA, Salmonson KL, Ganesan GS, Burns MW, Mithell ME. The syndrome of dysuria and hematuria in pediatric urinary reconstruction with stomach. J Urol. 1993;150:707.
41. Gosalbez Jr R, Woodard JR, Broecker BH, Warshaw B. Metabolic complication of the use of stomach for urinary reconstruction. J Urol. 1993;150:710.
42. Vemulakonda VM, Lendvay TS, Shnorhavorian M, Joyner BD, Kaplan H, Mitchell ME, Grady RW. Metastatic adenocarcinoma after augmentation gastrocystoplasty. J Urol. 2008;179:1094–7.
43. Castellan M, Gosalbez R, Perez-Brayfield M, Healey P, McDonald R, Labbie A, Lendvay T. Tumor in bladder reservoir after gastrocystoplasty. J Urol. 2007;178: 1771–4.
44. Austin JC. Long-term risks of bladder augmentation in pediatric patients. Curr Opin Urol. 2008;18:408–12.
45. Colvert III JR, Kropp BP, Cheng EY, Pope IV JC, et al. The use of small intestinal submucosa as an off-the-shelf urethral sling material for pediatric urinary incontinence. J Urol. 2002;168:1872–6.
46. Elder JS. Periurethral and pubovaginal sling repair for incontinence in patients with myelodysplasia. J Urol. 1990;144:434.
47. Castellan M, Gosalbez R, Labbie A, Ibrahim E, DiSandro M. Bladder neck sling for treatment of neurogenic incontinence in children with augmentation cystoplasty: long-term results. J Urol. 2005;173: 2128–31.

48. Levesque PE, Bauer SB, Atala A, Zurakowski D, Colodny A, Peters C, Retik AB. Ten-year experience with artificial urinary sphincters in children. J Urol. 1996;156:625–8.
49. Catti M, Lortat-Jacob S, Morineau M, Lottmann H. Artificial urinary sphincter in children-voiding or emptying? An evaluation of functional results in 44 patients. J Urol. 2008;180:690–3.
50. Roth DR, Vyas PR, Kroovan RL, Perlmutter AD. Urinary tract deterioration associated with the artificial urinary sphincter. J Urol. 1986;135:528.
51. Bauer SB, Reda EF, Colodny AH, Retik AB. Detrusor instability. A delayed complication in association with the artificial sphincter. J Urol. 1986;135:1212–5.
52. Mitrofanoff P. Cystometric continente trans-appendiculaire dans le traitement de vessies neurologiques. Chir Pediatr. 1980;21:297.
53. MacNeily AE, Morrell J, Secord S. Lower urinary tract reconstruction for spina bifida—does it improve health related quality of life? J Urol. 2005;174:1637–43.
54. Woodhouse CRJ, Malone PR, Cumming J, Reilly TM. The Mitrofanoff principle for continent urinary diversion. Br J Urol. 1989;63:53.
55. Montie PR, Lara RC, Dutra MA, DeCarvalho JR. New techniques for construction of efferent conduits based on the Mitrofanoff Principle. Urology. 1997;49:112.
56. Gerharz EW, Tassadaq T, Pickard RS, Shah P, Julian R, Woodhouse CRJ, Ransley PG. Transverse retubularized ileum: early clinical experience with a new second line Mitrofanoff tube. J Urol. 1998;159: 525–8.
57. Harris CF, Cooper CS, Hutcheson JC, Snyder III HM. Appendicovesicostomy: the Mitrofanoff procedure-A 15 year perspective. J Urol. 2000;163:1922–6.
58. Atala A, Bauer SB, Soker S, Yoo JJ, Retik AB. Tissue-engineered autologous bladders for patients needing cystoplasty. Lancet. 2006;367:1241–6.
59. Krogh K, Lie HR, Bilenber N, et al. 2003 Bowel function in Danish children with myelomeningocele. APMIS Suppl. 2003;(109):81.
60. Loening-Baucke V, Deach L, Wolraich M. Biofeedback training for patients with myelomeningocele and fecal incontinence. Dev Med Child Neurol. 1988; 30:781.
61. Griffiths DM, Malone PS. The Malone antegrade continence enema. J Pediatr Surg. 1995;30:68–71.
62. Squire R, Kiely EM, Carr B, et al. The clinical application of the Malone antegrade colonic enema. J Pediatr Surg. 1993;28:1012–5.
63. Gerharz EW, Vik V, Webb G, et al. The in situ appendix in the Malone antegrade continent enema procedure for faecal incontinence. Br J Urol. 1997;79:985.
64. Yerkes EB, Rink RC, Cain MP, Casale AJ. Use of a Monti channel for administration of antegrade continent enemas. J Urol. 2002;168:1883–5.
65. Bau MO, Younes S, Aupy A, Bernuy M, Rouffet MJ, Yepremian D, Lottmann HB. The Malone antegrade colonic enema isolated or associated with urological incontinence procedures: evaluation from patient point of view. J Urol. 2001;165:2399–403.
66. Aksnes G, Diseth TH, Helseth A, et al. Appendicostomy for antegrade enema: effects on somatic and psychosocial functioning in children with myelomeningocele. Pediatrics. 2002;109:484.
67. Bomalaski MD, Teague JL, Brooks B. The long-term impact of urologic management on the quality of life in children with spina bifida. J Urol. 1995;156:778.
68. Palmer JS, Kaplan WE, Firlit CF. Erectile dysfunction in patients with spina bifida is a treatable condition. J Urol. 2000;164:958–61.
69. Cass AS, Bloom BA, Luxenberg M. Sexual function in adults with myelomeningocele. J Urol. 1986;136:425.
70. Arata M, Grover S, Dunne K, Bryan D. Pregnancy outcome and complications in women with spina bifida. J Reprod Med. 2000;45:743–8.
71. Lassmann J, Garibay Gonzalez F, Melchionni JB, Pasquariello Jr PS, Snyder III HM. Sexual function in adult patients with spina bifida and its impact on quality of life. J Urol. 2007;178:1611–4.
72. Woodhouse CRJ. Myelomeningocele in young adults. BJU Int. 2005;95:223–30.
73. Gamé X, Moscovici J, Gamé L, Sarramon JP, Rischmann P, Malavaud B. Evaluation of sexual function in young men with spina bifida and myelomeningocele using the International Index of Erectile Function. Urology. 2006;67:566–70.
74. Decter RM, Furness PD, Nguyen TA, et al. Reproductive understanding, sexual functioning and testosterone levels in men with spina bifida. J Urol. 1997;157:1466–8.
75. Bruce DA, Schut L. Spinal lipomas in infancy and childhood. Brain. 1979;5:192–203.
76. Pierre-Kahn A, Zerah M, Renier D, Cinalli G, Sainte-Rose C, Lellouch-Tubiana A, Brunelle F, Le Merrer M, Giudicelli Y, Pichon J, Kleinknecht B, Nataf F. Congenital lumbosacral lipomas. Childs Nerv Syst. 1997;13:298–334.
77. Mandell J, Bauer SB, Hallett M, Khoshbin S, Dyro FM, Colodny AH, Retik AB. Occult spinal dysraphism: a rare but detectable cause of voiding dysfunction. Urol Clin North Am. 1980;7:349–56.
78. Koyanagi I, Iwasaki Y, Hida K, Abe H, Isu T, Akino M. Surgical treatment supposed natural history of the tethered cord with occult spinal dysraphism. Childs Nerv Syst. 1987;13:268–74.
79. Sarica K, Erbagci A, Yagci F, Yurtseven C. Multidisciplinary evaluation of occult spinal dysraphism in 47 children. Scand J Urol Nephrol. 2003;37:329–34.
80. Satar N, Bauer SB, Shefner J, Kelly MD, Darbey MM. The effects of delayed diagnosis and treatment in patients with an occult spinal dysraphism. J Urol. 1995;154:754–8.
81. Keating MA, Rink RC, Bauer SB, Krarup C, Dyro FM, Winston KR, Shillito J, Fischer EG, Retik AB. Neuro-urologic implications of changing approach in management of occult spinal lesions. J Urol. 1998; 140:1299.
82. Yamada S, Won DJ, Yamada SM. Pathophysiology of tethered cord syndrome: correlation with symptomatology. Neurosurg Focus. 2004;16:E6.

83. Henderson FC, Geddes JF, Vaccaro AR, Eric W, Berry KJ, Benzel EC. Stretch-associated injury in cervical spondylotic myelopathy. Neurosurgery. 2005;56: 1101–3.
84. Nogueira M, Greenfield SP, Wan J, Wan J, Santana A, Li V. Tethered cord in children: a clinical classification with urodynamic correlation. J Urol. 2004;172: 1677–80.
85. Satar N, Bauer SB, Scott RM, Shefner J, Kelly M, Darbey M. Late effects of early surgery on lipoma and lipomeningocele in children less than two years old. J Urol. 1997;157:1434–7.
86. Cornette L, Verpoorten C, Lagae L, Van Calenbergh F, Plets C, Vereecken R, Casaer P. Tethered spinal cord in occult spinal dysraphism: timing and outcome of surgical release. Neurology. 1998;50:1761–5.
87. Proctor M, Bauer SB, Scott MR. The effect of surgery for the split spinal cord malformation on neurologic and urologic function. Pediatr Neurosurg. 2000;32: 13–9.
88. Wilmshurst JM, Kelly R, Borzyskowski M. Presentation and outcome of sacral agenesis: 20 years' experience. Dev Med Child Neurol. 1999;41:806–12.
89. Papapetrou C, Drummond F, Reardon W, Winter R, Spitz L, Edwards YH. A genetic study of the human T gene and its exclusion as a major candidate gene for sacral agenesis with anorectal atresia. J Med Genet. 1999;36:208–13.
90. Ross AJ, Ruiz-Perez V, Wang Y, Hagan DM, Scherer S, Lynch SA, Lindsay S, Custard E, Belloni E, Wilson DI, Wadey R, Goodman F, Orstavik KH, Monclair T, Robson S, Reardon W, Burn J, Scambler P, Strachan T. A homeobox gene, HLXB9, is the major locus for dominantly inherited sacral agenesis. Nat Genet. 1998;20:358–61.
91. Kochling J, Karbasiyan M, Reis A. Spectrum of mutations and genotype-phenotype analysis in Currarino syndrome. Eur J Hum Genet. 2001;9:599–605.
92. Hagan DM, Ross AJ, Strachan T, Lynch SA, Ruiz-Perez V, Wang YM, Scambler P, Custard E, Reardon W, Hassan S, Nixon P, Papapetrou C, Winter RM, Edwards Y, Morrison K, Barrow M, Cordier-Alex MP, Correia P, Galvin-Parton PA, Gaskill S, Gaskin KJ, Garcia-Minaur S, Gereige R, Hayward R, Homfray T. Mutation analysis and embryonic expression of the HLXB9 Currarino syndrome gene. Am J Hum Genet. 2000;66:1504–14.
93. Lynch SA, Wang Y, Strachan T, Burn J, Lindsay S. Autosomal dominant sacral agenesis: Currarino syndrome. J Med Genet. 2000;37:561–6.
94. Bernbeck B, Schurfeld-Furstenberg K, Ketteler K, Kemperdick H, Schroten H. Unilateral pulmonary atresia with total sacral agenesis and other congenital defects. Clin Dysmorphol. 2004;13:47–8.
95. Guzman L, Bauer SB, Hallet M, Khoshbin S, Colodny AH, Retik AB. The evaluation and management of children with sacral agenesis. Urology. 1983;23:506–10.
96. De Biasio P, Ginocchio G, Aicardi G, Ravera G, Venturini PL, Vignolo M. Ossification timing of sacral vertebrae by ultrasound in the mid-second trimester of pregnancy. Prenat Diagn. 2003;23:1056–9.
97. Boemers TM, Van Gool JD, deJong TP, Bax KMA. Urodynamic evaluation of children with caudal regression syndrome (caudal dysplasia sequence). J Urol. 1994;151:1038–40.

# Continent Urinary Diversion

# 36

Rosalia Misseri and Richard C. Rink

Children with neuropathic voiding dysfunction, congenital anomalies of the lower urinary tract, and pelvic malignances may require urinary tract reconstruction. In these children the bladder may be absent due to surgical removal or being small and hypercontractile or hypocontractile. As a consequence, the child may develop vesicoureteral reflux or hydronephrosis secondary to high intravesical pressure, incontinence, or urinary retention. Overall, the goals of reconstruction are to maintain and preserve renal function, achieve urinary continence, and limit urinary infection. Terminology can be confusing but "incontinent diversion" refers to surgery that results in the need for an external collection bag such as an ileal conduit. Continent urinary diversion refers to a surgically constructed internal reservoir that does not require a bag but generally requires intermittent catheterization to empty. These reconstructions should create a low-pressure, acontractile or minimally contractile, capacious reservoir. In children, these reservoirs are most often created by adding an intestinal segment to the native bladder in order to "augment" the bladder. In cases where the bladder has been entirely resected, an entire new reservoir for urine may be fashioned from bowel alone and is termed a "continent urinary reservoir" (CUR).

The majority of children with bladder substitutions or augmented bladders are unable to void spontaneously and need a way to reliably empty the bladder. Catheterization through the native urethra or through a catheterizable channel created with a segment of bowel allows for bladder emptying. In children with low-pressure bladder outlets (low sphincter pressures), additional surgery on the bladder neck may be necessary to provide adequate outflow resistance to prevent urinary incontinence. Children with neuropathic bladders due to myelomeningocele may have an incompetent bladder neck causing continuous leakage of urine at low bladder volumes and low bladder pressures. Patients with bladder exstrophy, epispadias, or bilateral ectopic ureters have a poorly formed bladder and/or absent bladder necks and similarly may require surgery to increase bladder outlet resistance.

Regardless of the procedure performed, the most important aspect of lower urinary tract reconstruction is the preoperative evaluation of the patient. Both medical and social issues must be addressed fully. A thorough history should be obtained and a physical examination should be performed. Particular attention to past surgeries including cystectomy, bowel surgery, previous pelvic radiation, and history of renal disease is crucial. All patients should have a thorough

R. Misseri, M.D. (✉)
James Whitcomb Riley Hospital for Children, Indiana University School of Medicine, 705 Riley Hospital Drive, ROC4230, Indianapolis, IN 46202, USA
e-mail: rmisseri@iupui.edu

R.C. Rink, M.D.
James Whitcomb Riley Hospital for Children, Indiana University School of Medicine, Indianapolis, IN, USA

R. Rabinowitz et al. (eds.), *Pediatric Urology for the Primary Care Physician*, Current Clinical Urology,
DOI 10.1007/978-1-60327-243-8_36, © Springer Science+Business Media New York 2015

evaluation of the upper urinary tract beginning with renal ultrasonography. All patients with a bladder should undergo preoperative urodynamics to evaluate bladder capacity, bladder compliance, and outlet resistance. When fluoroscopy is used during urodynamics (videourodynamics or fluorourodynamics), one may also evaluate for vesicoureteral reflux and gain additional information regarding the bladder outlet and leakage per urethra. If urodynamics are performed without fluoroscopy, a voiding cystourethrogram should be obtained to evaluate for vesicoureteral reflux. Nuclear renography is used to evaluate renal function and rule out upper urinary tract obstruction when renal asymmetry or hydronephrosis has been identified on renal ultrasound. Preoperative assessment of renal function and nutritional status is also important for surgical planning and may dictate the type of reservoir that is created.

The patient and his/her caregivers must be totally committed to maintaining a healthy urinary tract. Stable family life and dedicated caregivers are essential to the success of the surgery. They must realize that catheterization is a lifelong commitment and that failure to catheterize in a timely fashion may result in potentially life-threatening consequences such as bladder perforation, infections, stone formation, and upper urinary tract deterioration. A child's physical and mental limitations should be considered as they may affect his/her ability and willingness to catheterize.

## Bladder Augmentation

Bladder augmentation is a major surgical procedure aimed at creating a more compliant, capacious bladder. Several surgical techniques to achieve this goal have been described over the last 30 years. The native bladder is bivalved to allow for the anastomosis of the gastrointestinal segment. If bowel is used, the intestinal segment is opened on the antimesenteric border and reconfigured in order to reduce intravesical pressure and contractions. This is done such that a spherical shape is created when the bowel is anastomosed to the bladder. This results in an augmented bladder with increased capacity, improved compliance, and fewer uninhibited contractions. A catheterizable channel (see below) is usually created in conjunction with this procedure. Several segments including the stomach, ileum, cecum, sigmoid, and the ileocecal segment have been used for bladder augmentation. Today, the most commonly performed surgical procedure is the ileocystoplasty; however, many interesting alternatives are on the horizon.

### Ileocystoplasty

The ileum is the least contractile segment of the gastrointestinal tract and therefore remains the segment most commonly used. In general, 20–30 cm of bowel 15–20 cm proximal to the ileocecal valve is isolated and an ileoileostomy is performed. The bowel segment is then opened, reconfigured in an S or W shape, and anastomosed to the bivalved bladder.

### Gastrocystoplasty

A gastrocystoplasty may be quite advantageous in children with short gut or in patients with renal insufficiency and metabolic acidosis that will not soon be transplanted. Though successfully used to augment the bladder, the used stomach is significantly limited due to hematuria-dysuria syndrome (HDS). HDS is particularly limiting in patients with sensate urethras. Ultimate bladder capacity when using a gastric segment may not be as large than that of an ileocystoplasty.

## Complications

### Metabolic Consequences

The particular metabolic derangements that occur after bladder augmentation are dependent on the segment of bowel used for the reconstruction. Hyperchloremic metabolic acidosis is associated with the use of colon or ileum. The colon and ileum maintain their secretory and absorptive properties after being incorporated into the urinary tract. In an exchange mechanism, chloride from the urine is absorbed by the bowel mucosa while bicarbonate is secreted. Ammonium, hydrogen, and organic acids are also reabsorbed by the bowel mucosa. The normal mechanism for buffering a chronic acid load is not possible as ammonium is reabsorbed across the intestinal segment. Therefore, in order to handle the increased acid load, inorganic salts and bony buffers are liberated. This may lead to bone demineralization that may lead to a decrease in linear growth. The metabolic acidosis may be mild, requiring no intervention, or severe and chronic requiring therapy. Limiting the time that urine remains in contact with the intestinal segment may improve metabolic abnormalities. Patients with chronic metabolic acidosis should be treated with oral alkaline therapy.

Additional problems related to the absorptive properties of the intestinal segment also occur. The intestinal segment of the augmented bladder may absorb drugs, notably phenytoin, and doses may require adjustment. The intestinal segment may also absorb urinary glucose, and therefore urinary glucose spot checks in diabetics may be inaccurate. Urine pregnancy tests have also been reported to be inaccurate in this population.

Gastrocystoplasty is responsible for nearly the opposite metabolic derangements. Hypokalemic, hypochloremic metabolic alkalosis may occur after gastrocystoplasty as hydrogen and chloride ions are secreted across the gastric mucosa. Stretching of the gastric segment of the augmented bladder may stimulate further acid secretion. Patients with a gastrocystoplasty and chronic or recurrent electrolyte abnormalities may require salt supplementation and/or H-2 blockers. Refractory cases may require proton pump inhibitors while others may require removal of the gastric segment or addition of an ileal patch to counteract existing electrolyte abnormalities.

## Mucus Production

All intestinal segments maintain their intrinsic properties including the production of mucus. Mucus production continues for years after augmentation though it may diminish with time. Mucus in the augmented bladder increases the risk of urinary tract infection and may interfere with the ability to empty the bladder completely using clean intermittent catheterization (CIC). Daily bladder irrigations are recommended to help eliminate mucus and decrease the risk of urinary tract infection and stone formation associated with retained mucus. Mucus produced by the intestinal segment may also be responsible for false-positives in women using commercially available urinary pregnancy tests.

## Stones

The risk of stone formation after enterocystoplasty has been reported to be as high as 52 % but in our hands has occurred in approximately 15 %. Potential factors that may lead to bladder stone formation after augmentation include urinary stasis, chronic bacteriuria, mucus production, abnormal urinary pH, and poor bladder emptying. Chronic bacteriuria with urea-splitting organisms such as *Klebsiella* and *Proteus* species is implicated in the formation of magnesium ammonium phosphate (struvite) calculi after augment. Patients with bladder outlet procedures and abdominal wall stomas are at increased risk likely related to increased difficulty emptying urine and mucus from the base of the bladder. Calculi may be removed endoscopically or via an open cystolithotomy.

## Urinary Tract Infection

A high incidence of bacteriuria after enterocystoplasty is likely related to urinary stasis, CIC, and urine pH. Nearly all patients with intestine in their urinary tract and on CIC will develop an infection at some time. Treatment of asymptomatic bacteriuria in patients that perform CIC is not typically indicated. If the patient has complaints of hematuria, suprapubic pain, foul odor, worsening incontinence, increased mucus production, or growth of urea-splitting organisms that predispose to stone formation, treatment is indicated. Urea-splitting organisms include bacteria from the *Proteus*, *Ureaplasma*, *Staphylococcus*, *Klebsiella*, *Pseudomonas*, and *Providencia* species.

## Bowel Obstruction

As with any major abdominal surgery, intra-abdominal adhesions and mechanical bowel obstruction may occur after augmentation cystoplasty. In the Indiana series bowel obstruction occurred in 3 %. In neurologically impaired patients bowel obstruction may present with atypical signs. Suspicion for obstruction should remain high in patients with nausea, vomiting, bloating, or pain.

## Bladder Perforation

Spontaneous perforation is a serious and potentially lethal complication of augmentation cystoplasty that has been reported in up to 10 % of patients. The site of perforation is typically within 1 cm of enterovesical anastomosis. At presentation the patient may be critically ill particularly as early symptoms may be masked in neurologically impaired individuals. There should be a high index of suspicion in any augmented patient that presents with abdominal pain, poor drainage, fever, or hemodynamic instability. Computed tomography of the abdomen and pelvis with a cystogram is the preferred radiographic evaluation. Images should be obtained with both the bladder full and empty. Standard cystograms may have up to a 33 % false-negative rate. While the patient is being evaluated radiographically, broad-spectrum antibiotics should be started, intravenous fluids should be administered, and a catheter should be anchored to allow for continuous bladder drainage.

The risk of fatal sepsis due to perforation increases with delays in diagnosis and treatment. If there is a strong clinical suspicion despite a negative radiographic evaluation or if radiographic evaluation cannot be completed in a timely fashion, urgent surgical exploration may be warranted.

Standard therapy involves surgical exploration, debridement of the perforated area, and closure of the perforation. The peritoneal cavity should be well irrigated. If the patient has a ventriculoperitoneal shunt, a neurosurgical consultation should be obtained. Conservative management with continuous bladder drainage, parenteral antibiotics, and serial abdominal examinations has been successful in carefully selected patients.

## Malignancy

Concern exists regarding the increased risk of tumor formation in augmented bladders. Various tumors have been described in the augmented bladder including adenocarcinomas, transitional cell carcinomas, and rare signet cell tumors. These tumors have been described in all gastrointestinal segments. The exact etiology is unknown; however, bacterial growth, urinary N-nitrosamines, chronic inflammation secondary to catheterization, and infection may be involved. The current risk of tumor in the augmented bladder remains unknown but an increased risk is apparent. It is currently our recommendation that all patients undergo a yearly cytology and cystoscopy beginning 7 years after augmentation cystoplasty.

## Alternatives

Though the intestinocystoplasty has been successful in creating a compliant, large capacity organ for the storage of urine, it is associated with numerous complications. The ideal augmented bladder would be lined with urothelium to prevent metabolic changes and mucus production. Many attempts have been made to create a metabolically neutral reservoir with and without the addition of gastrointestinal tissue. Though infrequently used, each variation has unique advantages and disadvantages.

### Gastrointestinal Composite Augment

Composite augments (intestine and stomach segments) are most often used to achieve electrolyte neutrality. As previously discussed, the metabolic changes associated with intestinal augment and gastric augment essentially oppose each other. This is an advantageous procedure in patients with preexisting metabolic acidosis or short gut syndromes. The disadvantages include longer operative times related to the need for two distinct anastomoses.

### Autoaugmentation

In autoaugmentation the muscularis of the bladder dome is excised leaving the urothelium to bulge similar to a diverticulum. This results in an increased bladder capacity and decreased bladder pressures. The advantages of this procedure over intestinocystoplasty include decreased risks of stones, tumors, and metabolic anomalies since the entire bladder is lined with urothelium without intestinal mucosa. The applicability is limited as few patients achieve adequate capacity with autoaugmentation alone.

### Ureterocystoplasty

The ureter is an ideal tissue with which to augment the bladder. The ureter may be sufficiently dilated due to high-pressure reflux that it may be used in to augment the bladder. Massively dilated ureters may be associated with nonfunctioning kidneys and in these cases the renal pelvis may also be used. Though an ideal autologous tissue, it is rare to find massively dilated ureters with nonfunctioning kidneys in children with neurogenic bladders that have been properly been followed and cared for since birth.

### Seromuscular Segments with Urothelial Lining

In this procedure a demucosalized colonic or gastric segment is placed over the bulging urothelium after a procedure similar to an autoaugmentation. Theoretically this should eliminate contracture seen commonly after autoaugmentation and preserve a urothelial bladder lining. Disadvantages include long operative times, greater reoperation rates, and poor knowledge of stromal–epithelial interaction.

### The Future

Much research is currently dedicated to the development of a tissue-engineered bladder. The goals remain the same as those of enterocystoplasty, i.e., to develop a large, compliant reservoir for urine. If successful, these technologies may eliminate many of the complications associated with the use of gastric and intestinal segments. Two major technologies exist: (1) unseeded and (2) seeded. In the unseeded tissue matrix grafts may be biodegradable, acellular, collagen based, autologous, or xenogeneic. These grafts then allow for cell growth and tissue generation. In the seeded group cells are cultured from the patient's bladder and are then placed on biodegradable scaffolds. Once seeded the graft is transplanted onto the host's native bladder. Though each technology has been used in human subjects, long-term data is lacking.

## Bladder Substitution

Ideally, reconstructive efforts should be directed at preservation of native urinary bladder; however, this is not always possible. Cystectomy may become necessary in children with pelvic malignancy or in a child with bladder exstrophy and a diseased bladder plate. In these cases, a bladder substitution is offered as an alternative to an ileal conduit that drains continuously into a urostomy bag or a ureterosigmoidostomy. In a ureterosigmoidostomy the ureters are anastomosed to the sigmoid and urine is evacuated along with feces through the rectum. Once popular, ureterosigmoidostomies are rarely used today amidst concern with the development of adenocarcinoma.

Bladder substitutions may be divided into two broad categories: (1) orthotopic and (2) non-orthotopic. Orthotopic bladder substitutions are rarely used in pediatric patients, as there are few diseases that require removal of the entire bladder while leaving the urethra with its sphincteric mechanism intact. Non-orthotopic substitutions do not rely on the urethra as a catheterizable conduit or the urethral sphincter as a continence mechanism. We refer to non-orthotopic bladder substitution as continent urinary reservoir (CUR).

A true CUR implies a reservoir that stores urine at low pressures and is emptied using CIC through the abdominal wall. Over the past 25 years nearly 50 different ways to construct CURs have been described. The goals are the same regardless of the technique used. The surgeon seeks to create a high-capacity, low-pressure reservoir with a reliable antireflux mechanism and an easily catheterizable channel. As in bladder augmentation, the segment of bowel selected will have metabolic consequences. Additionally, different bowel segments will have different contractile properties. Cecal and ileocecal segments are the most widely used for CUR construction. The reservoirs that use these segments are often referred to by names of the institution where they were first described, e.g., the Indiana pouch, Florida pouch, Mainz pouch, and Penn pouch.

As with any bladder reconstruction, parent and patient compliance is most important. Sufficient renal function is also important given potential metabolic derangements.

## Bladder Neck Reconstruction

Numerous techniques of variable technical difficulty and success have been described to increase bladder outlet resistance and aid in developing urinary continence for patients with poor outlet resistance. These techniques are often referred to as "bladder neck repairs." The most commonly used techniques aim to narrow the outlet without completely obstructing it. As bladder neck repair is often performed in conjunction with bladder augmentation, it is important to provide a "pop-off" valve in the event the patient is unable to catheterize and the bladder overdistends. Tightening the bladder neck also leads to increased difficulty in the endoscopic management of bladder and upper urinary tract calculi and endoscopic surveillance of the augmented bladder for tumor.

Techniques described include surgeries to narrow the bladder neck as in the Young-Dees-Leadbetter repair or surgeries to tubularize the bladder neck creating a flap valve mechanism as in the Kropp and Pippi-Salle repairs. Bladder neck sling procedures using autologous fascia, allogeneic grafts, synthetic grafts, and off-the-shelf materials such as small intestinal submucosa are commonly performed. Artificial urinary sphincters (AUS) are best suited for children that retain the ability to void spontaneously and thus do not require CIC. While the AUS is an excellent device, it must be remembered that it is a mechanical foreign body and may become infected, erode, or malfunction. Endoscopic bulking agents, including collagen, cartilage, polytetrafluoroethylene, polydimethylsiloxane, and dextranomer/hyaluronic acid, have all been used to coapt the open or lax bladder neck with varying durability and success. When all other surgical procedures have failed to provide social continence, bladder neck division with closure may be considered. With bladder neck division it is imperative to remember the risk of bladder perforation, as the potential for urinary leakage per urethra acting as a "pop-off" mechanism is no longer available. Patients in whom division is considered should be counseled on the increased risk of perforation if the bladder is not drained on a regular basis or if the bladder cannot be drained through the catheterizable channel.

## Catheterizable Channel

Following bladder augmentation or creation of a continent urinary reservoir spontaneous voiding is usually not possible. Therefore, CIC to empty the bladder is usually required. Nearly every child who has had an augmentation cystoplasty and all children with CURs are committed to a lifetime of CIC.

Catheterization through a catheterizable abdominal wall stoma is more convenient than catheterizing per urethra given the easily accessible location of the stoma. Additionally, patients in wheelchairs, obese patients, and those with limited manual dexterity may find it difficult to catheterize per urethra. Catheterizing per urethra is extremely difficult in patients that have had surgery to narrow the bladder neck to achieve continence. In these patients the urethra is narrowed significantly and will rarely allow passage of a catheter 8 French or larger. These patients rely almost entirely on catheterization through an abdominal wall stoma to ensure adequate bladder emptying.

A catheterizable channel may be created by anastomosing the appendix to the bladder after it has been removed from continuity with the cecum. The mesentery of the appendix is left intact. In the absence of the appendix, various tissues most notably tapered ileum and reconfigured ileum as in the Monti-Yang procedure. A flap valve is created to ensure continence of the channel. The channel is maintained as short as possible to avoid kinking and difficulties with catheterizations. It is brought out at the umbilicus or right lower quadrant. When creating a channel the goal is to be able to catheterize with a 12 French or 14 French catheter to allow for more rapid bladder drainage. Continent catheterizable channels are often referred to as a "Mitrofanoff" channel. Specifically, when made from appendix they are known as an appendicovesicostomy and when made from ileum they are known as a Monti channel.

Potential problems include difficulties catheterizing due to stomal stenosis, kinking of the channel beneath the skin, outpouchings, or narrowing along the course of the channel. If a child experiences difficulty catheterizing but is able to catheterize it is advisable to leave a catheter in place to allow for continuous drainage until the channel may be assessed by a urologist experienced with such reconstructions. If there is stomal stenosis, which occurs in 10–20 %, placement of a catheter and application of a steroid cream around the stoma may help to avoid surgical revision. If a catheter cannot be placed through the channel and the bladder outlet has not been revised, the patient should be catheterized per urethra. It is very important to ask the patient and his/her family if a bladder neck procedure has been performed, as using a large catheter to attempt to drain the bladder per urethra may destroy the continence mechanism at the bladder outlet. If a bladder neck repair has been performed and the child's bladder is overdistended, gentle attempts to drain the bladder per urethra using an 8F catheter may be made. If these attempts fail and the child is uncomfortable, suprapubic aspiration may be performed. Occasionally, the channel may be catheterizable once the bladder has been partially drained. In this scenario, the catheter should be placed in the channel and secured to the skin with an adhesive dressing until seen by a urologist.

## Suggested Reading

Filipas D, Stein R, Fisch M. Orthotopic and nonorthotopic bladder substitution. In: Gearhart JP, Rink RC, Mouriquand PDE, editors. Pediatric urology. Philadelphia: WB Saunders; 2001. p. 956–60.

Kennedy WA, Hensle TW. Bladder replacement in children and young adults. In: Libertino JA, editor. Reconstructive urologic surgery. 3rd ed. St. Louis: Mosby-Year Book; 1998. p. 307–18.

Kropp BP, Cheng EY. Bladder augmentation: current and future techniques. In: Docimo SG, Canning DA, Khoury AE, editors. Clinical pediatric urology. London: Informa Healthcare; 2007. p. 871–910.

Metcalfe PD, Rink RC. Bladder augmentation: complications in the pediatric population. Curr Urol Rep. 2007;8(2):152–6.

Rink RC, Yerkes EB, Adams MC. Augmentation cystoplasty. In: Gearhart JP, Rink RC, Mouriquand PDE, editors. Pediatric urology. Philadelphia: WB Saunders; 2001. p. 961–79.

# Pediatric Lower Urinary Tract Dysfunction and Associated Constipation

37

Nathan Ballek, Joel Koenig, and Patrick McKenna

## Introduction and Background

Lower urinary tract dysfunction (LUTD) is one of the most common problems seen in pediatric urology, affecting an estimated 20–30 % of children [1, 2]. An estimated 40 % of all clinic visits to pediatric urologists are related to symptoms caused by dysfunctional voiding [3, 4]. LUTD incorporates a variety of disorders of the lower urinary tract manifested by symptoms of incontinence, urgency, frequency, vesicoureteral reflux, and urinary tract infections. LUTD is also often associated with constipation.

LUTD has typically been categorized as nonneuropathic, neuropathic, and anatomic. Based on symptoms, the International Children's Continence Society has attempted to standardize LUTD terminology into various symptom groups including giggle incontinence, post-void dribbling, daytime urinary frequency (increased or decreased), and nocturnal enuresis [5]. Dysfunctional elimination syndrome (DES) is a term often used to describe contraction of the pelvic floor causing constipation as well as dysfunctional voiding. All effort should be made to use proper specific terminology when possible and avoid broad terms that may cause confusion.

Proper understanding of this disorder involves a review of the normal micturition cycle in infants and children. The bladder is a complex organ that receives innervation from autonomic and somatic sources resulting in functions of both storage and voiding of urine. Due to this complex innervation, voiding involves an intricate interplay of voluntary and involuntary control. The bladder wall consists of three layers: the mucosa, the detrusor, and the adventitia. The detrusor is composed of smooth muscle arranged in an interlaced pattern that allows contraction at varying levels of bladder filling. This also allows the bladder to be compliant and ensure low filling pressures. The bladder sphincter is composed of both an internal and external component. The external sphincter is composed of smooth and striated muscles while the internal sphincter is composed of smooth muscle. Storage therefore is a result of inactivity of the detrusor and the contraction of the sphincters. This is largely mediated by sympathetic nervous system. Voiding is under the influence of parasympathetic nervous system and consists of contraction of the detrusor and relaxation of the external and internal sphincters.

Bladder function is considerably different in children than adults. Frequency is much higher in

N. Ballek, M.D. (✉)
Lee's Summit, Missouri, MO, USA
e-mail: nballek@siumed.edu

J. Koenig, M.D.
Division of Urology, Department of Surgery, Southern Illinois University School of Medicine, 301 North 8th Street, PO Box 9665, Springfield, IL 62794, USA

P. McKenna, M.D., F.A.A.P., F.A.C.S.
American Family Children's Hospital, University of Wisconsin, Madison, WI, USA

R. Rabinowitz et al. (eds.), *Pediatric Urology for the Primary Care Physician*, Current Clinical Urology, DOI 10.1007/978-1-60327-243-8_37, © Springer Science+Business Media New York 2015

infants than adults. As children age the bladder capacity increases as does voluntary control of the external sphincter. This results in a decrease in frequency from up to 24 times a day in infants to around 4–6 times in normal adults. This change to adult voiding patterns usually occurs around age four [6].

Micturition control is determined by higher brain centers. In normal full-term infants conscious brain activity is required to void and results in no micturition while asleep. Voluntary control does not occur until around 2–3 years old. This occurs with teaching of socially acceptable times to void, further development of detrusor-sphincter mechanism, and increased bladder capacity. Around 4 years old, children develop near-adult levels of bladder control.

## Etiology and Pathophysiology

LUTD can be categorized into non-neuropathic, neuropathic, and anatomic. Non-neuropathic LUTD refers to any disturbance of normal micturition without an organic cause. Neuropathic LUTD is caused by a neurologic condition affecting the normal neural pathways. Anatomic abnormalities can result in voiding dysfunction by obstructing the normal flow of urine during voiding. Distinct entities will be discussed under evaluation.

## Constipation and LUTD

Bowel and bladder function share an integral link that is often overlooked by parents and physicians. One study found that a full one-third of children with enuresis also suffered from constipation despite only 14 % of parents reporting difficulty with stooling [7]. Constipation, as defined by the North American Society for Pediatric Gastroenterology, Hepatology, and Nutrition (NASPGHAN), is "a delay or difficulty in defecation, present for 2 weeks or more, and sufficient to cause significant distress to the patient [8]." However, in our experience, physicians should have a lower threshold for suspicion and treatment in any child with LUTD. Bowel and voiding issues need to be evaluated, managed, and followed up together. Addressing one may significantly improve the other and conversely, ignoring one may make successfully treating the other much more difficult [9–12]. This link is likely due in part to a closely related embryologic development within the pelvic floor and a shared innervation by the sacral spinal nerves as well as their close physical proximity.

## Differential of Lower Urinary Tract Dysfunction

### Non-neuropathic Bladder-Sphincter Dysfunction

#### Syndromes Related to Bladder Filling

##### Overactive Bladder

This entity is caused by detrusor overactivity in the setting of small urine volumes. This syndrome is more common in girls and is manifested as a burning sensation to urinate throughout the day. This syndrome may also cause constipation symptoms due to constant pelvic floor contraction [13].

##### Functional Urinary Incontinence

This disorder is the result of a functional loss of the normal ability of the sphincter to prevent the leakage of urine. Leakage of urine occurs during times of increased abdominal pressure. This is very uncommon in normal children and seen almost exclusively in females.

##### Giggle Incontinence

This uncommon disorder is seen predominately in young girls. Typical of this syndrome is involuntary leakage of urine during laughter. Giggle incontinence is differentiated from stress incontinence in that episodes may involve larger volumes and can amount to emptying of the entire bladder. Also, incontinence episodes occur during laughter only with normal continence at other times [14].

#### Syndromes Related to Bladder Emptying

##### Staccato and Fractionated Voiding

Both entities are manifested by quick bursts of urine in succession. Staccato voiding is caused by the inability of the pelvic floor to relax during voiding and periodic contraction leads to the interrupted

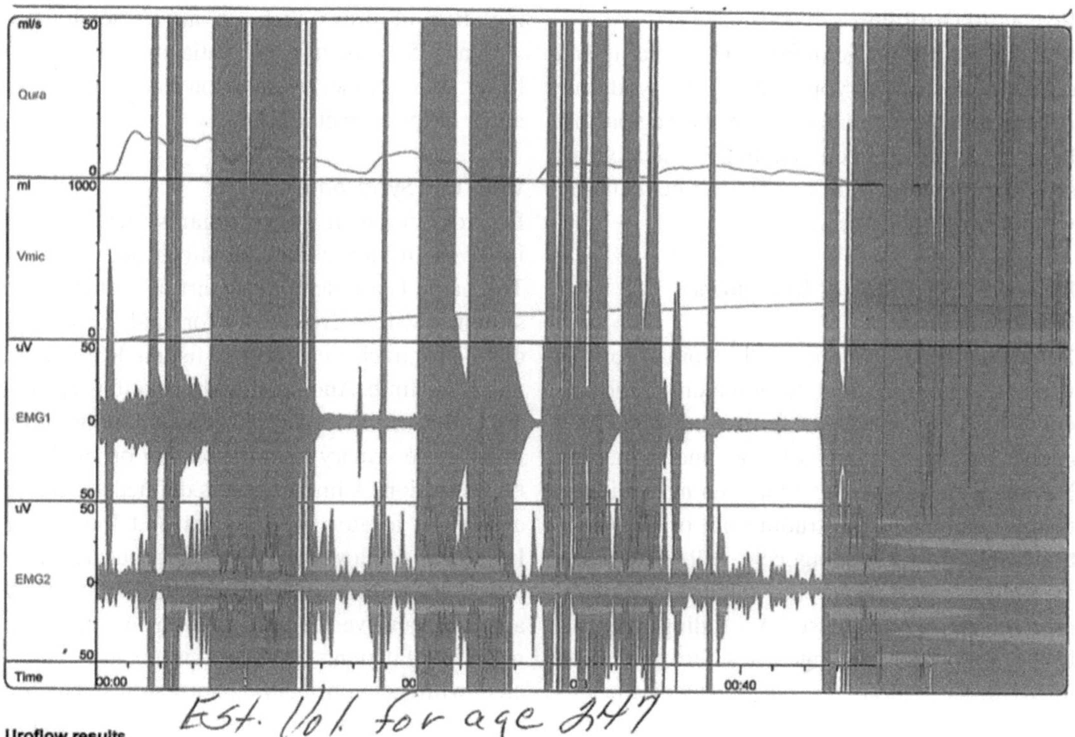


**Uroflow results**

| | |
|---|---|
| Peak flowrate | 15 ml/s |
| Time to peak flow | 2 s |
| Voided volume | 259 ml |
| Flow time | 46 s |
| Voiding time | 48 s |
| Average flowrate | 6 ml/s |
| Residual urine | 110 ml |

**Fig. 37.1** Uroflowmetry EMG study showing low flow rate, high EMG activity, and a large post-void residual

voiding pattern. Fractionated voiding has a similar pattern of small bursts of urine, but is caused by the inactivity of the detrusor muscle. Abdominal straining during voiding is common as well as elevated post-void residual urine. See Fig. 37.1.

## Infrequent Voiding and "Lazy Bladder" Syndrome

Most commonly occur in females. Both entities involve the same process in which the signal to urinate is depressed resulting in infrequent voiding. Over time this can lead to an increase in capacity and large post-void residual volumes. Urinary tract infections may result from the inability to void completely.

## Hinman's Syndrome or Occult Neuropathic Bladder

Thought to result from a bladder-sphincter dysfunction in which incontinence, urinary infections, and incomplete emptying occur. This syndrome represents full decompensation of the voiding mechanism and is the most severe of those listed [15]. Also there is significant bowel dysfunction with encopresis, constipation, and fecal impaction being common. The degree of bladder dysfunction can be similar to that of a neurogenic bladder with significant renal damage and failure in the most severe forms [16]. Early recognition and treatment is essential to prevent renal damage.

### Post-void Dribbling

Manifested by leakage of urine after voiding and occurs exclusively in young girls. This syndrome is caused by urine collecting in the vagina that leads to dribbling upon standing. Typically this syndrome resolves with age but can be managed with voiding maneuvers.

## Neuropathic Bladder Disorders

### Myelodysplasia

Refers to the conditions of the spinal cord in which there is abnormal development of the spinal cord. The lesions can further be subdivided based on the degree of the malformation. Meningoceles involve just the meninges with no neural components protruding out of the vertebral canal. Myelomeningocele will include the meninges as well as varying degrees of involvement of the nervous tissue protruding from the lesion. Lipomyelomeningocele refers to a lesion involving fatty tissue that develops with the nervous tissue and is also included with the nervous tissue and meninges. Myelomeningocele makes up the large majority of the lesions. The lesions most commonly occur at the level of the lumbar spine but can also occur at the sacral, thoracic, and cervical levels as well. The most common etiology of this disorder is low maternal intake of folate.

### Occult Spinal Dysraphisms

Refers to lesions that affect the spinal column, but are not open lesions as in myelodysplasia. Around ninety percent of patients will have a cutaneous abnormality over the back at the site of the lesion. Around one-third of infants with this syndrome have lower urinary tract dysfunction. This rate increases with age, and around 80–90 % will develop lower urinary tract dysfunction. The increase of dysfunction with age is due to tethering of the cord and stretching or compression of the cord by a lipoma or lipomeningocele.

### Sacral Agenesis

Disorder in which there is failure of two or more lower vertebral bodies to develop. A number of factors have been linked to the development of this disorder including maternal insulin-dependent diabetes, a deletion on chromosome 7, and maternal ingestion of drugs that can act as teratogens. Around 75 % of affected patients will develop lower urinary tract dysfunction due to either an upper or lower tract lesion.

### VACTERL Syndrome

Disorder in which several organ systems can be involved in various combinations and severity. The name is a mnemonic referring to the organ systems: V for vertebral, A for anal, C for cardiac, T for tracheoesophageal fistula, R for renal, and L for limb. Anorectal malformations associated with this disorder or occurring alone often involve the urinary tract depending on the location of lesion. A high lesion is defined as ending above the levator ani muscles and low if the lesion ends below the levator ani muscle. High lesions have been associated with fistula, renal agenesis, and vesicoureteral reflux in the large majority of patients. Low lesions are also associated with genitourinary abnormalities, but are much less common than in high lesion. Neurogenic bladder can occur with this syndrome usually in conjunction with a spinal abnormality and is more common with high anorectal lesions.

### Cerebral Palsy

Results from perinatal injury to the central nervous system usually caused by sepsis or anoxia. Virtually all patients will have some upper motor neuron injury resulting in detrusor-sphincter dyssynergia, exaggerated sacral reflexes, or detrusor overactivity. Incontinence is common, but depending on the degree of injury patients may or may not have complete control of voiding.

### Traumatic Spinal Injuries

Traumatic spinal injuries are very rare in infants and toddlers but incidence increases with age. Motor vehicle accidents and falls account for most injuries in infants and small children. Sports injuries account for a larger percentage of injuries in older children. With cervical and upper thoracic injuries, there is significant risk of renal damage due to increased pressure in the bladder due to detrusor-sphincter dyssynergia. With sacral injuries the somatic innervation is disrupted to the external sphincter and incontinence due to low-pressure leakage. In this setting renal damage does not occur due to the low bladder pressure.

### Anatomic Etiologies of Elimination Dysfunction

#### Posterior Urethral Valves (PUV)

Cause obstruction of the lower urinary tract due to an aberrant growth of tissue in the urethra. This obstruction can be devastating to all of the urinary tract proximal to the valves. In neonates the condition can be life threatening secondary to pulmonary hypoplasia. Less severe forms of PUV may be found later in life and are manifested by daytime incontinence or frequency. They may be the underlying cause of up to 20 % of overactive bladder symptoms in boys [17]. Voiding patterns on uroflowmetry will show low flow without pelvic floor activity on EMG. Ultrasound may show a thickened bladder wall. See Fig. 37.2.

#### Uncommon Urethral Anomalies

Include anterior urethral valves, urethral polyps, congenital urethral strictures, and urethral duplication. These entities are less common than posterior urethral valves but can cause similar damage to the upper and lower urinary tract in severe cases.

## Evaluation

### History

Typical presentation of children with non-neuropathic bladder-sphincter dysfunction starts soon after toilet training. Children will often continue to have daytime or nighttime incontinence or both. Initial history should focus on relevant questions pertaining to frequency, daily patterns of voids, volume of voids, and symptoms of urgency. History of urinary tract infections and vesicoureteral reflux is also relevant. Bowel dysfunction is a common finding in certain types of non-neuropathic bladder-sphincter dysfunction [18]. Relevant question pertaining to constipation, fecal impaction, and encopresis should be asked.

In children with neuropathic bladder dysfunction not diagnosed in infancy, a detailed history of voiding symptoms may reveal a progressive pattern. Urinary tract infections may also be a presenting complaint. Similarly children with posterior urethral valves not diagnosed in infancy can present with symptoms of elimination dysfunction, incontinence, and urinary tract infections.

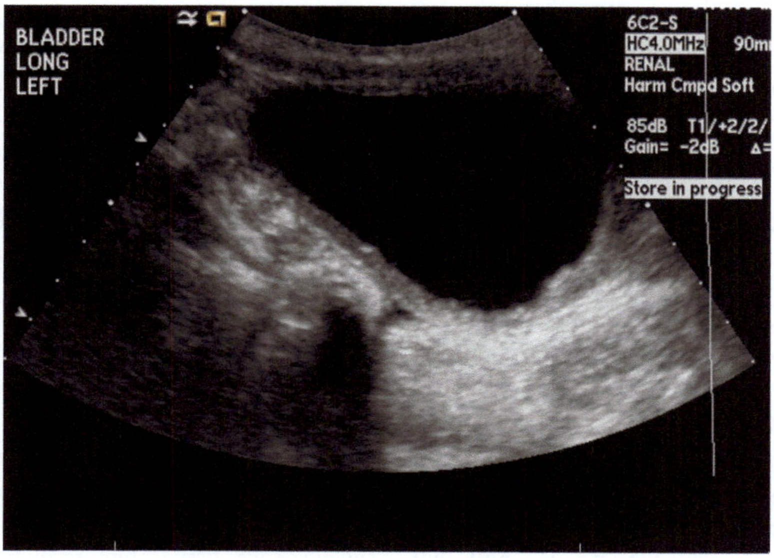


**Fig. 37.2** Ultrasound showing thickened bladder wall despite distention

Useful in the evaluation is a voiding diary to record daily volumes of intake and output. This includes timing of voids as well as frequency. It is also necessary to record symptoms of urgency and any occurrence of incontinence throughout the day.

## Physical Examination

Children with non-neuropathic bladder-sphincter dysfunction will typically have a normal physical exam. An examination of the buttocks, back, spine, and gait as well as a thorough neurologic exam should be performed to rule out spinal dysraphisms and neurologic lesions. An exam to the external genitalia should be performed to rule out any obvious anatomic cause of the dysfunction.

## Laboratory Studies

Laboratory studies are not routinely performed in non-neuropathic bladder-sphincter dysfunction unless there is suspicion of a urinary tract infection. For neuropathic bladder dysfunction laboratory studies useful for initial evaluation are urinalysis with culture and serum creatinine. For antenatally and perinatally detected anatomic abnormalities, routine labs are not performed for initial evaluation due to the effects of the maternal circulation on creatinine and urea nitrogen. Forty-eight hour may be needed to accurately assess intrinsic renal function in the newborn.

## Urodynamics and Other Functional Studies

The first-line studies used by a pediatric urologist are noninvasive studies without the use of an indwelling catheter. They include uroflowmetry, perineal electromyography, and post-void residual measurement. The child will come to the urologist's office with a full bladder and have an ultrasound performed to make sure bladder volume is appropriate. He will then have surface electrodes placed on his abdomen and perineum and void normally but through a device that measures the flow rate. Muscle activity will simultaneously be measured using the electrodes. After the child is done, a post-void residual will be measured with ultrasound. These provide adequate information for screening most new patients and assessing response to treatments.

Full urodynamic studies are only indicated in children with neurogenic causes of dysfunctional voiding, severe dysfunctional voiding, or symptoms that do not improve with therapy. The tests begin with insertion of a catheter transurethrally or suprapubically to measure intravesical pressure and placement of a catheter in the rectum to measure the abdominal pressure. EMG electrodes are applied to determine sphincter activity. The bladder is then filled gently via the catheter and the child is asked to void. During filling the child is asked when the first sensation to void occurs. Important information can be ascertained from these tests including bladder capacity, compliance, and voiding pressures in the bladder and abdomen. Detrusor pressure can then be determined by subtracting the abdominal pressure from the intravesical pressure. EMG can determine detrusor-sphincter activity during filling, storage, and voiding. Uroflowmetry is also recorded before urodynamic studies.

The importance of urodynamics is especially apparent for neurogenic LUTD. Neurogenic diseases are typically dynamic processes that require regular monitoring with urodynamics to properly manage. Urodynamic studies are used for monitoring bladder pressures and determining when conservative management is ineffective in preserving upper urinary tract function.

## Imaging Studies

### Ultrasonography

Ultrasonography is a cost-effective and safe modality for imaging the kidneys, bladder, and pelvic floor in infants and children. Due to the paucity of subcutaneous tissue, high-resolution ultrasound can be used to visualize the organs of the urinary system without the use of harmful radiation.

Ultrasound is useful for initial evaluation and monitoring in LUTD and constipation. It is highly accurate in detecting upper and lower urinary tract changes. Ultrasound can also be used for quantifying the degree of constipation and the response to treatment by measuring rectal diameter [7, 19]. Because of its low cost and minimal side effects, it can be used to screen for these changes over time and guide management.

Fetal ultrasound has become the primary mode for diagnosing posterior urethral valves. Although the actual diagnosis cannot be made in utero, it is suspected if there are hydronephrosis and a full bladder with a thickened wall. The use of maternal ultrasound has increased in recent years and has led to an increase in earlier detection of this condition. Timing is important in diagnosis of posterior valves since they are largely undetectable by ultrasound prior to 24 weeks gestation.

In addition to providing detailed anatomic images, ultrasonography is able to provide functional information. This is particularly useful in children with non-neuropathic voiding dysfunction in which up to one-third will show paradoxical movements of the pelvic floor with voiding.

#### Voiding Cystourethrogram

Voiding cystourethrogram (VCUG) is an imaging modality that utilizes radio-opaque dye inserted through a catheter and images are taken during filling and micturating. This is useful to screen for reflux and provide important anatomic information. VCUG is indicated in patients under the age of 5 with a documented UTI. Vesicoureteral reflux is present in more than 20 % of patients.

#### Magnetic Resonance Imaging

Magnetic resonance imaging (MRI) is indicated when there are findings consistent with spinal dysraphism (i.e., sacral dimple, hair patch). Although expensive, this provides the most detailed images of neural lesions of the spine and should be included in the initial evaluation when indicated.

## Management and Timing of Referral

In general, the management of LUTD requires early education, hydration, treatment of constipation, and postural changes. These measures should be instituted before any pharmacologic therapy. Referral to a pediatric urologist should be obtained in the setting of febrile urinary tract infections or symptoms that do not improve with education, early conservative measures, and resolution of constipation. Conditions such as occult neuropathic bladder (Hinman's syndrome), neuropathic conditions, and posterior urethral valves can be life threatening. Early recognition and intervention are essential to prevent renal damage or failure.

### Management of Non-neuropathic Bladder-Sphincter Dysfunction and Constipation

Recently the management of LUTD has moved away from early pharmacologic therapy and antibiotics to education, hydration, treatment of constipation, and pelvic floor muscle retraining (PFMR) (Fig. 37.3). Initial education should emphasize timed voiding, proper posture, and hygiene. In one study 60 % of patients showed improvement for up to 5 years after undergoing a conservative education-based therapy [20]. These approaches should be started before any pharmacologic therapy is begun.

Education can be started in the primary care setting and should include timed voiding every 2–3 h and proper posture to reduce abdominal straining. Proper sitting with foot and hip support will accommodate relaxation of the pelvic floor and reduce abdominal straining [21]. Proper hygiene is essential to reduce inflammation that may cause dysuria which will cause holding maneuvers. In this way early education will facilitate proper relaxation of the pelvic floor during voiding.

Early diagnosis and treatment of constipation is essential in children with suspected LUTD. Children should have at least one bulky soft bowel

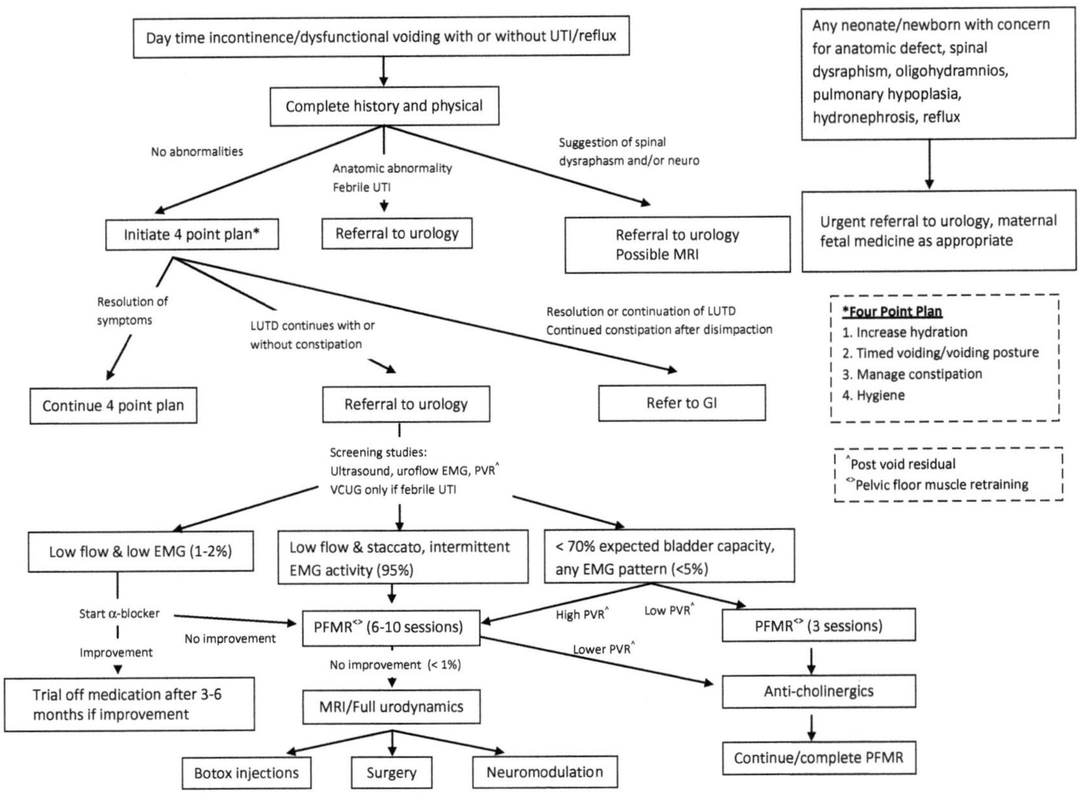


**Fig. 37.3** Algorithm for the evaluation and management of LUTD

movement per day. Resolution of constipation alone can facilitate normal voiding and reduce recurrent urinary tract infections [11, 22]. Early recognition and treatment of constipation and fecal impaction is an essential component of conservative therapy [9, 10, 23]. According to the NASPGN early disimpaction with laxatives or enemas is necessary to facilitate normal defecation. After initial therapy normal stooling should be maintained with the use of fiber supplementation and bulking agents, such as MiraLAX®, with the goal of one bulky bowel movement a day. If bowel habits cannot be managed with these conservative measures, consultation with a pediatric gastroenterologist should be considered.

Intensive nonsurgical urotherapy is the first-line therapy for non-neuropathic bladder-sphincter dysfunction that does not respond with conservative measures. The goal is to normalize voiding patterns and prevent functional changes of the lower urinary tract. Biofeedback has been established as an essential, effective, and well-tolerated therapy in children with non-neuropathic voiding dysfunction [24]. It consists of uroflowmetry and real-time EMG biofeedback on the quality of voiding the child is able to achieve. Recently video games combining this concept have been applied to biofeedback therapy with good results. Biofeedback and pelvic floor muscle retraining (PFMR) may provide durable resolution of LUTD symptoms in up to 80 % of patients without the use of any medications [25].

Medications aim to modulate the lower urinary tract in accordance with the functional disturbance. Antimuscarinics are the first-line medication in overactive bladders by reducing involuntary contractions. Alpha-adrenergic blockers act on the bladder neck to cause relaxation during voiding. Tricyclic antidepressants such as imipramine cause increase in storage through relaxation of the detrusor and increase in sphincter tone. Medical therapy may be used as a complementary therapy with biofeedback, but due to side effects, should be used cautiously as part of a larger dysfunctional voiding plan and should not be a first-line treatment [26, 27].

When conservative management has failed, more invasive therapy may be necessary to prevent upper urinary tract deterioration. Rarely, clean intermittent catheterization may be used in conjunction with other therapies or as a temporizing measure before other treatments reach full effect. It may allow easier retraining of normal micturition pattern, improve continence rates, and decrease UTIs [28, 29]. Surgery remains a last resort if more conservative management has failed. The principle of these interventions is to achieve a low-pressure system by increasing bladder volume. Often this is achieved by using bowel to augment the bladder thus increasing capacity.

## Management of Neurogenic Elimination Dysfunction

Newborns with myelodysplasia and other causes of neurogenic elimination dysfunction require early recognition and prophylactic measures to prevent upper tract deterioration. Early initiation of clean intermittent catheterization alone or in combination with anticholinergic is recommended to prevent harmful bladder pressures. Bowel regimens to soften stool and promotion of regular evacuation with enemas are recommended. The neurologic lesions are expected to change over time; surveillance with post-void residuals, VCUG, urodynamics, and renal ultrasound are recommended on a regular basis.

Reflux is present in up to 5 % of individuals with myelodysplasia and management is very similar to children without neurologic lesions. Adequate drainage is necessary possibly requiring clean intermittent catheterization (CIC) to prevent reflux and prophylactic antibiotics are used to prevent urinary tract infections. Antireflux surgery indications include recurrent urinary tract infections while on antibiotics, persistent upper tract dilation with puberty, and persistent hydroureteronephrosis despite adequate drainage, and when outlet resistance surgeries are planned.

Continence can be achieved for most individuals without surgery using CIC and medication. If incontinence persists despite conservative measures, surgery is indicated. Principles of continence surgery consist of increasing bladder outlet resistance and increasing bladder capacity to lower bladder pressure.

## Management of Anatomic Causes of LUTD

Anatomic causes of LUTD, such as urethral valves, can present anywhere along a spectrum of symptoms, degree of obstruction, and associated abnormalities. The spectrum of treatments parallels the severity of disease. Severe cases of valves are often detected prenatally or immediately after birth. They require early catheterization and drainage as well as respiratory support, correction of metabolic abnormalities, and intensive care services at experienced specialized centers. Definitive diagnosis and treatment of valves can then be carried out later when the child is medically stable.

Children with valves may present at any age with less severe cases presenting later in life as LUTD including dysfunctional voiding and UTIs. If symptoms do not improve with conservative measures or they have breakthrough febrile UTIs, these patients should undergo cystoscopic evaluation with possible concomitant endoscopic valve ablation.

Valve ablation can be achieved under direct vision with age-appropriate endoscopic instruments, including neonatal cystoscopes. Principles of ablation have changed over time to focus on disrupting the valves rather than completely resecting the valves. If the infant is too small for instrumentation, diversion with either a vesicostomy or upper tract diversion is an alternative. This will eventually be reversed when the valves can be ablated.

Long-term management of patients with posterior urethral valves is necessary since a large portion suffer with persistent incontinence into childhood. This is due to several factors including upper tract damage, decreased concentrating ability of the kidneys, bladder insensitivity, and detrusor instability. Children diagnosed at school age often suffer from milder symptoms but can still have persistent voiding difficulty and incontinence.

## Conclusion

Lower urinary tract dysfunction (LUTD) and associated constipation are complex issues that require a concerted effort by the patient, family members, primary care physicians, and specialists to properly manage. With early recognition and proper management, both in the office and at home, children can avoid some of the more devastating complications due to this common disorder.

## References

1. Whelan CM, McKenna PH. Urologic applications of biofeedback therapy. Contemp Urol. 2004;58:23–34.
2. Hellstrom AL, Hanson E, Hansson S, et al. Micturition habits and incontinence in 7-year-old Swedish school entrants. Eur J Pediatr. 1990;149:434–7.
3. Farhat W, Bagli D, Capolicchio G, et al. The dysfunctional voiding scoring system: quantitative standardization of dysfunctional voiding symptoms in children. J Urol. 2000;164:1011.
4. Rushton HG. Wetting and functional voiding disorders. Urol Clin North Am. 1995;22:75–93.
5. Nevéus T, von Gontard A, Hoebeke P, et al. The standardization of terminology of lower urinary tract function in children and adolescents: report from the Standardization Committee of the International Children's Continence Society. J Urol. 2006;176: 314–24.
6. Bauer SB, Yeung CK, Sihoe JD. Voiding dysfunction in children: neurogenic and non-neurogenic. In: Kavoussi LR, Novick AC, Partin AW, Peters CA, Wein AJ, editors. Campbell's urology. 9th ed. Philadelphia: WB Saunders; 2007. p. 3604–55.
7. McGrath KH, Caldwell PH, Jones MP. The frequency of constipation in children with nocturnal enuresis: a comparison with parental reporting. J Paediatr Child Health. 2008;44:19–27.
8. Baker SS, Liptak GS, Colletti RB, et al. Constipation in infants and children: evaluation and treatment. J Pediatr Gastroenterol Nutr. 1999;29:612–26.
9. Silva JMP, Diniz JSS, Lima EM, Vergara RM, Oliveira EA. Predictive factors of resolution of primary vesico-ureteric reflux: a multivariate analysis. BJU Int. 2006;97(5):1063–8.
10. Upadhyay J, Bolduc S, Bagli DJ, et al. Use of the dysfunctional voiding symptom score to predict resolution of vesicoureteral reflux in children with voiding dysfunction. J Urol. 2003;169:1842–6.
11. Zoppi G, Cinquetti M, Luciano A, et al. The intestinal ecosystem in chronic functional constipation. Acta Paediatr. 1998;87(8):152–4.
12. Dohil R, Roberts E, Jones KV, et al. Constipation and reversible urinary tract abnormalities. Arch Dis Child. 1994;70:56–7.
13. Bauer SB. Special considerations of the overactive bladder in children. Urology. 2002;60(Suppl 5A): 43–8.
14. Berry AK, Zderic S, Carr M. Methylphenidate in giggle incontinence. J Urol. 2009;182(4):2028–32.
15. Hinman F. Nonneurogenic neurogenic bladder (the Hinman syndrome)—15 years later. J Urol. 1986;136: 769–77.
16. Jakobsson B, Jacobson SH, Hjalmås K. Vesico-ureteric reflux and other risk factors for renal damage: identification of high- and low-risk children. Acta Paediatr Suppl. 1999;88(431):31–9.
17. Miller J, McKenna PH. Uroflowmetric parameters and symptomatologic outcomes in boy with overactive bladders. In: Programs and abstracts of the 83rd Annual Meeting of the North Central Section of the AUA, Arizona; 2009.
18. Bijos AM, Czerwionka-Szaflarska M, Mazur A, et al. The usefulness of ultrasound examination of the bowel as a method of assessment of functional chronic constipation in children. Pediatr Radiol. 2007;37: 1247–52.
19. Joensson IM, Siggard C, Rittig S, et al. Transabdominal ultrasound of the rectum as a diagnostic tool in childhood constipation. J Urol. 2008;179:1997–2002.
20. Wiener JS, Scales MT, Hampton J, et al. Long term efficacy of simple behavioral therapy for daytime wetting in children. J Urol. 2000;164:786–90.
21. Wennergren H, Oberg B, Sandstedt P. The importance of leg support for relaxation of the pelvic floor muscles: a surface electromyography study in healthy girls. Scand J Urol Nephrol. 1991;25:205–13.
22. Loening-Bauche V. Urinary incontinence and urinary tract infection and their resolution with treatment of chronic constipation of childhood. Pediatrics. 1997; 100:228.
23. Whelan CM, McKenna PH. Dysfunctional voiding as a co-factor of recurrent UTI. Contemp Urol. 2004; 16:58–73.

24. Herndon CDA, Decambre M, McKenna PH. Changing concepts concerning the management of vesicoureteral reflux. J Urol. 2001;166:1439–43.
25. Herndon CD, Decambre M, McKenna PH. Interactive computer games for treatment of pelvic floor dysfunction. J Urol. 2001;166:1893–8.
26. Bauer SB, Retic AB, Colodny AH, et al. The unstable bladder of childhood. Urol Clin North Am. 1980;7: 321–36.
27. Bolduc S, Moore K, Lebel S, et al. Double anticholinergic therapy for refractory overactive bladder. J Urol. 2009;182:2033–9.
28. Pohl HG, Bauer SB, Borer JG, et al. The outcome of voiding dysfunction managed with clean intermittent catheterization in neurologically and anatomically normal children. BJU Int. 2002;89(9):923–7.
29. van Gool JD, de Jonge GA. Urge syndrome and urge incontinence. Arch Dis Child. 1989;64:1629–34.

# Pyelonephritis

# 38

Richard W. Grady

## Introduction

Urinary tract infections (UTIs) are among the most common bacterial infections in children. Up to 8 % of children will experience at least one UTI between the ages of 1 month and 11 years.

The clinical spectrum ranges from minimally symptomatic lower urinary tract infections to potentially life-threatening pyelonephritis. Fortunately, in the current antibiotic era, the vast majority of these infections are treatable. It is difficult to imagine that 100 years ago, childhood kidney infections carried a mortality of up to 25 % and left many children with chronic kidney disease. At the turn of the century, Goppert-Kattewitz noted the acute mortality of pyelonephritis in young children at 20 %. Another 20 % failed to recover completely and subsequently died presumably secondary to renal failure [1]. After sulfonamide antibiotics became available in the 1940s, mortality dropped to 2 % in children hospitalized for nonobstructive UTI [2]. Currently, mortality secondary to UTI approaches 0 % for children in the United States.

This chapter will focus on the diagnosis, evaluation, and management of pyelonephritis in children. The consequences of urinary tract infections differ significantly between adults and children. Children appear more prone to renal scarring secondary to kidney infections. As a consequence current management of pyelonephritis focuses on prompt diagnosis and treatment to accomplish:

- Elimination of the acute symptoms of infection
- Prevention of recurrent UTI
- Prevention of renal scarring
- Correction of associated urologic abnormalities

Considerable variation exists in the evaluation, treatment, and management of children with UTI despite proposals to achieve a consensus approach. The American Academy of Pediatrics (AAP) created a subcommittee to address this. Their findings were published in 1999 and represent the consensus opinion of the AAP [3]. Since this time, the management of children with pyelonephritis has continued to change. This chapter will discuss modern management and point out where current evidence varies from AAP UTI guidelines.

## Etiology

The underlying pathophysiology of UTI between adults and children is the same. UTI commonly occurs as the result of an ascending route of infection. Adhesin attachment to the urinary tract

R.W. Grady, M.D. (✉)
Department of Urology, The University of Washington School of Medicine, Seattle, WA, USA

Division of Pediatric Urology, Children's Hospital & Regional Medical Center, Seattle, WA, USA
e-mail: richard.grady@seattlechildrens.org

R. Rabinowitz et al. (eds.), *Pediatric Urology for the Primary Care Physician*, Current Clinical Urology,
DOI 10.1007/978-1-60327-243-8_38, 

initiates UTI. Enteric flora ascends from the periurethral area up the urethra into the bladder to cause cystitis. Bacterial adherence to the cell surface of urothelium is the first step to initiate UTI [4]. Bacteria that cause UTI express adhesins that facilitate this binding.

The most common pathogen causing UTI in children is *Escherichia coli. E. coli* causes up to 80 % of urinary tract infections in children. Enteric pathogens such as *Klebsiella* organisms, *Enterobacteriaceae*, *Enterococci*, etc., cause most of the remaining infections. Gram-positive organisms cause 5–7 % of UTI in children. Some species such as *Proteus mirabilis* are found more commonly in boys (approximately 30 % of cases) [5, 6]. In the newborn period, *Group A* or *B streptococci* are common UTI pathogens. Hospital-acquired organisms often tend to be more aggressive (i.e., *Klebsiella* or *Serratia*) or represent opportunistic organisms (i.e., *Pseudomonas aeruginosa*) [3].

Given sufficient bacterial virulence characteristics (i.e., P fimbriae) or host anatomic abnormalities (i.e., vesicoureteral reflux or obstructive uropathies), uropathogenic bacteria can ascend to the upper urinary tract to cause pyelonephritis. Importantly, children are more likely to have an underlying anatomic abnormality increasing their susceptibility to UTI. This is especially true of young children. For older children, dysfunctional voiding and constipation represent risk factors that place them at risk of UTI.

In summary, common factors associated with an increased risk for UTI in children include:

- Vesicoureteral reflux (VUR)
- Foreskin (in infancy)
- Obstructive uropathies
- Disorders of elimination (voiding dysfunction and constipation)

## Diagnosis

### Signs and Symptoms

Infants and young children cannot localize infections. Furthermore, perhaps because of possible delay in diagnosis or other increased susceptibility, they also appear to be at increased risk of renal scarring secondary to infection. Most UTI diagnosed in this age group are kidney infections recognized during an evaluation for fever. Concomitant signs may include hematuria, foul-smelling and/or cloudy urine, malaise, jaundice, decreased appetite, and irritability. Symptoms of a poor urinary stream, intermittent voiding, or straining to urinate can indicate urethral obstruction.

Older children are able to more effectively localize the symptoms and signs of UTI. Some of the most common symptoms include dysuria, new-onset urinary incontinence, and urinary urgency. It is quite uncommon for a UTI to involve the kidneys in the absence of high fever such that fever in the presence of a urinary tract infection is a sine qua non for pyelonephritis. Nausea can also be associated with pyelonephritis.

### Physical Examination

In infants, physical examination may reveal a palpable flank mass due to ureteropelvic junction obstruction, a palpable suprapubic mass secondary to posterior urethral valves or other causes of bladder outlet obstruction such as a neurogenic bladder. A back examination may reveal stigmata of an underlying spinal dysraphism. Male infants should also be checked for the presence of a foreskin. In female infants, an introital examination may reveal labial adhesions or a mass whose differential includes hydrometrocolpos, an ectopic ureter, or prolapsing ureterocele. These anatomic anomalies can predispose an infant to pyelonephritis.

In older children, physical examination may reveal costovertebral angle tenderness. Flank masses become more difficult to palpate in older children. Lower abdominal examination can be augmented with ultrasonographic bladder scanning to determine if the child can empty his/her bladder.

### Differential Diagnosis

In infants, the practitioner should include meningitis, gastroenteritis, and hematogenous infections in the diagnostic differential. In adolescents and children, the differential will also include renal calculi, renal infarction, and malignancy.

## Laboratory Testing

### Urinalysis and Urine Culture

Urinalysis and urine culture are important elements in the diagnosis of pyelonephritis. Urinalysis in a young child may reveal red blood cells and leukocytes (indicated by hemoglobin and leukocyte esterase on dipstick evaluation). Infants and young children test positive less commonly for nitrites because they void so frequently that the nitrites that bacteria produce often do not accumulate to a detectable level.

A bacterial UTI is defined by the presence of bacteria in a urine culture. In older children, a growth of more than $10^5$ colony-forming units is considered a positive culture from a clean midstream-voided specimen. Urine collection from children prior to toilet training is problematic. To obtain the most accurate specimen, one must obtain it either from urethral catheterization or suprapubic aspiration (SPA). Colony counts of $10^3$ from urethral specimens are significant. Any growth from a specimen obtained by SPA is considered clinically important. Urine-bagged specimens are commonly obtained for newborns or toddlers because of increased ease compared to SPA or urethral catheterization. Unfortunately, these specimens are more frequently contaminated by skin flora and periurethral flora.

### Infant Urine Collection

The American Academy of Pediatrics issued guidelines regarding UTI management in 1999 to address variation in evaluation and management. Because of the nonspecific presentation of pyelonephritis in infants, these guidelines specifically stated that practitioners evaluating unexplained fever in infants and young children 2 months to 2 years should strongly consider the possibility of UTI [3]. Most emergency department protocols routinely include a urinalysis as part of a fever evaluation protocol for children in this age group. Obtaining a urine specimen from infants can be challenging. AAP guidelines state:

> If the child (2 months to 2 years of age) is ill enough to warrant immediate antibiotic usage, the urine specimen should be obtained by SPA or urethral catheterization—not a "bagged" specimen. If an infant or young child 2 months to 2 years of age with unexplained fever is assessed as not being so ill as to require immediate antibiotic therapy, there are two options; (1) Obtain and culture a urine specimen collected by SPA or transurethral bladder catheterization, (2) Obtain a urine specimen by the most convenient means and perform a urinalysis. If the urinalysis suggests a UTI, obtain and culture a urine specimen collected by SPA or transurethral bladder catheterization; if urinalysis does not suggest a UTI, it is reasonable to follow the clinical course without initiating antimicrobial therapy, recognizing that a negative urinalysis does not rule out a UTI [3].

In practice, many practitioners obtain a first urine specimen using a bagged technique. To optimize the results from a bagged specimen, the genital skin should be cleaned meticulously before bag application and repeated if no voided specimen results within 3 h of bag application. Urine bags must also be removed within 15–20 min after the child voids to reduce the chance of false-positive results. For patient practitioners, a clean-voided sample is possible to obtain from pre-toilet-trained infants and toddlers but may not be practical in a busy clinic or emergency department setting.

### Older Children: Urine Collection

After toilet training, most children can provide a clean midstream catch with the assistance and supervision of their parents or caregivers. Interpretation of urine specimens from uncircumcised boys who cannot retract the foreskin can be confounded by specimen contamination from the large numbers of bacteria in the preputial folds. Urine specimens should be cooled immediately after voiding to improve the accuracy of urine culture results by reducing bacterial growth prior to inoculation on culture media.

## Other Studies

Adjunctive hematologic studies such as a peripheral white blood cell (WBC) count, C-reactive protein (CRP), and erythrocyte sedimentation rate (ESR) may be useful in some cases. These studies are too nonspecific to diagnose a child with a UTI but can help gauge the severity of the infection and response to therapy [5].

### Radiographic Studies

Recommendations from the AAP based on their 1999 guidelines include the evaluation of all children after febrile UTI with a renal and bladder ultrasound (RUSN) examination and a voiding cystourethrography (VCUG). These recommendations have come under increased scrutiny based on the relatively low yield of renal and bladder ultrasonography to identify anatomic anomalies that have increased the risk for pyelonephritis. A normal third trimester prenatal ultrasound examination, however, does not carry a strong-enough negative predictive value to discount the use of renal ultrasound examination in the evaluation of pediatric pyelonephritis. Similarly, significant debate is ongoing regarding the utility of voiding cystourethrography (VCUG) to identify clinically important vesicoureteral reflux. Several clinical research studies are underway including the National Institutes of Health (NIH)-funded RIVUR study that may shed further knowledge on the use of these imaging modalities. Current recommendations include the use of both renal and bladder ultrasound examinations and VCUG in the evaluation of children after an episode of pyelonephritis [6].

In select situations where the diagnosis of pyelonephritis remains in question, an intravenous contrast-enhanced computed tomographic (CT) scan or [99mTc]-DMSA (dimercaptosuccinic acid) scan can assist in the diagnosis; these studies will demonstrate a focal area of low uptake in the setting of pyelonephritis. [99mTc]-DMSA renal scanning may be useful in the diagnosis of pyelonephritis and in the evaluation of renal scarring. In particular, the role of DMSA scans in the management of patients with febrile UTI varies from institution to institution and regionally. DMSA scanning provides the most sensitive method to assess renal scarring and damage. Acute uptake defects are detectable by DMSA scanning in 50–80 % of children with febrile UTI. 40–50 % of these defects remain on follow-up imaging studies—indicating scar formation.

## Treatment

Children who present with a febrile UTI should be treated without delay. Several retrospective studies provided evidence that a delay in treatment of greater than 4 days resulted in higher rates of renal scarring [7]. In contrast, initiation of treatment after only 24 h of fever has not been shown to cause an increased rate of long-term renal scarring. So, a slight delay in therapy appears equivalent to immediate treatment. Therapy can be initiated empirically. Antibiotic therapy can be tailored later according to the urine culture results when they become available. The initial choice of antibiotic will vary according to region. Treating physicians should be cognizant of the antibiotic resistance patterns in their geographic area and choose accordingly since bacterial resistance patterns vary by region due to differences in the use of various antibiotics. Only a few comparative, randomized studies have evaluated the safety and efficacy of antibiotics to treat children for UTI. As a consequence, the choice of antibiotic may vary by region and by treating facility. However, in many regions of the world, including the United States, ampicillin and other aminopenicillins are no longer clinically effective against many of the common bacterial pathogens that cause UTI in children [8].

Historically, most children with febrile UTI were admitted for initial inpatient therapy with intravenous antibiotics. Ampicillin and gentamicin function synergistically and have a therapeutic spectrum that covers almost all of the common bacterial pathogens that cause UTI. As a consequence, this antibiotic combination is frequently used for initial empiric antibiotic therapy. More recently, clinical trials have demonstrated that outpatient oral antibiotic therapy can be effective for children with no difference in short-term treatment efficacy or long-term renal scarring compared to intravenous therapy [9]. Effective oral agents include cefixime, ceftibuten, and amoxicillin/clavulanic acid [10]. As a result, many health-care providers now treat children with febrile UTI as outpatients.

In contrast, children who appear toxic, septic, and dehydrated or are unable to maintain adequate oral intake of fluids should be admitted for inpatient antimicrobial therapy and intravenous hydration. The 1999 AAP guidelines on UTI currently recommend inpatient treatment for febrile UTI. They specifically recommend hospital admission for treatment until the children appear clinically improved. At that time, antibiotic therapy may be converted to an appropriate oral agent. Current reviews published in the Cochrane database suggest that a short course (2–4 days) of intravenous antibiotics followed by a course of oral antibiotics can be equally effective to a complete course of intravenous antibiotic therapy and that once-daily gentamicin therapy is as effective as therapy delivered every 8 h [10].

Current systematic reviews of the literature support a treatment course of 7–10 days duration. Treatment courses shorter than this (1–4 days) demonstrated lower cure rates. Longer courses of therapy result in improved outcomes in 5–21 % of cases. A test of cure (urine culture) may be performed after completion of therapy to demonstrate efficacy of therapy [11].

## Indications for Referral

In the acute setting, if a child fails to respond to treatment within 24–48 h, consultation with a pediatric urologist or pediatric nephrologist is suggested. If an anatomic abnormality is identified during subsequent imaging evaluation or if a child is noted to have significant voiding dysfunction (as indicated by urinary incontinence and/or urinary retention), consultation with a pediatric urologist is also recommended.

## References


1. Goppert-Kattewitz F. Uber die eitrigen Erkrankungen der Harnwege im Kindersalter. Ergebinesse uber innern Medizin und Kinderheilkund. 1908;2:30–73.
2. Lindblad B, Ekengren K. The long-term prognosis of non-obstructive urinary tract infection in infancy and childhood after the advent of sulphonamides. Acta Peadiatr Scand. 1969;58:25–32.
3. Roberts KB. A synopsis of the American Academy of Pediatrics' practice parameter on the diagnosis, treatment, and evaluation of the initial urinary tract infection in febrile infants and young children. Pediatr Rev. 1999;20(10):344–7.
4. Winberg J, Andersen HJ, Bergstrom T, Jacobsson B, Larson H, Lincoln K. Epidemiology of symptomatic urinary tract infection in childhood. Acta Peadiatr Scand Suppl. 1974;252:1–20.
5. Naber K, Bergman B, Bishop MC, Bjerlund-Johansen TE, Botto H, Lobel B, Jimenez Cruz F, Selvaggi FP. EAU Guidelines for the management of urinary and male genital tract infections. Urinary Tract Infection (UTI) Working Group of the Health Care Office (HCO) of the European Association of Urology (EAU). Eur Urol. 2001;40(5):576–88.
6. Keren R. Imaging and treatment strategies for children after first urinary tract infection. Curr Opin Pediatr. 2007;19(6):705–10.
7. Dick P, Feldman W. Routine diagnostic imaging for childhood urinary tract infections: a systematic overview. J Pediatr. 1996;128:15–22.
8. Tullus K, Winberg J. Urinary tract infections in childhood. In: Brumfitt W, Hamilton-Miller J, Bailey R, editors. Urinary tract infections. London: Chapman & Hall Medical; 1998. p. 175–97.
9. Hoberman A, et al. Oral versus initial intravenous therapy for urinary tract infections in young febrile children. Pediatrics. 1999;104(1 Pt 1):79–86.
10. Jepson R, Craig J. Cranberries for preventing urinary tract infections. Cochrane Database Syst Rev. 2008;1.
11. Moffatt M, Embree J, Grimm P, Law B. Short-course antibiotic therapy for urinary tract infections in children. A methodological review of the literature. Am J Dis Child. 1988;142(1):57–61.

# Nephrologic Aspects of Urologic Disease

# 39

James A. Listman and Scott Schurman

## Introduction

The fields of urology and nephrology are inextricably linked in the pediatric population.

Approximately one third of patients with renal failure have congenital renal disease, a significant proportion of which is related to obstruction and/or vesicoureteric reflux.

While we expect that many of these cases will be detected by prenatal ultrasound, there still exist those unusual patients who defy our expectations and come to our doorsteps with often time's dramatic presentations right from the textbook. Failure to thrive in infants, growth failure, and bone pain from rickets/renal osteodystrophy constitute some of these unusual presentations.

Some acquired disease processes may also have both medical and surgical needs.

Nephrolithiasis is perhaps the most common emerging problem in this category. Finally, there are those patients who have abnormal screening tests (hematuria and proteinuria being the commonest) that perhaps create the most confusion for the primary care physician primarily because it may not be clear who best to refer such patients or if referral is even necessary at all. Established referral patterns and availability of subspecialists likely determine where one starts.

In practice, requests for consultation by the nephrologist often breaks down into two distinct categories: patients with abnormal screening tests (meaning they will likely be asymptomatic) and those with discrete complaints that are referable to the GU tract. This distinction is important because the former is unlikely to have bona fide disease and one can spend inordinate amounts of time and money—not to mention the parental anxiety induced—that comes with over-testing for diseases that are not likely present or for which there are likely to be no treatments that dramatically change the outcome. Asking the right questions and performing the correct tests will exclude the exotic diseases. For symptomatic patients, the dictum that the history is 90 % of the diagnosis (at least in verbal patients) rings true, and the workup should proceed in a staged manner where one weighs the risks and benefits of each test and anticipates the findings rather than blindly shooting darts. With these concepts in mind, the discussion that follows will break problems down by how they were discovered—asymptomatic patient with an abnormal screening test or the symptomatic patient—so that the primary care physician can more easily formulate a management plan.

J.A. Listman, M.D. (✉)
Bernard and Millie Duker Children's Hospital at Albany Medical Center, 47 New Scotland Avenue, Albany, NY 12208, USA
e-mail: ListmaJ@mail.amc.edu

S. Schurman, M.D.
Upstate Golisano Children's Hospital, 750 E. Adams Street, Syracuse, NY 13210, USA

R. Rabinowitz et al. (eds.), *Pediatric Urology for the Primary Care Physician*, Current Clinical Urology, DOI 10.1007/978-1-60327-243-8_39, © Springer Science+Business Media New York 2015

## Clinical Scenarios

### Asymptomatic Patients with Abnormal GU Screening Tests

#### Microscopic Hematuria

##### History

Ostensibly all patients referred for this problem are asymptomatic. The microhematuria is detected during a routine physical or school sports physical. Notably, there are no other abnormal findings on the dipstick (isolated hematuria). Pertinent ROS should focus on recent history or trauma, episodic gross hematuria (red or dark urine) in the past, or GU referable complaints. Importantly, a family history of renal disease (Alport syndrome or polycystic kidney disease) or sickle cell disease/trait (sometimes also noted on routine newborn screens) should be sought out. Any positive findings may immediately point to the cause. Finally, a family history of hematuria in the absence of renal failure following an autosomal dominant pattern may point to familial hematuria (thin basement membranes), a benign condition if present in only one parent.

##### Exam Findings

The exam is generally normal.

##### How to Evaluate

Assuming a negative history, exam, and absence of coexisting proteinuria, one can be reassured that the likelihood of a serious disease is low [1]. In fact, most cases of isolated microhematuria are transient and 75 % resolve by the third test (done weeks apart). Quantification by microscopic exam can also be reassuring as most nephrologists consider less than 5 rbc/hpf insignificant in terms of potential for underlying disease (there is a poor correlation between the strength of the dipstick reading and the microscopic exam). Therefore, only patients with persistent microhematuria should be considered for further testing. The differential diagnosis is large, but the vast majority of patients will not have anything treatable uncovered. For example, the likelihood of uncovering a low-grade glomerulonephritis such as IgA nephropathy is low if there is no history of gross hematuria [2]. Furthermore, in the absence of proteinuria, therapy would almost certainly not be entertained. The only disease type of significance that would have devastating consequences if missed would be the extremely rare case of a renal or bladder wall tumor. These would include Wilms tumor (in young children) and renal cell carcinoma (in teenagers) of the kidney and rhabdomyosarcoma of the bladder wall. Many patients will have familial benign hematuria (thin basement membrane disease). This can be sought out by screening the parents, siblings, and, ideally, the grandparents of affected individuals to show three-generation involvement (again verifying a negative family history or renal failure).

Screening tests for persistent microhematuria could include UA testing in parents and other siblings, CBC, renal function tests, and renal/bladder US (Fig. 39.1). Urine culture is not necessary in asymptomatic patients and is susceptible to false-positive results. In selected cases, an evaluation for a hemoglobinopathy may be indicated.

##### When to Refer

Referral is not necessarily warranted if a thorough history is taken, the hematuria is transient, or if persistent, the remainder of the workup, including the imaging, is negative. If any of these is suspect or there is parental anxiety, a referral can be useful. Cystoscopy is not warranted for the evaluation of children with asymptomatic microhematuria. To be absolutely sure a low-grade glomerulonephritis does not progress, prudence would dictate follow-up urinalysis and monitoring of blood pressure at routine physical examinations to monitor for onset of proteinuria or hypertension—both signs of nephritis.

#### Proteinuria

##### History

A urine dipstick is clearly indicated in a child who presents with periorbital edema, gross hematuria, hypertension, or growth failure.

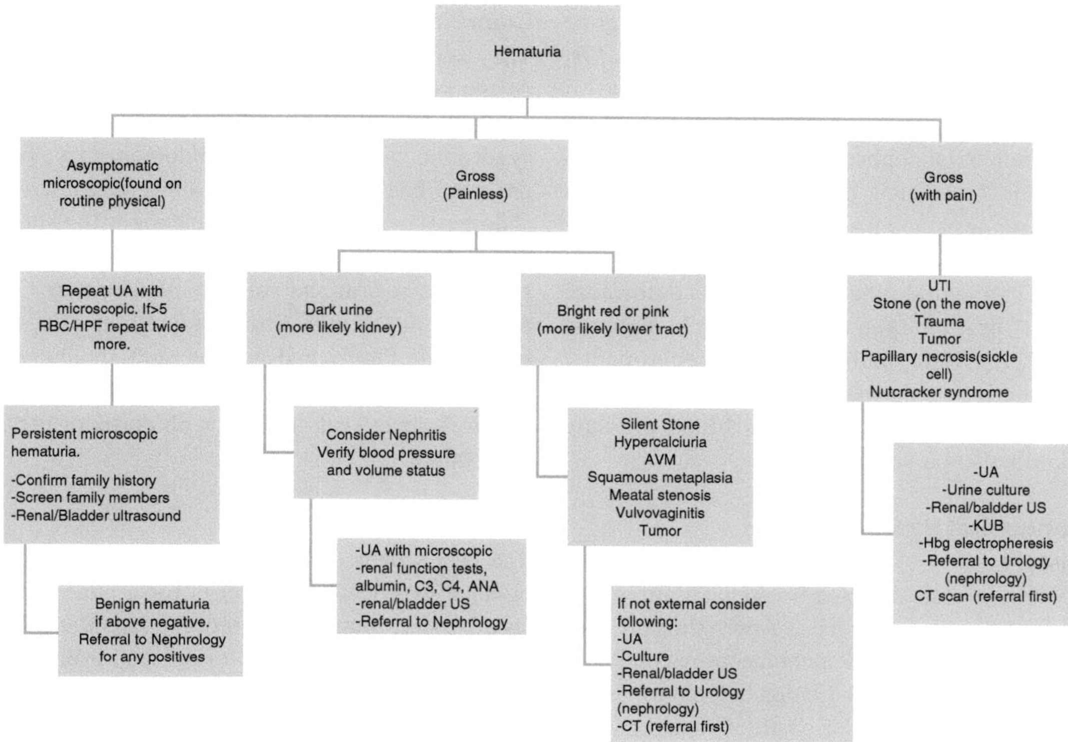


**Fig. 39.1** Evaluation of hematuria

Nephrotic syndrome, acute/chronic glomerulonephritis, and chronic kidney disease from congenital renal anomalies can all cause excessive protein in the urine among other findings. However, when proteinuria is detected during a routine physical examination in the absence of symptoms, the specificity for detecting a renal disease is very low. Factors such as hydration typically come into play so that even normal amounts of protein excretion can result in a low-positive dipstick reading when the urine is concentrated. Furthermore, upwards of 20 % of children, particularly older boys with a high BMI, have orthostatic proteinuria—a benign condition [3].

## Exam Findings

The exam is normal in asymptomatic patients.

## How to Evaluate

Frequently the primary physician jumps to a 24 h urine collection to better quantify asymptomatic proteinuria. Much more useful is to screen first morning urine samples to look for evidence of orthostatic proteinuria, a normal physiologic variant not associated with underlying renal disease (Table 39.1). If the morning samples remain positive, the proteinuria is referred to as fixed proteinuria to indicate that it is not due to an orthostatic mechanism. As a benign condition, it

**Table 39.1** Evaluation of orthostatic proteinuria

| |
|---|
| Patient should void prior to bedtime to eliminate daytime urine |
| Immediately after morning arousal, void into sample container, store in refrigerator, and repeat collection the following day |
| Test in office by dipstick or send to lab for total protein/creatinine ratio (Tp/Cr). If dipstick ≤1 (30 mg/dl), send for Tp/Cr |
| If Tp/Cr ≤ 0.2, patient has orthostatic proteinuria. Can stop evaluation and monitor blood pressure and repeat urine screens using AM urine samples at yearly physicals |
| If Tp/Cr ≥ 0.2: |
| Verify blood pressure |
| Obtain renal function tests and serum albumin |
| Renal US |
| Refer |

does not require any follow-up, but if future urine testing is performed, it is best done from first morning samples to avoid confusion.

Patients with fixed proteinuria should be referred to a nephrologist. The consultation will be facilitated by obtaining basic renal function tests and a serum albumin and having the patient undergo a renal ultrasound to rule out a congenital renal disease that could cause hyperfiltration injury from reduced nephron number. These include reflux nephropathy/obstructive nephropathy, renal hypoplasia, or renal dysplasia. The patient's blood pressure should also be verified.

## Congenital Hydronephrosis

### History

Hydronephrosis detected by prenatal ultrasound is a common occurrence. Approximately one half of these will show spontaneous resolution or improvement to trivial dilation before birth while others have a variety of obstructive and nonobstructive anomalies. Some of these may require evaluation by the pediatric urologist, but many will not. The problem, of course, is that there is no generally applied standard to quantifying this entity and the ultrasound report is generally vague. Fortunately, the clinical significance for many of these infants is nil so that identifying those at risk becomes the challenge. Furthermore, newer data questioning the utility of UTI prophylaxis in children with vesicoureteric reflux calls into question the necessity of preemptive identification of such infants particularly if there is no evidence of reflux nephropathy by ultrasound. The key historical factors to identify are unilateral vs bilateral dilation (the later having potentially more significant implications for renal dysfunction), the severity (mild is better than severe), a determination of ureteric or bladder involvement (less likely benign), association with other congenital anomalies (of which the kidney may be of least importance), and family history of individuals with conductive hearing loss with outer ear anomalies and/or renal failure as seen in the branchio-oto-renal syndrome, an autosomal dominant disease of variable phenotype within families.

### Exam Findings

The exam is normal in the majority of cases. Attention to facial dysmorphisms and preauricular pits/tags may provide a clue to an underlying syndrome. A protuberant abdomen may be present when the hydronephrosis is severe. Lax abdominal musculature in association with undescended testes in males will point to prune-belly syndrome. A firm and palpable bladder may be found in males with posterior urethral valves. Finally, the family and nursing staff should be queried about the urinary stream in male infants, which is often weak in those with posterior urethral valves.

### How to Evaluate

The best scheme for evaluating newborns with prenatal hydronephrosis comes for a large prospective study done in Belgium [4]. All infants in this study who met criteria for prenatal hydronephrosis underwent a series of ultrasounds, a VCUG, and renal scan at predetermined intervals and were followed for 2 years. The investigators determined that if the following criteria were met, there was only a 3 % chance of missing a nonobstuctive uropathy (vesicoureteral reflux or low-grade posterior urethral valve), none of which required surgical intervention: (1) the newborn and 1-month ultrasound screenings showed pelvic dilation under 7 mm at the midpole pelvic region in the anterior-posterior (AP) dimension; (2) there was no evidence of significant calyceal dilation, renal parenchymal defects, or dilated ureter. Therefore, if these criteria are met, ongoing investigation with VCUG and renal scans is not justified. Babies with AP diameter between 7 and 10 mm had significant risk for some uropathy and above 1 cm all babies had a uropathy identified. The investigators conclude that measurement of the AP diameter at the midpole region of hydronephrosis by renal ultrasound could distinguish between infants with low or high risk for having any identifiable anatomic disease. Therefore, a renal ultrasound prior to discharge is reasonable. Renal function tests are indicated in babies with bilateral disease and may need to be repeated as an outpatient once feedings are established.

### When to Refer

The triaging of newborns with prenatal hydronephrosis requires special attention to quantifying the hydronephrosis as noted above. Many radiographic programs do not do this. Therefore, referral may be necessary for an expert opinion. Certainly, babies labeled with bilateral disease, findings of a dilated ureter(s), or small kidneys should undergo consultation by an expert before discharge from the nursery. Babies with unilateral moderate to severe hydronephrosis (or AP diameter $\geq 7$ mm) might benefit from prophylactic antibiotic to lower risk of UTI should they have vesicoureteral reflux. Keflex 10 mg/kg once daily is suitable for this purpose (sulfa drugs are contraindicated in newborns and for the first few months of life). At least a phone conversation with an expert prior to discharge is suggested to facilitate the outpatient follow-up plan. Babies with mild hydronephrosis (AP diameter $< 7$ mm) should be scheduled for a repeat renal/bladder ultrasound around 1 month of age. If the repeat ultrasound shows AP diameter $< 7$ mm, the baby can discontinue prophylaxis and no further workup is necessary.

## Symptomatic Patients with GU Disease

### Gross Hematuria

#### History and Physical

Gross hematuria is a relatively common presentation to the office or emergency room.

Historical events may be very helpful to help identify the cause. A history of trauma should always be sought after even when the patient is not initially forthcoming. Associated pain will help to localize the source of the bleeding along the urinary tract. Acute onset of flank pain with hematuria is seen with trauma, stone disease, sickle cell disease/trait, or a rare tumor. Suprapubic or low back pain that is gradual in onset may point to cystitis or bladder pathology. Dysuria points to a bladder, urethral, or external source. Pain and hematuria following exertion can be seen in stone disease or sickle cell disease.

Glomerulonephritis is more likely when the urine is tea colored or rusty and occurs in the face of an intercurrent illness, sometimes with vague complaints of abdominal or flank pain. Hypertension and other signs of fluid overload should be sought after in this circumstance.

Painless gross hematuria can be trickier if not impossible to isolate particularly when it is transient in nature. The color and timing may be helpful. Bright red or pink urine generally localizes the bleeding to below the renal parenchyma, while brown urine originates from the glomerulus. The brown color results from exposure of hemoglobin to a low urine pH and is time dependent. NB: this is not a perfect association. A very active IgA nephropathy can yield red urine, while urine tinged with blood from the bladder can look brown if hours pass between the bleeding event and voiding. Terminal hematuria is relatively common and localizes the source of bleeding to the urethra in males or urethra/vulvas in girls. Meatal stenosis is a common cause in younger circumcised males, and the boys may admit to blood-tinged stains on their underwear in the past. Girls with vulvovaginitis may note blood-tinged streaks on toilet tissue along with drips or streaks of blood mixed in yellow urine on directed questioning. The physical exam may be revealing in this regard, although, not always depending on the timing. A silent kidney stone (one that has not yet dislodged to obstruct the ureter) or hypercalciuria are other relatively common causes of painless hematuria. Finally, a rare renal or bladder wall tumor may manifest with painless gross hematuria.

#### How to Evaluate

Evaluation will be directed by where you suspect the source of bleeding is and its cause.

In all cases, a complete urinalysis with microscopic examination is useful for a variety of reasons including: verification that blood is the cause for the color change (for example, myoglobinuria will cause heme positive dipstick with brown urine but no blood on microscopic examination while heme negative results should point to bilirubin or other pigment such as a dye or drug that is excreted into the urine); presence of proteinuria, particularly at high levels will point to a glomerular disease; presence of leukocytes point to infection in patients with appropriate symptoms, but is also found in acute glomerulonephritis; presence of dysmorphic blood cells and cellular casts are classic features of glomerular disease. A urine culture should also be performed to exclude UTI as a source for hematuria especially when associated with other appropriate signs and symptoms of UTI. In suspected cases of GN, laboratory testing should include renal function tests, serum albumin, C3, C4, and ANA.

Imaging plays an essential role in the evaluation of hematuria. A traumatic injury will likely be directed to an emergency department and will require imaging by CT scan. In most other cases, a renal/bladder ultrasound is warranted to look for evidence of anatomical disease. Presence of echogenic kidneys is consistent with "medical renal disease" as with GN. Unilateral hydronephrosis associated with ipsilateral flank pain would suggest presence of a stone in the distal ureter causing obstruction and renal colic. A KUB may be useful for detecting such a stone, but is relatively insensitive. While CT scanning has been touted as the most sensitive diagnostic tool for stone disease, it is not the safest modality because of the exposure to ionizing radiation and should be reserved for diagnostic dilemmas.

### When to Refer

A solitary (one void) episode of gross hematuria may not require referral particularly if there are no symptoms or physical exam findings at the time of evaluation and the UA and renal/bladder ultrasound are normal. Prolonged hematuria or recurrent episodes should be referred to a nephrologist or urologist depending on the suspected diagnosis or availability.

## Chronic Kidney Disease (Congenital Renal Dysplasia/Hypoplasia and Obstructive/Reflux Nephropathy)

### History and Physical

Patients with congenital chronic kidney disease (CKD) may have a variety of signs and symptoms (Table 39.2). However, some may escape notice until the pubertal growth spurt when they present with ESRD. It is important to note that many infants and young children with CKD will have a normal creatinine, which belies their true renal condition and even older children with CKD may have a normal appearing urinalysis because dilute urine is nonspecific and can mask low-grade proteinuria. Small/dysplastic kidneys are easily seen by ultrasound using a pediatric probe while hydronephrosis may point to an obstructive or reflux cause for the disease. Therefore, when considering CKD in the differential of a problem patient, imaging with renal ultrasound is critical to exclude CKD from the differential diagnosis.

**Table 39.2** Signs and symptoms of CKD

| Finding | Cause |
|---|---|
| Failure to thrive and/or dehydration | Concentrating defect, malignant hypertension (in infants), RTA, uremia |
| Polyuria | Concentrating defect |
| Nausea/vomiting | Concentrating defect, RTA, uremia |
| Headache | Hypertension |
| Limp/bone pain | Rickets/renal osteodystrophy |
| Growth failure | CKD |
| Constipation | Concentrating defect |
| Flank/suprapubic pain | UTI |

*RTA* renal tubular acidosis, *CKD* chronic kidney disease, *UTI* urinary tract infection

Among the most common problems seen in CKD, particularly of the obstructive/reflux type is polyuria. This will not necessarily be obvious in a thriving infant. However, newborns are especially susceptible when feeding volumes are relatively small and the anticipated weight loss may be excessive and prolonged. The dehydration in and of itself can cause inanition fever and lead to multiple work ups for infection before the true nature of the patients problem is ascertained. Once properly hydrated, these infants can often times begin to feed and grow normally. Some will do better on a low renal solute formula (Similac PM 60/40). Intercurrent illnesses may be another vulnerable period when reduced oral intake leads to rapid dehydration. Older children with polyuria will be susceptible to dehydration in warmer climates and during physical exertion with sweating. Anticipating the need for vigorous hydration can prevent orthostatic symptoms and enhance physical performance.

### Evaluation

Most of the signs and symptoms of CKD are non-specific, and as such, this chapter cannot serve as a guide to evaluate thoroughly each and every one of these problems.

However, once CKD is considered in the differential diagnosis, the evaluation for CKD is straight forward and will include a urinalysis, renal function tests, and a renal/bladder ultrasound.

### When to Refer

Simple urinary tract infection is in the realm of the primary care physician. Other forms of anatomic disease should be vetted by a urologist and/or nephrologist depending on the suspected cause.

## References

1. Dodge WF, West EF, Smith EH, Bunce 3rd H. Proteinuria and hematuria in schoolchildren: epidemiology and early natural history. J Pediatr. 1976;88(2):327–47.
2. Trachtman H, Weiss RA, Bennett B, Greifer I. Isolated hematuria in children: indications for a renal biopsy. Kidney Int. 1984;25(1):94–9.
3. Brandt J, Jacobs A, Raissy H, et al. Orthostatic proteinuria and the spectrum of diurnal variability of urinary protein excretion in healthy children. Pediatr Nephrol. 2010;25(6):1131–7.
4. Ismaili K, Avni FE, Martin Wissing K, Hall M. On behalf of the Brussels Free University Perinatal Nephrology Study G. Long-term clinical outcome of infants with mild and moderate fetal pyelectasis: validation of neonatal ultrasound as a screening tool to detect significant nephrouropathies. J Pediatr. 2004;144(6):759.

# Pediatric Primary Nocturnal Enuresis (Bed-Wetting)

# 40

Dawn D. Saldano and Max Maizels

## Background

To this day, there remains controversy on how to manage bed-wetting or primary nocturnal enuresis (PNE) in children. We plan to identify controversial areas (Table 40.1) and provide you with practical insights so that you may address management using your own practice preferences. Finally we will present our successful approach used for more than 25 years, now known as the Try for Dry program.

The National Kidney Foundation estimates that about 5 million children wet their bed. The problem of bed-wetting is not just an issue for children and teens, as 1 % of adults also wet their bed at night. While this is a widespread problem, there have not been proactive treatments to get children dry. This in part may relate to the current state of medical research which does not identify a clear pathophysiology for the condition, and so directed treatments have not been amenable to prospective controlled trials [1]. The view that bed-wetting is a symptom and not a medical condition pervades society's perception of the disorder. It has been shown that successful treatment normalizes the low self-esteem of children who bed wet [2]. From this perspective, in this chapter, we present an *empiric* plan to treat bed-wetting.

D.D. Saldano, R.N., A.P.N., M.S.N.
M. Maizels, M.D., F.A.A.P., F.A.C.S. (✉)
Division of Urology, Ann and Robert H. Lurie Children's Hospital, Northwestern University Feinberg School of Medicine, 255 E. Chicago Avenue, Chicago, IL 60404, USA
e-mail: Max.maizels@gmail.com

## Etiology

The practitioner's ability to recognize the varied etiologies which contribute to PNE will facilitate the evaluation and management process. PNE can be regarded as a syndrome of bed-wetting, failure of sleep arousal (otherwise commonly referred to as deep sleep), and small bladder capacity, in an otherwise normal child. Additional features may include polyuria, bowel irregularity, attention deficit/hyperactivity disorder, and dietary sensitivities.

### Syndromic Features of PNE

#### Bed-Wetting

Bed-wetting is regarded as a symptom after 5 years of age. It consists of involuntary wetting during sleep. Bed-wetting may be due to a variety of causes, such as PNE, UTI, and constipation.

#### Failure of Sleep Arousal

Almost all children who bed wet show failure of sleep arousal. It is generally accepted that the

R. Rabinowitz et al. (eds.), *Pediatric Urology for the Primary Care Physician*, Current Clinical Urology,
DOI 10.1007/978-1-60327-243-8_40, © Springer Science+Business Media New York 2015

**Table 40.1** Topics in bed-wetting controversial to physicians and parents

| Topic | Perspective |
|---|---|
| When to treat | Bed-wetting is considered a pathological diagnosis after 5 years old and as such may be treated medically |
| Is medication needed to treat bed-wetting | Medication is not required to attain dryness. However, medication as used in the Try for Dry program [1] will halve the time to dryness from about 6 months to about 3 months. The rapid attainment of dryness fosters compliance with treatments. Such compliance is less likely when non-Try for Dry programs are used [2] |
| Bed-wetting is not treatable | It is surprising how often parents have delayed seeking medical advice because of their perception that treatments are not done since the child will ultimately outgrow the wetting. This sentiment is further entrenched by diaper manufacturers who advertise that bed-wetting is not curable |
| Bed-wetting is a result of psychosocial problems (such as birth of a new sibling, move to a new home, divorce) | It is our position that while psychosocial concerns may be implicated in secondary nocturnal enuresis, our experience shows that children can be successfully treated with the TFD method without first addressing these everyday concerns. On the other hand, if treatment does not show the expected improvement in dryness, then it is worthwhile to consider pediatric urological and/or psychological consultation |
| Removing the tonsils / adenoid will stop bed-wetting | Children with obstructed airways due to enlarged tonsils/adenoid may experience sleep apnea. As deep sleep is a likely etiology to bed-wetting, then improving sleep patterns may reduce bed-wetting. There is no data to show that simple tonsillectomy is a reliable treatment for bed-wetting |

child's "sleeping" brain does not "get the message" from the full bladder that urination is urgent and imminent.

### Small Bladder Capacity

Almost all children with PNE show a small functional bladder capacity. Functional bladder capacity is defined as the largest volume of urine at which the bladder can function or empty at one time, as measured and recorded on a 3-day voiding diary (Fig. 40.1). A small bladder capacity is likely the explanation for the daytime symptoms (e.g., urgency, frequency, and wetting as damp underwear) which about 25 % of children with PNE in our practice also experience.

## Clinical Features Ancillary to the Syndrome of PNE

### Polyuria

Studies have shown that nocturnal urine output in PNE is increased in children who may show low levels of endogenous vaspressin [3]. The correlation of polyuria and bed-wetting in children is seen in cases of habitual water drinking and bed-wetting. However, polyuria alone does not explain why sleeping children with PNE do not arouse to a full bladder.

### Bowel Irregularity and/or Constipation

We regard defecation as irregular when defecation is only three times/week. Bowel irregularity is discerned from constipation which we regard as difficult passage of "hard" stools. In these circumstances the rectum dilates and thereby reflexly creates bladder spasticity, a loss of the accommodative function of the bladder to retain urine. Relieving bowel irregularity/constipation reduces detrusor spasticity. About 20 % of children with PNE show irregular bowel emptying/constipation.

### Attention Deficit/Hyperactivity Disorder

Children with ADHD have impaired sensory integration. In our practice approximately 25 % of children we evaluate for bed-wetting also show ADHD. Most of these children show day-wetting symptoms as well. We regard this association of ADHD with wetting as a form of impaired sensory integration that can manifest as the inability to quell an impending bladder contraction while awake or during sleep. When dealing with ADHD and the associated social problems it presents for a child in school and other social settings, we recommend that children optimize their treatment for ADHD prior to addressing the nighttime enuresis.

## TRY FOR DRY - VOIDING DIARY

Please use the enclosed form to keep a diary of your child's bladder and bowel habits. Please do not prompt your child to eliminate as the diary is meant to show your child's natural urine and bowel habits and behavior. Please keep the diary for three days. These need not be consecutive days, as they could be a Saturday and Sunday of one weekend and a Sunday of the following weekend. The record should record EVERY use of bathroom for bladder and bowel during the daytime (for example from when your child awakens, perhaps 8am to when your child retires, perhaps 9pm). It is very helpful to bring the completed diary to your child's appointment.

If this is your first visit with us we ask that you do not prompt your child to use the bathroom. We are attempting to gain a record of when your child uses the bathroom without reminders! If there are follow up visits, we may ask you to repeat the diary but now with prompting as directed by our treatments. Using such prompting may improve urinary\bowel difficulties. In this way we can evaluate your child's progress.

DATE:_______ day of the week ____________

| TIME | FOOD INTAKE | VOLUME OF FLUIDS DRANK (oz.) | VOLUME OF URINE PASSED (oz.) | Pants\skirt are: (circle one) | We Bed (circle one) | COMMENTS you would like to make such as: There was urgency to void, or bowel movement was hard) |
|---|---|---|---|---|---|---|
| | | | | Dry damp wet | Yes / No | |
| | | | | Dry damp wet | Yes / No | |
| | | | | Dry damp wet | Yes / No | |
| | | | | Dry damp wet | Yes / No | |
| | | | | Dry damp wet | Yes / No | |
| | | | | Dry damp wet | Yes / No | |
| | | | | Dry damp wet | Yes / No | |
| | | | | Dry damp wet | Yes / No | |
| | | | | Dry damp wet | Yes / No | |
| | | | | Dry damp wet | Yes / No | |
| | | | | Dry damp wet | Yes / No | |
| | | | | Dry damp wet | Yes / No | |
| | | | | Dry damp wet | Yes / No | |

______________________ ____________ ______________________

Patient Name Date of Birth Name of your child's doctor

**Fig. 40.1** How to do a voiding diary

## History Taking in the Child Who Wets

*Office evaluation.* History will help to establish if the symptom of bed-wetting represents PNE. Detailed toilet training and voiding habits:

- Is there a history of prematurity? Prematurity may be linked to developmental delay that can influence the time at which a child may accomplish developmental milestones.
- Age when the child was toilet trained (dry for at least 1 year) to determine if wetting represents primary (never been toilet trained) or secondary (successfully toilet trained but now secondarily experiences bed-wetting at least two times/month). While it is interesting to make this distinction on intake, treatment of PNE and secondary onset PNE are commonly the same.
- Is there bowel control? Lack of bowel control with associated wetting may signal the need for further neurological evaluation looking for neuropathic conditions such as a tethered cord.
- Day voiding pattern (assess with a voiding diary) (Fig. 40.1):

Voiding diary recording fluid intake and pattern of voiding, evaluating for presence of damp underpants, frequency, and urgency.

The diary results are used to check the functional bladder capacity, frequency of day urination, and excess fluid intake. Categorizing the capacity as reduced or not is needed to structure algorithm management (see Fig. 40.2). Diagnosis of urinary frequency (empirically defined as the inability to delay urination which occurs at least as often as every 2 h while awake).

### Night Wetting Pattern

"What is the common number of wet nights/week over a 2-week interval? Is the wetting nightly, or perhaps is episodic?"

Documenting the pattern of wetting can give clues to clinical management of PNE. For example, if the wetting is episodic, it is likely that as time passes, the episodes of dry intervals will be longer and medical treatment could be deferred.

Furthermore, episodic wetting could be triggered by instances of bowel irregularity, evening sports with associated tiredness, and overindulgence in sports drinks. On the other hand if the wetting is nightly, it is likely to remain nightly, unless episodes of dryness emerge. In this instance, medical treatment could be discussed with the family. An interesting scenario is the special circumstance in which a youngster wets nightly while sleeping at home, but on overnights, for example, at "grandma's," he is dry. From this scenario, it is reasonable to infer that deep sleep in the comfort of the home contributes to night wetting, but when there is a sleep over, there is a heightened awareness of the wetting potential, and sleep is "not so deep."

### Past Medical History

Is there a history of sleep apnea which may present as "deep sleep"?

Does the child snore, have nightmares, do teeth grinding, and sleepwalk? Such symptoms may be associated with sleep apnea which may cause a child to sleep poorly.

- Has the child experienced a UTI?
- Perineal problems? Such as vaginitis, labial adhesions, and phimosis/balanitis. These external genital irritations may exacerbate or induce bed-wetting.
- Psychosocial history. Information regarding such features as the occurrence of divorce, serious illness, impending family vacation, or lack of motivation may influence timing of starting treatment (such as waiting for stress of a recent divorce to resolve) or the success of the treatment (e.g., absent motivation may preclude successful treatment).

## Physical Exam

The physical examination is aimed at identifying signs and symptoms that could represent manifestations of urological problems which account for wetting (see Table 40.2).

## When to Refer for Acute/Elective Treatment or Evaluation

Bed-wetting is a disorder which may be treated exclusively by the primary care provider. When the guidelines presented here are followed but wetting still persists, referral to a pediatric

**Fig. 40.2** Try for Dry algorithm

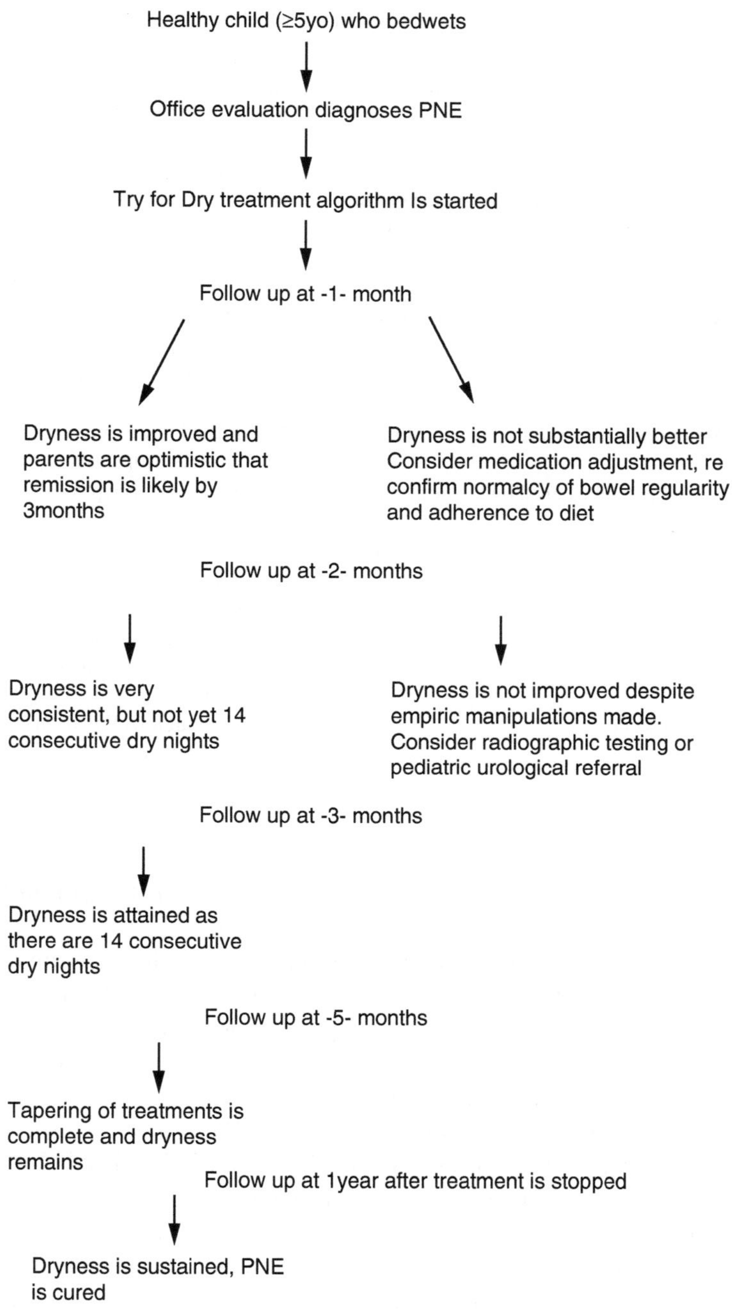


urologist is advised. This practice is distinguished from those cases of "bed-wetting" that masquerade as PNE but actually represent a pediatric urological condition (Table 40.2) which merits pediatric urological evaluation.

## When to Evaluate

It is reasonable to evaluate based on parental request and recognizing that the diagnosis of PNE is not made before 5 years of age.

**Table 40.2** Findings on physical examination which are stigmata of urological disorders which may cause wetting/bed-wetting

| | |
|---|---|
| Boys with a small urethral meatus | An obstructive meatus may cause bladder spasticity as prolonged time to void, dribbling post void, and urine infection may be noted. Boys with meatal stenosis who still wet after PNE treatment may improve to dryness after meatoplasty |
| Listening to the sound of the voided urine stream which is slow, weak, intermittent | Obstruction in boys at the prostatic urethra (posterior urethral valves) or meatus may cause symptoms as described in "boys with a small urethral meatus" |
| Sacral dimple | These findings may represent the external features of a tethered spinal cord |
| Asymmetric buttock crease/natal crease | |
| Feet show high arches | A neuropathic process, such as a tethered spinal cord, may imbalance innervation of the muscles of the foot to cause high arches and bladder muscles to cause neuropathic bladder |
| Abdominal exam shows palpable stool | Constipated bowel will "push" against the bladder and cause detrusor spasticity. Constipation may also be a sign of a neuropathic process |
| Female genital exam showing urine leaking from introitus | An ectopic ureter bypasses the bladder and drains directly onto the introitus |
| *Suspicious findings which are not stigmata* | |
| UTI | Uncommon in PNE. Suspect vesicoureteral reflux or enlarged bladder capacity as the cause |
| Enlarged functional bladder capacity in a youth | Youths with PNE typically show a reduced bladder capacity. If they show large capacity and infrequent voiding, redirect to urological evaluation |
| Day soaking | While children with PNE may show dampness, or frequency, outright soaking merits urological evaluation |

The child must be cooperative, for example, children under 5 years old are commonly frightened by the noise made by the moisture alarm excluding its use. The level of motivation is a key indicator to a positive outcome. Children under 5 years of age are not commonly motivated to cooperate with treatment modalities. However, parents can be instructed on simple measures to help the child be dry at night. These measures include: simple nightly routine of assuring the child to empty the bladder before bed and nightly lifting of the young child to keep the child dry as a temporizing treatment until the bedwetting is resolved.

## How to Evaluate

Office exam to exclude items in Table 40.2.

## Goals of Evaluation

The goals are to exclude the likelihood of a urological condition causing PNE and thereby permit the primary practitioner to apply the treatment to resolve bed-wetting.

## Goals of Management

*Getting to Dry*. The authors regard the goal of management of PNE as remission of wetting, 14 consecutive dry days and nights. This view differs from the common perspective presented in the medical literature which describes "management successes" as simply a *significant* reduction in the number of wet nights.

*Life after got Dry*. Parents often ask, once dryness is attained, how will my child behave during sleep? We find that about 80 % of children now sleep through the night dry; the remainder arouse themselves to toilet at night during sleep. We will discuss remission, relapse, and cure of PNE below in treatment outcomes.

## Treatment

Conventional treatment of PNE will be presented and then compared with the TFD algorithm method.

Conventional treatments consist of the use of single modality treatment: alarm, desmopressin, or psychological counseling. Less frequently used treatments include osteopathic manipulation or acupuncture which while they purport effectiveness will not be discussed in this chapter.

- Enuresis alarm (Fig. 40.3). The alarm is used in the following manner. The alarm sensor is worn on the outside of the underwear front panel, such that as soon as urine moistens the sensor, the alarm sounds. The parent is instructed to serve as a "sentry" who listens for the first sounding of the alarm. Upon sounding, the parent rouses the child and assists the child to ambulate to the toilet to finish voiding.

*Basis for alarm use*. Alarm use is reserved for families who have failed other treatments such as restricting liquids or positive practice (see below). The practice of scheduled lifting is also a consideration, namely, as most children who bed wet do so at about 10 pm, 2 am, and/or 5 am, and lifting the child to toilet, preemptively, before an episode of bed-wetting has occurred may remedy the wetting. Should these practices fail, wearing an enuresis alarm is considered as a next treatment. The alarm, which sounds to the first drops of urine, is expected to alert a parent to lift the child to toilet so the urine remaining in the bladder can empty into the toilet. This practice does not require awakening the sleeping child. How these treatments promote night acquiring dryness is unknown.

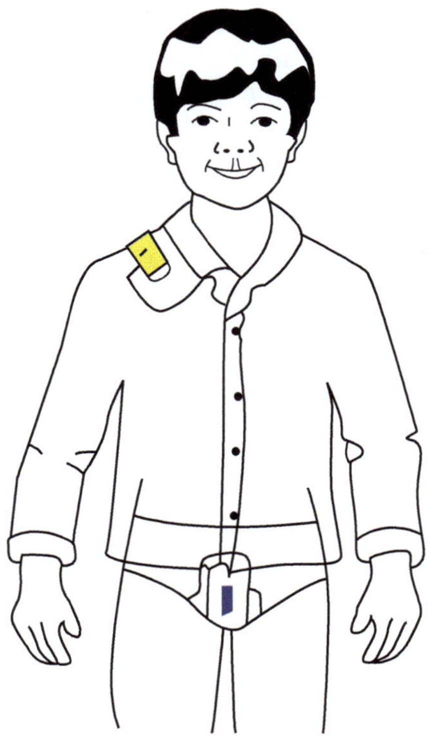

**Fig. 40.3** Drawing of alarm

*Effectiveness of alarm use*. The alarm is reported to be 50–70 % successful for PNE [4]. This statistic may overestimate alarm success as it does not include the 30 % of children who drop out.

Of the many available moisture alarms, we focus on alarms which respond quickly to moisture and sounds loud enough to alert the parent. It is implicit that alarms which respond to urine by vibration are not *widely* suitable to PNE treatment, since it does not alert anyone else other than child wearing the alarm.

*Safety*. The conventional alarms are viewed as safe. Old alarms which permit continual discharge of electricity in response to urine wetting have been associated with electrical burns. Entanglement of the child by wires is a concern that has not been reported. Some parents hesitate applying mechanical devices to the child's genital area, being fearful of psychological consequences in later years.

In summary, alarm-alone treatment can remit PNE; it is not a practical treatment as the need for long duration of treatment frustrates families and so treatment is discontinued.

## Desmopressin (DDAVP)

*Basis of treatment.* Desmopressin, a synthetic analogue of the naturally occurring hormone vasopressin, reduces the volume of urine. Research shows that some children with PNE have an obligatory nocturnal polyuria which may be reduced by DDAVP treatment. The polyuria is likely an inherited characteristic which explains why PNE may "run in families." The use of DDAVP to treat PNE regards polyuria as the main pathophysiological process which accounts for the wetting. There has yet to be research to assess if polyuria remains reduced after DDAVP treatment.

*Effectiveness of DDAVP treatment.* Research reports show that while dryness achievement ranges between 50 and 90 % of patients while medication is administered, the relapse rate of PNE after medication is discontinued is about 90 % of patients. When used as standalone treatment, DDAVP is commonly administered nightly for 3 months followed by a 1-week hiatus to evaluate for relapse of PNE. If PNE recurs, then the DDAVP is restarted.

## Safety

DDAVP has been regarded as safe until recent FDA reports on death in adults associated with use of the nasal spray as a vehicle to administer DDAVP. We advise that in hot weather, the medication should be used cautioning against overdrinking. Children with PNE and cystic fibrosis should not use the medication.

In summary, DDAVP as a standalone treatment can remit PNE, but it is not a practical treatment as relapse is frequent.

## Psychological Issues to Consider When Beginning PNE Treatment

We do not advise routine counseling to address behavior problems prior to starting treatment for PNE, but if the family chooses to do this, the basis of psychological treatment is considered below.

It is widely recognized that children with PNE do not show higher incidence of psychological issues than children who do not wet. We discuss the basis of psychological treatment from this framework.

Psychological treatment in a *normal well-adjusted* child may effect dryness, but clinical trials to better define these results remain to be done [9]. It is recognized that frequent, weekly, office visits of the child with PNE with the family doctor will enhance the awareness of the wetting and help effect dryness. The effectiveness of this treatment is unknown.

- Psychological treatment in a child with *psychosocial stresses*. The Try for Dry method does not involve itself with psychological/psychiatric treatment of children with PNE, but expect the family's healthcare provider will judge the need for this.
- ADHD is a condition which has shown comorbidity with PNE.
- Children with low self-esteem. Children with PNE may experience feelings of shame believing that they are different from other children who do not bed wet. Because PNE is often not discussed in the family in a positive manner, children with PNE often avoid activities in which they would like to participate, such as sleepovers and overnight camps. The issue of low self-esteem may progress to the point that the children refuse to participate in treatment for PNE because they express apathy. We regard the level of motivation of the child as important to PNE treatment, and if the parents cannot motivate the child, consider involving a psychologist to assist in this matter.
- Once motivation to get to dry is established, then TFD treatment can begin.

In summary, psychological evaluation/treatment is done to assess if there is a basis for poor compliance with PNE treatment. Such issues merit resolution before beginning the PNE treatment.

## Try for Dry Method

*Basis of the treatment.* The foundation of the Try for Dry treatment program is largely derived from our clinical observations in pediatric urology practice. The following three vignettes below describe our experiences that have led to incorporation of various components in the TFD method.

1. Children with PNE who were recovering from bladder surgery and were receiving oxybutynin as an anticholinergic to address spastic bladder symptoms
2. Boys with PNE who were recovering from orchiopexy and who required laxatives to manage constipation
3. Respecting parents observations on the effects of certain dietary food/beverage intakes which were regarded as exacerbating bed-wetting

The method incorporates these three observations to synthesize a holistic approach to PNE, namely, combination therapy. As an overview, the method involves algorithm treatment which is structured by categorizing age, bladder capacity, and bowel regularity. The method combines treatments used to target the syndromic and ancillary features of PNE. This strategy provides the most effective results to remit PNE (see algorithm).

The treatments which are combined include: alarm with motivation rewards, medication (oxybutynin, DDAVP), bowel regulation, and elimination diet [5].

## Alarm

The alarm is used in the TFD method as it is described above. However, the method mandates that the parents *understand* how the alarm is used. It is important for the parent to understand that she/he is to listen for the alarm sounding. This is because the child who shows failure of sleep arousal will not respond to the initial sounding of the alarm. Parents are advised to allow the child to handle the alarm prior to wearing it as this helps alleviate fear of the device.

After the alarm sounds, the parent's job is to get to the child's room as soon as possible and assist the child to the bathroom, where urination is completed in the toilet. The child returns to bed, fresh clothing with a dry sensor is donned, and the alarm is reattached. The alarm is worn every night until the child is dry for 14 nights consecutively.

## Medication (Oxybutynin, DDAVP)

Oxybutynin is used to treat a small functional bladder capacity. A 3-day home diary is used to ascertain the functional bladder capacity (see diary). The normal functional bladder capacity can be predicted by the formula, normal capacity (in oz.) = age (in years) ± 2 (as ounces). For example, a 9-year-old boy should have a bladder capacity 11 oz., but most 9-year-olds with PNE show a reduced functional capacity at less than 9 oz. Our experience shows that oxybutynin when used in conjunction with an enuresis alarm decreases the number of times the alarm sounds during the night; thereby there are fewer needed lifting, so compliance is improved. We use an algorithm for initial dosing of oxybutynin (see Table 40.3). Should dryness not be shown as expected, tailoring the dose to the child's individual needs is done.

*Desmopressin (DDAVP).* The ancillary feature of polyuria is addressed with DDAVP. We have come to appreciate that the medication is not routinely needed for children <8-year-old. For children ≥8-year-old, the dose initially prescribed is subtherapeutic dose (0.1 mg). This is intentionally done so as not to remit wetting but rather simply to decrease the volume of urine produced. This reduction of urine output is seen in both reductions in the number of times the child wets at night and so reduces the efforts with alarm use.

**Table 40.3** Try for dry—treatment algorithm

| Try for dry treatments | Age of child | | | | | | | | |
|---|---|---|---|---|---|---|---|---|---|
| | <8 years old | | | 8–13 years old | | | >13 years old | | |
| ALARM | Yes | | | Yes | | | Yes | | |
| OXYBUTYNIN DOSE | AM (mg) | PM (mg) | HS (mg) | AM (mg) | PM (mg) | HS (mg) | AM (mg) | PM (mg) | HS (mg) |
| Bladder capacity reduced | 2.5 | 2.5 | 2.5 | 2.5 | 2.5 | 5 | 2.5 | 2.5 | 7.5 |
| Bladder capacity not reduced | 0 | 0 | 2.5 | 0 | 0 | 5 | 0 | 0 | 7.5 |
| DESMOPRESSIN DOSE | 0 | 0 | 0 | 0 | 0 | 0.1 | 0 | 0 | 0.2 |
| ELIMINATION DIET | Yes | | | Yes | | | Yes | | |
| INDUCEMENTS | Yes | | | Yes | | | Yes | | |
| BOWEL PROGRAM | Yes | | | Yes | | | Yes | | |

## Ancillary Treatments

### Bowel Regulation

In the Try for Dry program, bowel irregularity/constipation is managed with laxatives such as senna, stool softeners such as mineral oil, or high fiber such as Miralax. If the child is severely constipated, enema may be used as initial bowel cleanout before starting the laxative. Once a bowel program is established that works well for the child, the combined use of the alarm and medications is started.

### Elimination Diet

In the Try for Dry program, the empiric use of elimination diet is implemented for 2 weeks which focuses mainly on an elimination of dairy products, caffeinated liquids, citric products, and heavily sugared foods. Following this diet appears to facilitate dryness in about 10 % of children treated by the TFD method. The parent is given a list and asked to eliminate those products for 2 weeks, and other acceptable liquids are listed to substitute during this interval. At the end of 2 weeks, eliminated items are gradually reintroduced. The empiric use of this diet eliminates the child's exposure to items which may restrict getting to dry.

### Motivation/Rewards

The use of a star chart is encouraged to track dry nights and wet nights on a calendar using "star stickers." There should be an agreed upon reward for a number of dry nights (anywhere from 1 to a few dry nights), cooperation with alarm use, adherence to diet, and taking the medication(s).

## Follow-Up/Evaluation of Treatment

Using the Try for Dry treatment program, the expectation is for night wetting to remit by 3 months after beginning treatment.

A smooth result to dryness is seen in about 80 % of families who follow the TFD method. Specifically, at 1 month after starting TFD treatment, the majority of families should have noted a 50 % improvement in night wetting, by 2 months a 75 % improvement in night wetting, and 3 months remission in wetting (14 consecutive nights dry).

For the remainder dryness is not attained according to this tempo. Should a child not show timely acquisition of dryness, then adjustments can be made addressing the following concerns. Insufficient medication administration can be addressed by increasing titrated dosage of oxybutynin/DDAVP administered before bed. Concerns regarding noncompliance may impact on treatment success; compliant use of the alarm should be reviewed as this can be a source of frustration for the family. Concerns regarding constipation should be addressed by clear confirmation that bowel emptying is regular. Following up on such charting may show that child originally considered to have regular defection.

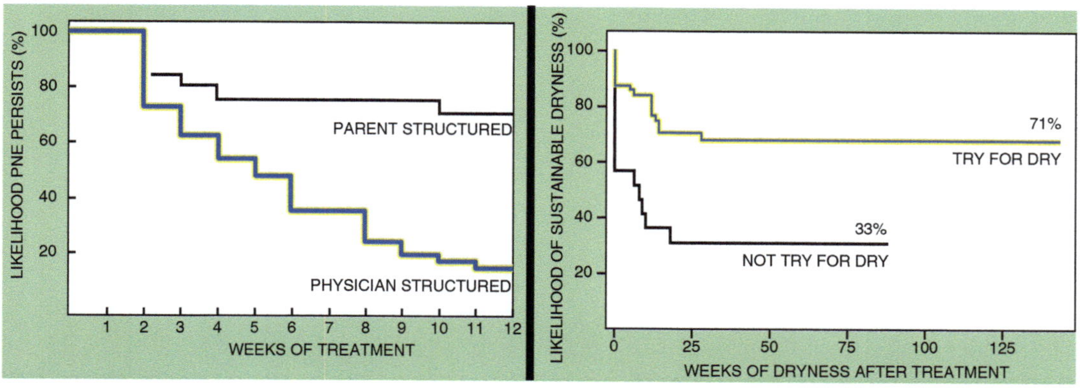


**Fig. 40.4** (*Left panel*) Kaplan–Meier curve compares probabilities of remission of PNE in two treatment groups, one which is structured by physician as Try for Dry or one which is structured by a parent not following the TFD method. At the end of 12 weeks of treatment, the TFD group (*solid blue line*) shows 88 % remission in PNE, while the parent chosen treatment group (*black line*) shows 29 % remission in PNE ($p<0.0001$). Adapted from Saldano et al. [6]. (*Right panel*) Kaplan–Meier curve comparing probabilities of sustaining dryness in the treatment groups. The Try for Dry group (*solid blue line*) shows 71 % sustainable dryness, while the non-Try for Dry treatment group (*solid black line*) shows 33 % sustainable dryness ($p<0.0005$). Adapted from Saldano et al. [7]

Tapering of treatment once PNE is resolved. Try for Dry suggests a structured tapering of the alarm and medication use. Tapering treatment seems to yield better success at permanent remission than sudden discontinuation of treatment. TFD plans involve tapering the alarm use first (every other night, to three times/week, to twice/week, then stop) and then tapering medication (oxybutynin and desmopressin reduce dose/day and then reduce dosing weekly). We have noted that up to 20 % of children will experience relapse in night wetting. The recurrence of wetting is addressed by TFD again. If wetting relapses a second time and if wetting does not remit, then urological work-up is done.

## Treatment Outcomes

In a recent study children treated with the Try for Dry program for PNE showed earlier remission of bed-wetting. Eighty percent of the children in this study who followed the TFD treatment were dry by the end of 12 % weeks (see Fig. 40.4a). A follow-up study looking at long-term remission in the aforementioned group showed that children who were used to the TFD program had sustained dryness and lower relapse (29 %) than the comparison group with a relapse of 67 % (see Fig. 40.4b). Cure of primary nocturnal enuresis is considered to be remission of wetting for 2 or more years.

## References


1. Austin P, Ferguson G, Yan Y, et al. Combination therapy in nonresponders to desmopressin for monosymptomatic nocturnal enuresis: a randomized, double-blind, placebo-control trial. J Urol. Pediatrics. 2008;122(5):1027–32. doi: 10.1542/peds.2007-3691.
2. Hafflof B, Andren O, et al. Self-esteem in children with nocturnal enuresis and urinary incontinence: improvement of self-esteem after treatment. Eur Urol. 1998;33 Suppl 3:16–9.
3. Aikawa T, Kasahara T, Uchiyama M. The arginine-vasopressin secretion profile of children with primary nocturnal enuresis. Eur Urol Suppl. 1998;33:41.
4. Monda J, Husmann DA. Primary nocturnal enuresis: a comparison among observation, imipramine, desmopressin acetate and bed-wetting alarm systems. J Urol. 1995;154(2):745–8.
5. Maizels M, Saldano DD. Childhood bed-wetting: the case for combination therapy. Contemp Urol. 2007;18:21–3.
6. Saldano D, Chaviano AH, Maizels M, Yerkes E, Cheng EY, Losavio J, Porten SP, Sullivan C, Zebold KF, Kaplan WE. Office management of pediatric primary nocturnal enuresis: a comparison of physician advised and parent chosen alternative treatment outcomes. J Urol. 2008;178:1758–62.
7. Saldano D, Chaviano AH, Maizels M. Sustainability of remission of pediatric primary nocturnal enuresis—comparison of remission using a TRY for DRY treatment plan vs. other plans. Urol Nurs. 2008;28(4):263–6.

# Index



R. Rabinowitz et al. (eds.), *Pediatric Urology for the Primary Care Physician*, Current Clinical Urology,
DOI 10.1007/978-1-60327-243-8, © Springer Science+Business Media New York 2015

## M



## N



## O

MIX
Papier aus verantwortungsvollen Quellen
Paper from responsible sources
FSC® C105338

If you have any concerns about our products,
you can contact us on
**ProductSafety@springernature.com**

In case Publisher is established outside the EU,
the EU authorized representative is:
**Springer Nature Customer Service Center GmbH**
**Europaplatz 3, 69115 Heidelberg, Germany**

Printed by Libri Plureos GmbH
in Hamburg, Germany